The of
Human on

NCE

DATE			

The Biochemistry of Human Nutrition

A DESK REFERENCE

Eva May Nunnelley Hamilton

Sareen Annora Stepnick Gropper

FLORIDA STATE UNIVERSITY

WEST PUBLISHING COMPANY

St. Paul   New York   Los Angeles   San Francisco

Copyediting by Robert Bergad

Text Design by Rick Chafian

Artwork and Composition by Rolin Graphics

Cover by Theresa Jensen. Art is an abstraction
of a micrograph of glucose.

Library of Congress Cataloging-in-Publication Data

Hamilton, Eva May Nunnelley.
  The biochemistry of human nutrition.
  1. Nutrition—Handbooks, manuals, etc.
2. Biological chemistry—Handbooks, manuals, etc.
I. Gropper, Sareen Stepnick. II. Title.
[DNLM: 1. Biochemistry—handbooks, 2. Nutrition—
handbooks.   QU 39 H217b]
QP141.H338   1987   612'.3   86-28204
ISBN 0-314-29520-8

Contents in Brief

Table of Contents

Table of Contents

Table of Contents

Table of Contents

Preface

To understand the science of nutrition, biochemistry and its language must be learned. Insofar as it is possible, we have explained the concepts of biochemistry and nutrition in a language that most readers can understand. At the same time, however, we have written the topics so that readers can gradually become familiar or reacquaint themselves with precise biochemical terminology. In this way we hope that those who need to brush up on forgotten biochemical concepts in their profession as well as those who are learning biochemistry for the first time will be helped in their pursuit of nutrition knowledge.

In the selection of topics to discuss, we have chosen biochemical concepts that are necessary if nutrition science is to be understood. Some other biochemical concepts, not directly applicable to nutrition, are included but discussed briefly. We apologize to those who may not find their favorite topic included and we would appreciate suggestions for inclusion in subsequent editions.

The discussion provided under each topic is generally restricted to that which is accepted as true, as opposed to that which is controversial. We believe this approach is a more useful one for the intended audience. For those who want to read more recent research on a topic, we have listed references that we have found valuable although we may have chosen to exclude the ideas from our discussions.

The alphabetical format, while it facilitates locating the desired information, requires that each topic be written so that it can be understood without having to recall the preceding material. For this reason, redundancy may occur when multiple topics are reviewed.

We are grateful to Gary Woodruff for his advice and support in conceptualizing this book. In addition, we would like to thank those at West Publishing Company, especially Peter Marshall, Catherine Maggio and Rebecca Tollerson, and those professionals who reviewed the manuscript and provided valuable criticism and guidance. These professionals include: Ann Bock, New Mexico State; Merrill J. Christensen, Brigham Young University; Kay Franz, Brigham Young University; Nancy Green, Florida State University; Sara Hunt, Georgia State University; Carolyn Lara-Brand, University of Iowa; Susan Moore, California State Fullerton; Scott Pattison, California Polytechnic University; Patsy Reed, Northern Arizona University; David Straus, State University of New York; and Stan Winter, Golden West College.

We are especially appreciative of our family and many friends for their encouragement throughout the production of this book.

Eva May Nunnelley Hamilton
Sareen Annora Stepnick Gropper

Guide to Using This Book

GREEK LETTERS

Chemical terms that begin with Greek letters are alphabetized under the English spelling of the Greek word. For example, "β-alanine" is alphabetized as "beta alanine." The following Greek letters appear in this book:

α alpha	γ gamma	μ mu
β beta	Δ or δ delta	ω omega

SMALL CAPS

SMALL CAPS appearing within the discussion of a topic denote the exact title of another topic which the reader may wish to review. A topic is written in small caps only the first time it appears in a discussion. At the conclusion of a discussion, topics that enlarge or complete the present topic are listed.

ITALICS

Italics within the discussion of a topic indicate the names of enzymes. The names of classes of enzymes are not italicized.

PARENTHESES

Parentheses in a topic title enclose a chemical symbol, an abbreviation, and/or a synonym for the substance or process named in the title.

SUGGESTED READINGS

At the ends of many topics are suggested readings which direct the reader to more advanced material or to classic studies on the given topic.

acetaldehyde. An aldehyde formed from the oxidation of ethanol. An aldehyde contains a carbonyl group with only one hydrogen attached (formaldehyde, $H_2C{=}O$, is an exception). The terminal placement of the carbonyl group in acetaldehyde makes it more reactive than when it is buried within the molecule as it is in a KETONE BODY, such as acetone.

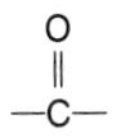

$$\begin{array}{c} O \\ \parallel \\ -C- \end{array}$$

Carbonyl group

CH$_3$—CH$_2$—OH $\xrightarrow[\text{dehydrogenase}]{\text{alcohol}}$ CH$_3$—CH
ethanol

$\overset{O}{\overset{\parallel}{}}$

NAD$^+$ NADH+H$^+$

acetaldehyde

H$_2$O   NAD$^+$

aldehyde
dehydrogenase

NADH+H$^+$

$$\begin{array}{c} O \\ \parallel \\ CH_3-C-O^- \end{array}$$
acetate

ATP

CoASH

acyl-CoA
synthetase

AMP+PP$_i$

$$\begin{array}{c} O \\ \parallel \\ CH_3-C-S-CoA \end{array}$$
acetyl-CoA

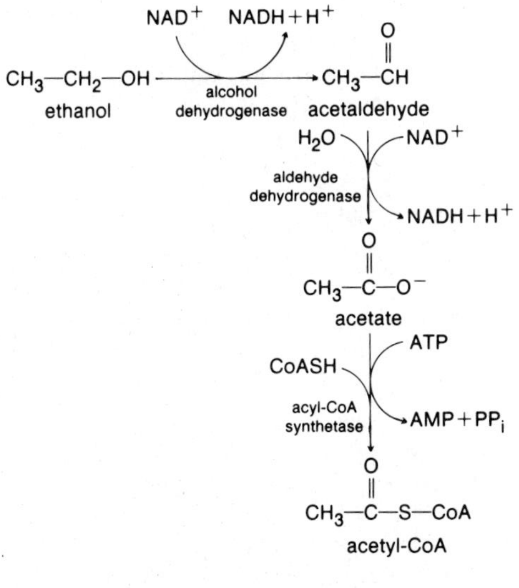

One pathway for the degradation of ethanol

Acetaldehyde results from the first step in the body's handling of beverage alcohol (ethanol) and, if allowed to accumulate, produces toxic results. The breakdown (oxidation) of ethanol occurs principally in liver cells and is catalyzed by *alcohol dehydrogenase* and NAD$^+$, generating NADH + H$^+$. The resulting acetaldehyde is then converted to acetate using another molecule of NAD$^+$ and producing more NADH + H$^+$. Acetate is then converted to ACETYL-COA by *acyl-CoA synthetase* in a reaction requiring COENZYME A and ATP.

The use of two molecules of NAD$^+$ for each molecule of alcohol converted to acetyl-CoA is at least partially responsible for the development of fatty liver in heavy users of beverage alcohol. The high level of NADH + H$^+$ produced by the reactions inhibits acetyl-CoA's entry into the TCA CYCLE and forces the conversion of acetyl-CoA into fat and other LIPIDS. Fat, however, cannot enter the blood unless it is wrapped in protein, but protein synthesis is depressed by the presence of alcohol. Consequently, fat accumulates in the intercellular spaces of the liver and blocks the flow of nutrients and oxygen into the cells and waste products out of the cells. See also: ACETYL-COA; NAD$^+$, NADP$^+$.

SUGGESTED READINGS

Boeker, E. A. 1980. Metabolism of ethanol. *J. Am. Diet. Assoc.* 76:550–554.

Eisenstein, A. B. 1982. Nutritional and metabolic effects of alcohol. *J. Am. Diet. Assoc.* 81:247–251.

Friedman, H. S., and C. S. Lieber. 1983. Alcohol and the heart. In *Nutrition and heart disease*, ed. E. B. Feldman, 145–164. New York: Churchill Livingstone.

Peters, T. J. 1982. Ethanol metabolism. *Br. Med. Bull.* 38:17–20.

Acetone, a ketone body

acetone. One of the KETONE BODIES that is present normally in the blood in small amounts but rises to toxic levels when there is not enough oxaloacetate to keep the TCA CYCLE functioning. See also: KETONE BODIES; KETOSIS; TCA CYCLE.

O
‖
CH$_3$—C—S—CoA

Acetyl-CoA
(acetyl-S-CoA)

acetyl-CoA. A two-carbon (acetyl) molecule made active by the attachment of COENZYME A. Acetyl-CoA is in a key position in the reclaiming of energy from fuel nutrients or in the synthesis of lipids derived from the consumption of excess fuel nutrients. One of the immediate precursors of acetyl-CoA is pyruvic acid, the three-carbon compound that is the end product of GLYCOLYSIS.

When glucose, some amino acid backbones, and glycerol from triacylglycerol (triglyceride) degradation are metabolized to pyruvic acid, there are several pathways through which this pyruvate may be degraded. From pyruvate, a reverse path may lead to the rebuilding of carbohydrate, protein, or glycerol for the synthesis of triacylglycerols. Alternatively, the reaction may proceed through the TCA CYCLE

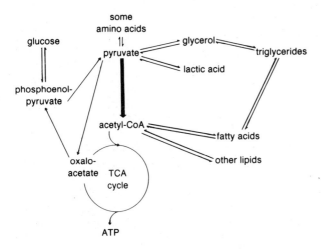

Pyruvate may follow several reversible pathways.
Path to acetyl-CoA is irreversible.

and RESPIRATORY CHAIN to carbon dioxide, water, and ATP.

Once the giant step leading from pyruvic acid to acetyl-CoA is taken, however, there are no reverse paths open. The major commitment is to the capture of energy in the bonds of ATP. If the ATP level is high, the route through the TCA cycle will be blocked. The acetyl groups still arriving from pyruvate will be diverted into FATTY ACID SYNTHESIS or synthesis of other lipids, such as CHOLESTEROL. Acetyl-CoA, then, can be thought of as a "fork in the road" leading either to ATP or to lipid synthesis.

The chemical reactions leading from pyruvate to acetyl-CoA form the link between the anaerobic (without oxygen) and aerobic (with oxygen) phases of catabolism, glycolysis and the TCA cycle, respectively. To make this transition a carbon must be removed from the pyruvate and coenzyme A must be attached to the remaining two-carbon fragment to activate it. The enzymes which catalyze these efforts are assembled into the pyruvate dehydrogenase complex that also contains the cofactors THIAMIN PYROPHOSPHATE (TPP), coenzyme A, lipoamide, FAD, and NAD^+, as well as MAGNESIUM (Mg^{++}) and CALCIUM (Ca^{++}) ions.

The complex steps from pyruvate to acetyl-CoA require the presence of many vitamins and minerals. Among these the vitamins THIAMIN and NIACIN are particularly critical to the capture of energy from food. During any sustained dietary regimen that deprives the body of thiamin and/or nia-

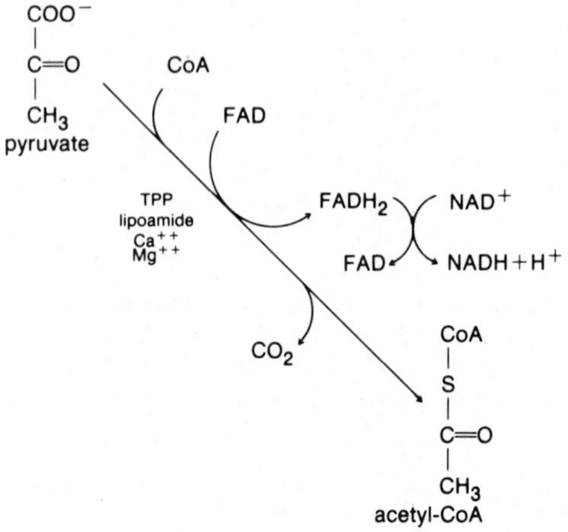

$$COO^-$$
$$|$$
$$C=O$$
$$|$$
$$CH_3$$

pyruvate

CoA

FAD

TPP
lipoamide
Ca^{++}
Mg^{++}

FADH$_2$ — NAD$^+$

FAD — NADH+H$^+$

CO_2

CoA
$|$
S
$|$
C=O
$|$
CH$_3$
acetyl-CoA

The conversion of pyruvate to acetyl-CoA
by the pyruvate dehydrogenase complex

cin, these steps can become blocked, resulting in a danger-ous buildup of acid (pyruvic and lactic) and in a lowered production of ATP. See also: COENZYME A; NIACIN; TCA CYCLE; THIAMIN; THIAMIN PYROPHOSPHATE.

acetyl coenzyme A.   See ACETYL-COA.

acid-base balance.   An optimal balance between the num-ber of acidic ions and basic ions in the fluid of a tissue. This is a requirement for the continuation of life processes since vital reactions can take place only when the PH is maintained within narrow limits. Both the respiratory and renal sys-tems contribute to the maintenance of the acid-base balance by excreting or conserving the acidic or basic ions under their control.

Most metabolic processes result in the production of acid that the tissues must handle or they will be destroyed. Car-bon dioxide, a volatile gas, is a principal end product of the oxidation of the fuel nutrients. Upon generation it is dis-solved in water and forms carbonic acid (H_2CO_3). Very lit-tle carbon dioxide is carried in this form, however, which is fortunate because of its lowering effect on pH. Instead, the carbonic acid is quickly ionized to a hydrogen ion (H^+) and a bicarbonate ion (HCO_3^-). The latter may combine with cations, especially SODIUM (Na^+) and POTASSIUM (K^+). A third way that carbon dioxide is carried is in combination with proteins, principally hemoglobin.

In order for the pH of the blood to remain at its optimum, the ratio of carbonic acid to bicarbonate ion must be main-

$$CO_2 + H_2O \rightleftharpoons H_2CO_3$$

carbon   water   carbonic
dioxide   acid

$$H_2CO_3 \rightleftharpoons H^+ + HCO_3^-$$

carbonic   hydrogen   bicarbonate
acid   ion   ion

tained at 1:20. Any increase or decrease in carbon dioxide entering the blood will affect this ratio and thus lower or raise the pH and call forth compensatory actions.

Simple compensatory actions owing to an increase of carbon dioxide are those of the lungs expelling the additional carbon dioxide through hyperventilation and of the kidneys excreting hydrogen ions. Both these actions raise the pH toward normal. With a decrease in carbon dioxide and the consequent rising of the pH, hypoventilation will retain the carbon dioxide and the kidneys will not reabsorb the bicarbonate ions. Under normal conditions, these compensatory actions tend to restore the 1:20 ratio and thus maintain normal pH. Compensations taken in the body are, of course, much more complex than this simple explanation suggests.

Organic acids, such as lactic, pyruvic, and others, as well as some inorganic acids, such as phosphoric (from the metabolism of phospholipids) and sulfuric (from the metabolism of sulfur-containing amino acids), are also formed during oxidations. In the kidneys, the exchange of sodium ions for hydrogen ions causes the pH of the urine to fall and conserves the cell's reserve of positive ions (cations). Another action the kidneys take is the production of ammonia, which is alkaline, from the metabolism of amino acids and the excretion of this ammonia at times when there is an increase in acid production.

Compounds that help maintain the optimum pH of cells are called BUFFERS. Buffers of blood are the plasma proteins, hemoglobin and oxyhemoglobin, as well as bicarbonates and phosphates.   See also: ACIDOSIS; ALKALOSIS; BUFFER; HENDERSON-HASSELBALCH EQUATION; PH.

acidic amino acids.   Amino acids whose side chains have an extra carboxyl ($—COO^-$) group. They are aspartic acid and glutamic acid, herein designated as ASPARTATE and GLUTAMATE to denote the ionized state in which they exist at the pH of the cells.

acidosis.   A set of conditions that would tend to lower the pH (increase the acidity) of blood if the body did not act to resist this change. Even with the compensatory actions that the body automatically takes, conditions sometimes result in a drop in pH. "Metabolic acidosis" refers to changes in the bicarbonate concentration of the plasma; "respiratory acidosis" refers to changes in the carbon dioxide pressure.

Some of the nutrition-related causes of metabolic acidosis include: dehydration, especially in infants; KETOSIS, which can result from starvation, anorexia nervosa, uncontrolled diabetes, or a low-carbohydrate diet; or accumulation of strong organic acid ions, such as sulfate and phosphate ions, during cardiac failure or pulmonary insufficiency. Pyruvic and lactic acids, especially, may accumulate if entry into the TCA CYCLE is blocked by vitamin deficiencies or by lack of the carbohydrate metabolities of the TCA cycle.

A compensatory action that the body may take, in addition to the normal actions of the buffering system, is an increase both in the respiration rate and in the depth of breathing. This faster and deeper breathing (hyperventilation) will lower the carbon dioxide content and help restore the pH to normal. In fact, hyperventilation is a useful clinical sign of the presence of metabolic acidosis.

Respiratory acidosis is due to the retention of carbon dioxide that could produce a drop in the blood pH if the body did not take compensatory action. Retention of carbon dioxide may result from any condition that obstructs the airways, such as pneumonia, asthma, or the presence of an object in the trachea.   See also: ACID-BASE BALANCE; ALKALOSIS; BUFFER; PH.

ACP.   See ACYL CARRIER PROTEIN.

active site.   A three-dimensional region of an enzyme molecule where substrates combine or are broken apart.   See also: ENZYME.

active transport.   Energy-requiring transport of a solute across a membrane in the direction of greater concentration or, in other words, against a concentration gradient. The usual, unassisted movement of molecules is by diffusion from a place of higher concentration to a place of lower concentration, a movement often noticed when an odor travels from the kitchen to the rest of the house. This motion does not require an input of energy. On the other hand, the work of active transport to maintain concentration gradients in the cells of a human at rest is so great that it may consume as much as 30–40 percent of the total input of energy.

MEMBRANES, by their nature, are barriers to most polar molecules. This quality is important in living cells since it keeps ionized vital components of the cell from leaking into the surrounding extra-cellular spaces. At the same time, the cell must import some polar molecules, such as sugars and amino acids, even though these may be at a greater concentration inside the cell; conversely, the cell must export some polar molecules even when they are at greater concentrations outside the cell. This characteristic of membranes—

unidirectional and selective flow of molecules—requires a large input of energy.

The hydrolysis of ATP to ADP and phosphate supplies the free energy to perform such work of actively transporting select molecules in one direction against a concentration gradient. A good example of such cellular work is performed across the plasma membrane of the parietal cells of the stomach. Gastric juice in the lumen of the stomach has a concentration of hydrogen ions from hydrochloric acid such that its pH is 1.0, but the concentration of H^+ ions in the parietal cells maintains a pH of about 7.0. Therefore the parietal cells must secrete H^+ ions against a concentration gradient of about a million to one—from a concentration of 10^{-1} M to 10^{-7} M. For every ATP hydrolyzed by the H^+-transporting *ATPase*, two H^+ ions are secreted to form gastric juice.

Active transport systems are available in the membranes for many import/export activities. These activities include maintenance of an optimal concentration of nutrients and volume of the cells; nerve transmission; optimal concentrations of electrolytes, especially of CALCIUM (Ca^{++}), POTASSIUM (K^+), and SODIUM (Na^+); absorptive and secretory functions of the kidney; and muscle contraction. See also: ATP, ADP, AMP; MEMBRANES; SODIUM PUMP.

acyl carrier protein (ACP). A protein that has pantothenic acid as its prosthetic group. It is active in the synthesis of fatty acids as it carries acyl groups that are bound to the pantothenic acid in a thioester (sulfur ester) linkage. See also: FATTY ACID OXIDATION.

adenine. A purine base. See also: PURINE, PYRIMIDINE BASES.

adenosine. A nucleoside composed of a purine (adenine) and ribose. See also: ATP, ADP, AMP; NUCLEOSIDES, NUCLEOTIDES.

adenosine diphosphate (ADP). A nucleotide composed of a purine (adenine), ribose, and two phosphates. See also: ATP, ADP, AMP.

adenosine monophosphate (adenylate, AMP). A nucleotide composed of a purine (adenine), ribose, and one phosphate. See also: ATP, ADP, AMP.

adenosine triphosphate (ATP). A nucleotide composed of a purine (adenine), ribose, and three phosphates. See also: ATP, ADP, AMP.

adenylate. See ADENOSINE MONOPHOSPHATE.

ADP. See ADENOSINE DIPHOSPHATE.

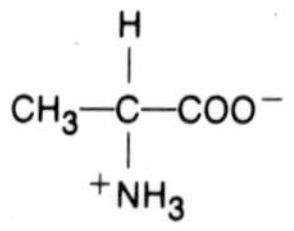

$$CH_3-\overset{\overset{\displaystyle H}{|}}{\underset{\underset{\displaystyle +NH_3}{|}}{C}}-COO^-$$

Alanine at
biological pH

aerobic reaction. A chemical reaction requiring oxygen. See also: BETA OXIDATION; TCA CYCLE.

alanine (Ala). A three-carbon, dietarily nonessential, glucogenic (glycogenic) α-amino acid which has a simple methyl group (CH_3) as its side chain.

Alanine can be synthesized in the body from pyruvate and GLUTAMATE. To accomplish this, the amino group of glutamate is transferred to the carbon skeleton of pyruvate by a VITAMIN B_6-dependent enzyme, *alanine transaminase,* also called *glutamate-pyruvate transaminase* (GPT). When glutamate loses its amino group it becomes α-ketoglutarate, a carbohydrate metabolite in the TCA CYCLE. It is both interesting and useful that in the same process by which alanine is synthesized, the TCA cycle is resupplied with a necessary metabolite.

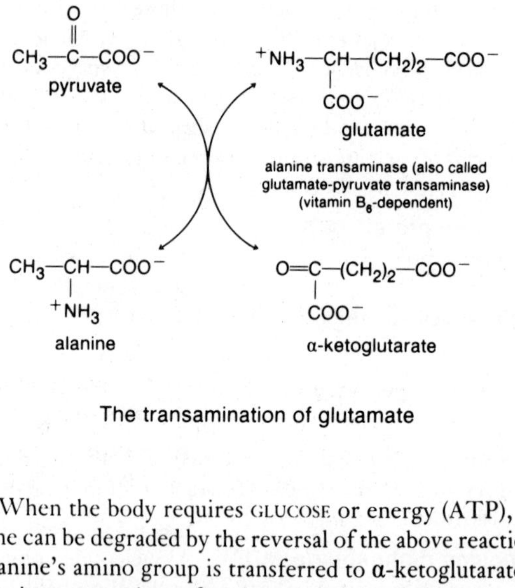

$$CH_3-\overset{\overset{\displaystyle O}{\|}}{C}-COO^-$$
pyruvate

$$^+NH_3-\underset{\underset{\displaystyle COO^-}{|}}{CH}-(CH_2)_2-COO^-$$
glutamate

alanine transaminase (also called
glutamate-pyruvate transaminase)
(vitamin B_6-dependent)

$$CH_3-\underset{\underset{\displaystyle +NH_3}{|}}{CH}-COO^-$$
alanine

$$O=\underset{\underset{\displaystyle COO^-}{|}}{C}-(CH_2)_2-COO^-$$
α-ketoglutarate

The transamination of glutamate

When the body requires GLUCOSE or energy (ATP), alanine can be degraded by the reversal of the above reactions. Alanine's amino group is transferred to α-ketoglutarate by *alanine transaminase,* forming pyruvate and glutamate. Pyruvate either is routed through phosphoenolpyruvate to form glucose, or is decarboxylated to ACETYL-CoA if the demand is for energy. Acetyl-CoA enters the TCA cycle after which its energy will be captured in ATP. The glutamate may participate in other transaminations, or be oxidatively deaminated by *glutamate dehydrogenase,* donating the hydrogens to NAD^+, which will carry them to the RESPIRATORY CHAIN. The ammonium ion (NH_4^+) released, if not used in other transaminations or for building nonprotein nitrogenous compounds, is incorporated into urea for excretion.

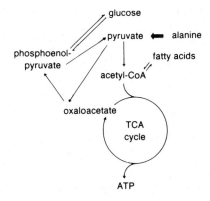

The carbons of alanine enter metabolic pathways

$CH_3—CH—COO^-$
$|$
$^+NH_3$

alanine

$O=C—(CH_2)_2—COO^-$
$|$
COO^-

α-ketoglutarate

alanine transaminase

$CH_3—\overset{\overset{O}{\|}}{C}—COO^-$

pyruvate

$^+NH_3—CH—(CH_2)_2—COO^-$
$|$
COO^-

glutamate

H_2O

NAD^+
(or $NADP^+$)

glutamate dehydrogenase

$NADH + H^+$
(or $NADPH + H^+$)

$NH_4^+ + O=C—(CH_2)_2—COO^-$
$|$
COO^-

α-ketoglutarate

The degradation of alanine and glutamate

Alanine plays an interesting role during STARVATION (fasting, famine, postsurgical food deprivation, or uncontrolled diabetes). During these times of food deficit, the branched-chain amino acids present in the muscles are selectively oxidized to their respective alpha keto acids. The released amino groups are then used to aminate pyruvate and thereby form alanine. The alanine is released into the blood. During a short-term deficit, the alanine levels in the serum rise, supplying the liver with a precursor for the synthesis of GLU-COSE. If starvation continues for more than a week, the tissues shift to the use of KETONE BODIES and FATTY ACIDS for fuel, diminishing the critical need for glucose. Consequently, muscle degradation lessens and serum alanine levels fall. See also: BETA ALANINE; CORI CYCLE; SGPT; INSULIN; STARVATION.

SUGGESTED READINGS

Cahill, G. F., Jr. 1970. Starvation in man. *N. Engl. J. Med.* 282:668–675.

Felig, P. 1973. The glucose-alanine cycle. *Metabolism* 22:179–207.

Kelts, D. G., et al. 1985. Studies on requirements for amino acids in infants with disorders of amino acid metabolism. I. Effect of alanine. *Pediatr. Res.* 19:86–91.

Kinney, J. M., and D. H. Elwyn. 1983. Protein metabolism and injury. *An. Rev. Nutr.* 3:433–466.

albinism. A rare, recessive, inherited disorder in which the enzyme, *tyrosinase*, normally found in the pigmented cells (melanocytes) is missing. Albinos have white hair, pale skin and pink eyes.

SUGGESTED READINGS

Witkop, C. J., W. C. Quevedo, and T. B. Fitzpatrick. 1983. Albinism and other disorders of pigment metabolism. In *The metabolic basis of inherited disease,* 5th ed., ed. J. B. Stanbury et al., 301–346. New York: McGraw Hill.

albumin. A serum globular protein that occurs in the highest concentration of the major serum proteins. Its single chain consists of 610 amino acids. Albumin is soluble both in water and salt solutions. Its importance relates to the maintenance of the osmotic pressure of intravascular spaces, and as a carrier in the blood of FATTY ACIDS, bilirubin, drugs, and trace elements.

alcohol. A hydrocarbon in which one or more of the hydrogens has been replaced by a hydroxyl (—OH) group. See also: ACETALDEHYDE for the metabolism of beverage alcohol, ethanol (C_2H_5OH).

SUGGESTED READINGS

See suggested readings for ACETALDEHYDE.

aliphatic. Belonging to that series of organic compounds characterized by open chains of carbon atoms rather than by rings.

aliphatic amino acids. Amino acids whose side chains are in strings of carbons (and sulfur) rather than rings. They are: ALANINE, CYSTEINE, GLYCINE, ISOLEUCINE, LEUCINE, METHIONINE, SERINE, THREONINE, and VALINE.

alkalosis. A set of conditions that would tend to raise the pH (increase the alkalinity) of the blood if the body did not act to resist this change. Sometimes, however, the normal actions of the body's renal, respiratory and buffering systems cannot reduce the pH when there has been an overload of base.

"Metabolic alkalosis" may be caused by (1) loss of body acid or chloride ion (Cl^-) as with vomiting, (2) an excess of base as from ingestion of antacids, peptic ulcer medications, or vegetable diets, or (3) a depletion of POTASSIUM resulting from diarrhea or use of diuretics. The kidneys compensate for this loss of acid ions by excreting bicarbonate ions (HCO_3^-), an action not without danger, for it may lead to dehydration and a further loss of potassium.

"Respiratory alkalosis" is a condition noted for its decrease in the partial pressure of carbon dioxide. With lower carbon dioxide pressure, less carbonic acid (H_2CO_3) is formed, and the pH rises. The lowering of carbon dioxide pressure is caused by hyperventilation, which occurs for various reasons, including pain and fear. Mild cases of respiratory alkalosis usually follow trauma, such as surgery. These will be corrected without any intervention by good cardiac and renal functions. However, severe respiratory alkalosis has a poor prognosis. See also: ACID-BASE BALANCE; ACIDOSIS; PH.

alkaptonuria. A genetic disease in which the enzyme, *homogentisic acid oxidase,* is lacking, causing an accumulation of homogentisic acid owing to the incomplete metabolism of TYROSINE and PHENYLALANINE. Alkaptonuria is detected by the darkening of the urine upon standing. The most serious complication is degenerative joint disease. See also: HOMOGENTISIC ACID.

SUGGESTED READINGS

See suggested readings for INBORN ERRORS OF METABOLISM.

amide bond. A generalized name for the bond in which the hydroxyl (OH) group of carboxylic acid is replaced by an amino (NH_2) group. Organic groups may be linked to the carbon and nitrogen atoms. When the amide bond links the carboxyl group of one amino acid to the amino group of another amino acid to form a dipeptide, it is called a peptide bond.

$$\begin{array}{c} O \\ \| \\ -C-NH_2 \end{array}$$

An amide bond

11

amides of acidic amino acids. Amino acids that have amide groups substituted for their carboxyl groups on the side chains. They are: ASPARAGINE, derived from ASPARTATE, and GLUTAMINE, derived from GLUTAMATE.

COO^-
$H_3N^+ —CH$
CH_2
C
O O^- carboxyl group

aspartate

COO^-
$H_3N^+ —CH$
CH_2
C
O NH_2 amide group

asparagine

COO^-
$H_3N^+ —CH$
$(CH_2)_2$
C
O O^- carboxyl group

glutamate

COO^-
$H_3N^+ —CH$
$(CH_2)_2$
C
O NH_2 amide group

glutamine

amino acid biosynthesis. The naturally occurring biological synthesis, or manufacture, of amino acids undertaken by all living organisms.

A testament to the simplicity of nature's organization lies in the fact that there are only seven compounds and three pathways that give rise to the twenty essential and nonessential amino acids, which, in turn, give rise to the possibly 5 million different proteins in the human body. These seven compounds are: 3-phosphoglycerate, pyruvate, α-ketoglutarate, oxaloacetate, phosphoenolpyruvate, ribose 5-phosphate, and erythrose 4-phosphate. The three pathways are GLYCOLYSIS, the PENTOSE PHOSPHATE PATHWAY, and the TCA CYCLE.

Four compounds are biosynthetic precursors of the NONESSENTIAL AMINO ACIDS in humans. From glycolysis are produced (1) 3-phosphoglycerate, the precursor of SERINE from which CYSTEINE and GLYCINE are produced, and (2) pyruvate, the precursor of ALANINE. From the TCA cycle are produced (3) α-ketoglutarate, which is responsible for GLUTAMATE from which GLUTAMINE and PROLINE are produced, and (4) oxaloacetate, which yields ASPARTATE from which ASPARAGINE is produced.

The pathways that lead to the biosynthesis of the ESSENTIAL AMINO ACIDS take place in some other part of the food chain but not in humans. Although humans can synthesize a few of the essential amino acids, the reactions do not occur rapidly enough or produce large enough quantities to support the protein synthesis needed for human growth and repair of tissues. In whatever species the biosynthesis of the essential amino acids occurs, the same processes provide six precursors, three of which (pyruvate, α-ketoglutarate, oxa-loacetate) have already been listed as precursors for the non-essential amino acids.

Glycolysis produces (1) phosphoenolpyruvate (PEP), which combines with erythrose 4-phosphate to synthesize TRYPTOPHAN as well as PHENYLALANINE that, in turn, leads to the synthesis of nonessential TYROSINE, and (2) pyruvate, which leads to the synthesis of valine and LEUCINE. The TCA cycle produces (3) α-ketoglutarate that is responsible for the production of the nonessential glutamate from which ARGININE is synthesized, and (4) oxaloacetate, which yields ASPARTATE from which LYSINE and METHIONINE are produced as well as THREONINE that, in turn, yields ISOLEUCINE. The pentose phosphate pathway produces (5) ribose 5-phosphate, which yields HISTIDINE, and (6) erythrose 4-phosphate, which combines with phosphoenolpyruvate to produce PHENYLALANINE, TRYPTOPHAN, and tyrosine.

An interesting part of the story of the synthesis of amino acids is the way inert nitrogen from the air and soil is recycled into protein in the food chain, providing a continuous supply of amino acids for growth and repair of human tissue. See also: NITROGEN.

SUGGESTED READINGS

Calvin, M. 1969. *Chemical evolution.* London: Oxford University Press.

Lehninger, A. L. 1982. *Principles of biochemistry. New York: Worth Publishers, p. 59–62.*

Ross, H. H. 1966. *Understanding evolution.* Englewood Cliffs, N.J.: Prentice-Hall, Inc. p. 29–37. A classic, easy-to-read, brief statement of how amino acids may have been formed.

Ponnamperuma, C. *Cosmos: Chemistry and origins of life.* College Park: University of Maryland.

amino acid degradation. Breaking apart of the amino acid into its amino group and carbon skeleton so that the parts may be used to synthesize other molecules, oxidized to provide energy, or converted into molecules that can be excreted. Degradation may be stimulated under the following circumstances: (1) when protein foods are eaten in excess of the need for amino acids for repair and replacement of tissues; (2) when a low-carbohydrate diet is eaten and the carbon skeletons of amino acids are used to resupply the TCA CYCLE with carbohydrate intermediates; and (3) when too few calories are supplied in the diet so that body proteins must be sacrificed and their amino acids are oxidized for fuel.

The first step in amino acid degradation is transamination or deamination. During transamination, the amino group is transferred to another carbon skeleton to form one of the NONESSENTIAL AMINO ACIDS. Transamination requires little energy and is accomplished by ENZYMES called transaminases, or aminotransferases, which use VITAMIN B$_6$ as coenzyme. These enzymes are specific for certain amino acids, for example, *alanine transaminase* transfers an amino group from another amino acid to pyruvate, forming ALANINE.

The liver is the major site of transamination for most of the amino acids except for the branched-chain amino acids (LEUCINE, ISOLEUCINE and VALINE), which are transaminated in the peripheral tissues, such as kidney and muscles.

If there is no demand for the amino group to form other amino acids or for NITROGEN for the synthesis of nonprotein nitrogenous molecules, the amino group may be transferred

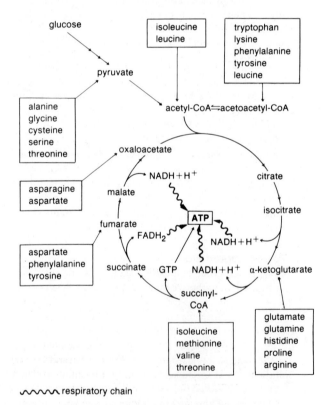

Entry of the carbon skeleton of amino acids into
common metabolic pathways

14

to α-ketoglutarate, forming GLUTAMATE. Glutamate then can be oxidatively deaminated by *glutamate dehydrogenase*, which uses NAD^+ as coenzyme. The resulting ammonium ion (NH_4^+) will be converted to urea and excreted.

The carbon skeleton that remains after deamination can enter the TCA cycle when the carbons have been incorporated into one of seven molecules: pyruvate, ACETYL-COA, acetoacetyl-CoA, α-ketoglutarate, succinyl-CoA, fumarate, or oxaloacetate. All seven molecules may lead to complete oxidation through the TCA cycle and the RESPIRATORY CHAIN, producing ATP, CO_2, and water. Alternatively, the carbons from the TCA cycle intermediates—α-ketoglutarate, succinyl-CoA, and fumarate—may exit the TCA cycle when they have been converted to oxaloacetate. In this case, the carbons may proceed through PEP (phosphoenolpyruvate) to generate GLUCOSE, a process termed GLUCONEOGENESIS. In another instance, the carbons may be converted to acetyl-CoA and then diverted from the TCA cycle to form triglycerides, to form sterols such as CHOLESTEROL, or to form KETONE BODIES. The major site of these conversions is the liver. Which path is followed is determined by the environment or the current needs of the cells.   See also: specific AMINO ACIDS for a discussion of individual degradative pathways; GLUCOGENIC AMINO ACIDS; KETOGENIC AMINO ACIDS; TCA CYCLE; UREA CYCLE.

amino acid pool.   The free amino acids present mainly in the cytosol and circulating blood. These amino acids may have joined the pool during either the digestion and absorption of protein-rich foods or the degradation of body proteins. The amino acids stand ready to be incorporated into protein or used for fuel. To keep this pool adequately supplied, ESSENTIAL AMINO ACIDS must be provided daily in the diet. In addition, a large enough supply of the NONESSENTIAL AMINO ACIDS must be present so that if one is needed, and not present, it can be made instantly from another nonessential amino acid by transamination without dismantling an essential amino acid. An ample supply of calories from carbohydrates and fats ensures that the pool will not be depleted by cells using amino acids for fuel.

amino acids.   Simple, organic, nitrogenous compounds that are the building blocks of peptides and proteins. In humans there may be as many as 5,000,000 different proteins and each one may contain one or more chains of 100 to 300 amino acids, yet all these widely differing proteins are constructed from only 20 amino acids plus several uncommon ones. The diversity of proteins, which can be assembled from 20 amino acids, has been compared to the millions of words in many languages that can be formed from the 26 letters of the English alphabet.

α-amino acids are the only kinds of amino acids in proteins. The alpha (α) refers to the central carbon to which are attached four different groups. Three of these are common to all the amino acids: a hydrogen atom (H—), a carboxyl (carboxylic acid) group (—COOH, $-\overset{\displaystyle \|}{\underset{\displaystyle O}{C}}$—OH, or —COO$^-$), and an amino group (—NH$_2$, —NH$_3^+$). The fourth group (R), referred to as a "side chain," is unique for each of the amino acids.

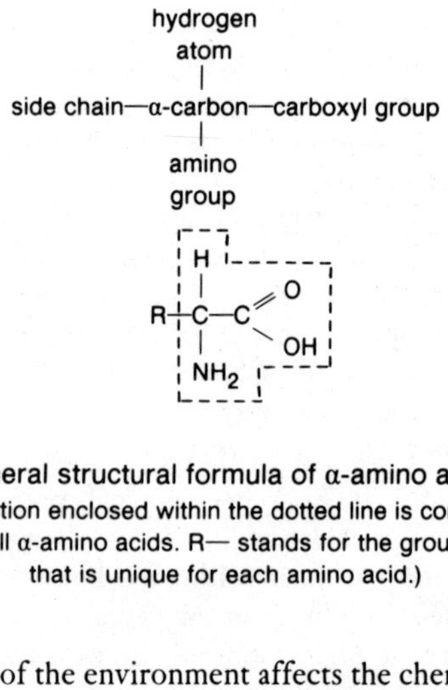

hydrogen
atom
|
side chain—α-carbon—carboxyl group
|
amino
group

General structural formula of α-amino acids
(The portion enclosed within the dotted line is common to all α-amino acids. R— stands for the group that is unique for each amino acid.)

The pH of the environment affects the chemical reactivity of the amino and carboxyl groups because pH affects the ionization states of these two groups. At biological pH of around 7, the amino group attracts an extra proton (is protonated), making it positively charged; therefore usually it is written "—NH$_3^+$." Also, at this pH the carboxyl group loses a proton (is dissociated), making it negatively charged; therefore usually it is written "—COO$^-$." The resulting dipolar ion is called a "zwitterion." In this text, structural formulas will show the compound as it exists at the pH of the tissues—the physiological pH.

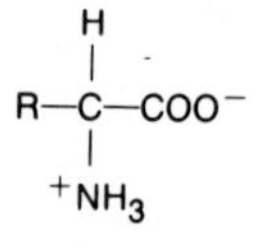

Of several ways of classifying α-amino acids, one divides them according to their essentiality. If a species is unable to synthesize an amino acid in sufficient quantity to support life and growth, the amino acid is said to be "essential" for that species. The individuals of that species must secure that amino acid preformed from food. Since all 20 of the amino acids are essential in the sense that they are necessary for

$$R-\overset{\displaystyle H}{\underset{\displaystyle ^+NH_3}{C}}-COO^-$$

Zwitterion

life and growth, a better term that is sometimes used in "dietarily essential." For adult humans, the essential amino acids are ARGININE, HISTIDINE , ISOLEUCINE, LEUCINE, LYSINE, ME-THIONINE, PHENYLALANINE, THREONINE, TRYPTOPHAN, and VALINE. The body cells can manufacture on demand enough of the remaining amino acids to meet their needs. Therefore those amino acids are called "nonessential" or "dietarily nonessential."

Another way of classifying amino acids is by the characteristics of their side chains which are unique for each amino acid. As the amino acids join together one after another during protein formation, the amino and carboxyl groups on the α-carbons of each amino acid form the backbone of the finished protein. After this bonding, these two groups exert no further chemical influence because they are covalently bonded in a peptide (amide) bond. However, the amino group at one end of the protein and the carboxyl group at the other end do ionize and contribute to the chemical properties of the protein. Moreover, because the side chains stick out from the backbone of the developing protein, they may interact with each other and determine the conformation of the protein.

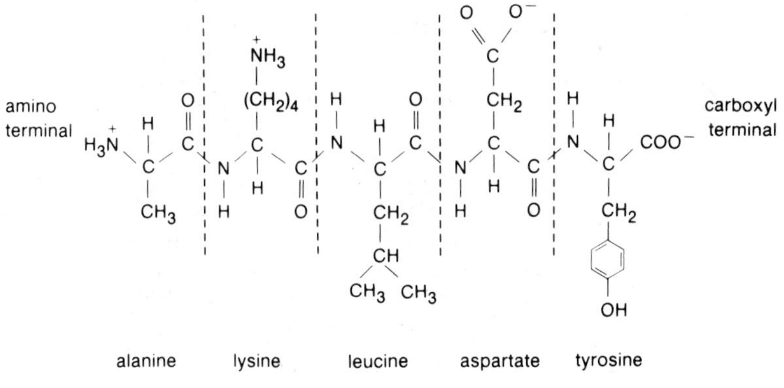

Alanyllysylleucylaspartyltyrosine
(Ala-Lys-Leu-Asp-Tyr)

It is by the conformation, or "shape," of the protein that it will be "recognized" by the tissues and be able to do its job. Consequently, knowledge of the chemical characteristics of the side chains is crucial to understanding proteins. Following are some groupings of amino acids based on the structure of their side chains.

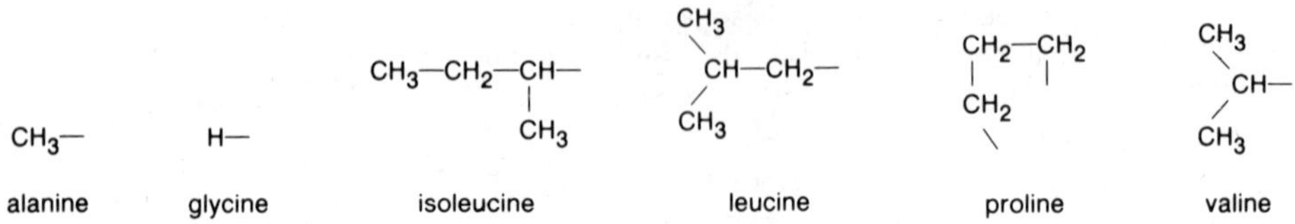

$$CH_3- \qquad H- \qquad CH_3-CH_2-\overset{\displaystyle |}{\underset{\displaystyle CH_3}{CH}}- \qquad \overset{\displaystyle CH_3}{\underset{\displaystyle CH_3}{\diagdown CH-CH_2-}} \qquad \overset{\displaystyle CH_2-CH_2}{\underset{\displaystyle CH_2}{| \qquad |}} \qquad \overset{\displaystyle CH_3}{\underset{\displaystyle CH_3}{\diagdown CH-}}$$

alanine   glycine   isoleucine   leucine   proline   valine

Side groups of aliphatic amino acids

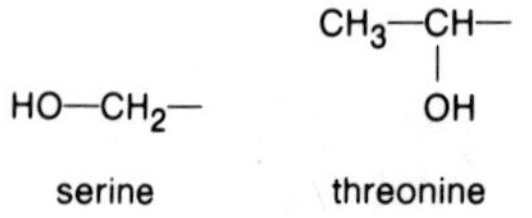

$$HO-CH_2- \qquad \overset{\displaystyle CH_3-CH-}{\underset{\displaystyle OH}{}}$$

serine   threonine

Amino acids with uncharged hydroxyl groups on their side chains

Six amino acids have uncharged aliphatic (hydrocarbon) side chains. These are ALANINE, GLYCINE, ISOLEUCINE, LEUCINE, PROLINE, and VALINE. Proline is different in that the amino group that is attached to the α-carbon is also linked to the side chain, creating a ring structure. Actually, this so-called "amino" group is an "imino" group (—NH). Valine, leucine, and isoleucine (shown above) have branched side chains, which give them special characteristics. These three are spoken of as the "branched-chain" amino acids. Two amino acids, SERINE and THREONINE, have uncharged hydroxyl groups on their side chains. Three amino acids PHENYLALANINE, TYROSINE, and TRYPTOPHAN, have uncharged aromatic side chains. The side chains of LYSINE, ARGININE, and HISTIDINE are positively charged at the pH of the cells.

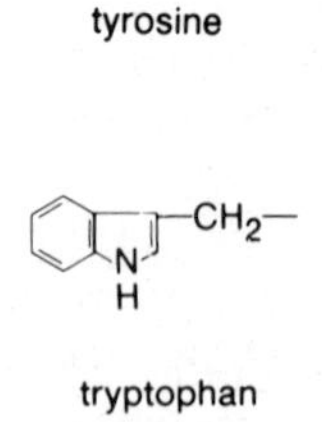

phenylalanine

lysine

$$\overset{+}{N}H_3-CH_2-CH_2-CH_2-CH_2-$$

tyrosine

arginine

$$\underset{\displaystyle NH_2-\overset{\displaystyle \overset{+}{N}H_2}{\underset{}{\overset{||}{C}}}-NH-CH_2-CH_2-CH_2-}{}$$

tryptophan

histidine

$$\underset{\displaystyle HN \quad NH}{\underset{\displaystyle \diagdown_{\displaystyle C}\diagup}{HC=C-CH_2-}}$$

Amino acids with uncharged, aromatic side chains 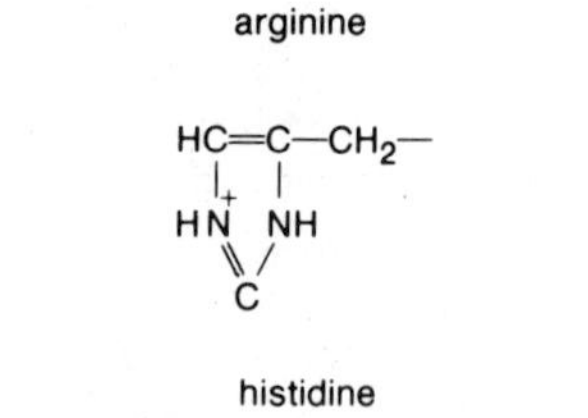   Amino acids with positively charged side chains

Histidine's side chain at times may be neutral, depending on its local environment. Two amino acids, cysteine and methionine have sulfur atoms in their side chains. The amino acids aspartate and glutamate have negatively charged carboxyl groups on their side chains. Each has a derivative in which an uncharged amide group replaces the carboxyl group on its side chain.

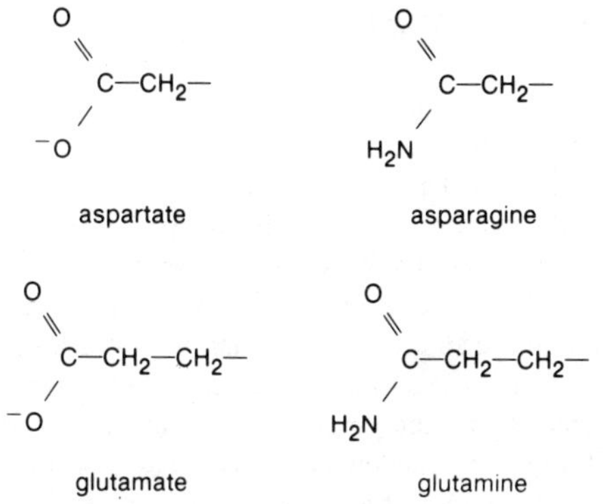

aspartate

asparagine

glutamate

glutamine

Amino acids with carboxyl group on their side chains and a derivative that has an uncharged amide group

HS—CH_2—

cysteine

CH_3—S—CH_2—CH_2—

methionine

Amino acids with sulfur in their side chains

All biologically active amino acids, except glycine, have an asymmetric carbon atom, termed an "anomeric" carbon. An asymmetric carbon is one having four different groups attached to it. These groups can be arranged in two different ways so that the two mirror-image forms cannot be superimposed on each other (in the same way that the left and right hands cannot be superimposed on each other.)

Compounds containing such asymmetric carbons are said to be "optically active" because they have the ability to rotate the plane of plane-polarized light. The two different forms of a parent compound are stereoisomers or enantiomers of each other. Threonine and isoleucine have two asymmetric carbons therefore they have four stereoisomers each. The other amino acids, except glycine, have one asymmetric carbon and thus two stereoisomers; one is referred to as the L-isomer and the other as the D-isomer.

The stereoisomers of a parent compound are identical in physical and chemical properties except that (1) they rotate the plane of plane-polarized light in opposite directions (L- and D-) and (2) they react differently with reagents which also have an asymmetric carbon. It is interesting to note that living tissues can distinguish between two stereoisomers. For example, L-amino acids, but not D-amino acids, can be incorporated into proteins.

The specific rotation of a single isomer can be determined; but it is more useful to relate the four groups around

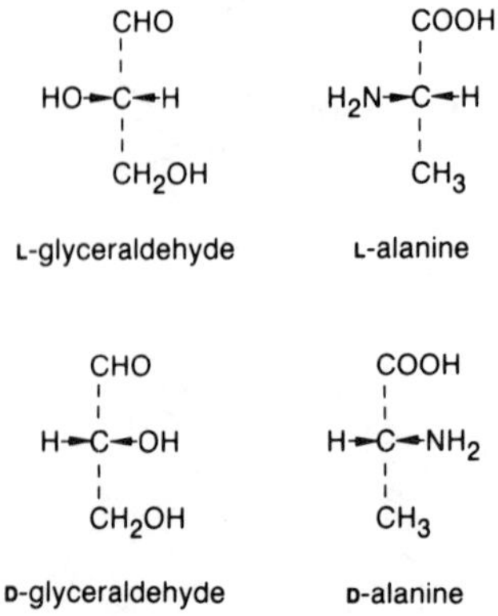

CHO
|
HO→C←H
|
CH₂OH

L-glyceraldehyde

COOH
|
H₂N→C←H
|
CH₃

L-alanine

CHO
|
H→C←OH
|
CH₂OH

D-glyceraldehyde

COOH
|
H→C←NH₂
|
CH₃

D-alanine

Stereoisomers of alanine
compared to the standard
stereoisomers of glyceraldehyde

the central carbon of an amino acid to the four groups around the central carbon of a reference compound. The compound chosen as the standard of reference for the absolute configuration of stereoisomers is glyceraldehyde—one isomer is labeled L-glyceraldehyde and the other is D-glyceraldehyde.

The figure at left shows the absolute configuration of the amino acid alanine. The horizontal wedges in the formulas indicate that the attached groups are oriented in space above the plane of the text page; the vertical dotted lines indicate those groups that extend below the plane of the text page. These formulas are known as "perspective formulas." Note that the amino group of alanine occupies a space that corresponds to the space occupied by the hydroxyl group of glyceraldehyde, the —COOH of alanine is related to the —CHO of glyceraldehyde, the —CH₃ of alanine is related to the —CH₂OH of glyceraldehyde, and the hydrogens of both compounds occupy the related spaces. In this way, the stereoisomers of the naturally occurring amino acids can be designated as D- or L- according to their relationship to D- or L-glyceraldehyde. The designation of D- or L- will be used rarely in this text since only L-amino acids are incorporated into proteins.

Sometimes amino acids are classified as glucogenic or ketogenic according to the destination of their carbon skeletons during degradation. The "skeleton" is the carbon-carbon portion of the amino acid that remains after the amino group has been removed. If the skeleton, or a portion of it, is changed into a compound that may lead to the production of GLUCOSE, the amino acid is said to be "glucogenic." (Many chemists think of glycogen rather than glucose as the end product of GLUCONEOGENESIS; therefore, they use the term "glycogenic." Both are correct.) These amino acids are useful in maintaining a normal BLOOD GLUCOSE LEVEL and in replenishing the carbohydrate metabolites of the TCA CYCLE. If the compound is one that could lead to the formation of KETONE BODIES, the amino acid is said to be "ketogenic." These amino acids would lead to the synthesis of fats, ketone bodies, and sterols. For a further discussion of this classification, see GLUCOGENIC AMINO ACIDS and KETOGENIC AMINO ACIDS. See also: AMINO ACID DEGRADATION; AMINO ACID BIOSYNTHESIS; ESSENTIAL AMINO ACIDS; PROTEIN STRUCTURE; individual amino acids.

SUGGESTED READINGS

Broquist, H. P. 1984. Amino acid metabolism. In *Present knowledge in nutrition*, 5th ed., 147–155. Washington, D. C.: The Nutrition Foundation, Inc.

Cooper, A. J. L. 1983. Biochemistry of sulfur-containing amino acids. *Ann. Rev. Biochem.* 52:187–222.

Jackson, A. A. 1983. Amino acids: Essential and nonessential? *Lancet* 2:1034–1037.

See suggested readings for: individual amino acids; ESSENTIAL AMINO ACIDS; BRANCHED-CHAIN AMINO ACIDS.

aminotransferases (transaminases). A group of VITAMIN B_6-dependent enzymes that catalyze the removal of the amino group ($-NH_2$) from an amino acid to produce the α-keto acid, and then reversibly transfer the $-NH_2$ to a second keto acid to yield a new amino acid. These enzymes carry the names of the pair of amino acids involved, such as *glutamate-alanine aminotransferase*. Normally the serum levels of aminotransferases are low, but if there is extensive damage to a tissue, the affected enzymes will be spilled into the blood stream where they become a diagnostic marker. For example, a rise in *serum glutamate-oxaloacetate aminotransferase* (SGOT) alerts the medical team to a possible myocardial infarct. See also: VITAMIN B_6.

ammonium ion (NH_4^+). A toxic substance released during the degradation of amino acids and some other nitrogenous substances. See also: UREA CYCLE for a description of the body's method of handling this ion.

ammonotelic. Organisms that excrete nitrogen as ammonia. Fish are ammonotelic organisms.

AMP. See ADENOSINE MONOPHOSPHATE.

amphipathic. The characteristic of a molecule possessing two regions of opposing solubility such that one end of the molecule is attracted to water (is hydrophilic) while the other end is not (is hydrophobic).

anabolism. The energy-requiring production of macromolecules from smaller molecules. See also: METABOLISM.

anaerobic reaction. A chemical process that does not require oxygen.

analbuminemia. A deficiency in the liver's capacity to synthesize the protein albumin, thus leading to a decrease in the plasma albumin. Albumins serve to maintain the osmotic pressure which helps water and nutrients to pass through capillary walls. Albumins are also important as carriers in the blood for a variety of drugs, bilirubin, fatty acids, and trace elements.

Andersen's disease (glycogen storage disease: type IV). A disease caused by a deficiency of the enzyme that produces the branches on glycogen, resulting in an accumulation of glycogen with abnormally long chains. Infants born with this disease generally die of cirrhosis and liver failure soon after birth.

SUGGESTED READINGS

Howell, R. R., and J. C. Williams. 1983. The glycogen storage diseases. In *The metabolic basis of inherited disease*, 5th ed., ed. J. B. Stanbury, et al., 141–166. New York: McGraw-Hill.

anomeric carbon. The carbon in AMINO ACIDS (and in other organic compounds) that has four different groups attached to it. This configuration confers optical activity on the amino acid. Amino acids with one anomeric carbon have two stereoisomers, those with two anomeric carbons have four stereoisomers. See also: AMINO ACIDS, for a more complete explanation of D-amino acids and L-amino acids.

antibody. A serum protein that is synthesized in response to the entry of a foreign substance (antigen). The antibody combines selectively with the foreign agent to neutralize its toxic effects. See also: IMMUNOPROTEIN.

anticodon. A sequence of three bases in transfer RNA that is complementary to a sequence of three bases (a codon) in messenger RNA. See also: GENETIC CODE; RNA.

antigen. A foreign substance, either free or combined, at the surface of a bacterial or tissue cell that elicits the formation of a specific antibody protein.

antimetabolite. A substance that bears a structural resemblance to a normal substrate or enzyme and thus competes with it in metabolism. Some antimetabolites are used therapeutically; for example, an antimetabolite of FOLACIN is used as an agent for slowing the growth of cancers, thus creating a folacin deficiency.

antioxidant. An agent that prevents or inhibits oxidation of a substance by combining with oxygen. In this way, the oxygen is tied up with the antioxidant and the desirable substance is protected. Vitamins C and E are antioxidants.

apoenzyme. The inactive, protein part of an enzyme that remains after the cofactor is removed. The replacement of the cofactor, either a coenzyme or a metallic ion, restores the activity of the enzyme.

arginine (Arg). A glucogenic (glycogenic), six-carbon α-amino acid that, along with HISTIDINE and LYSINE, has a positively charged side chain.

In addition to its role in many protein structures and in the production of creatine, arginine plays a key role in the

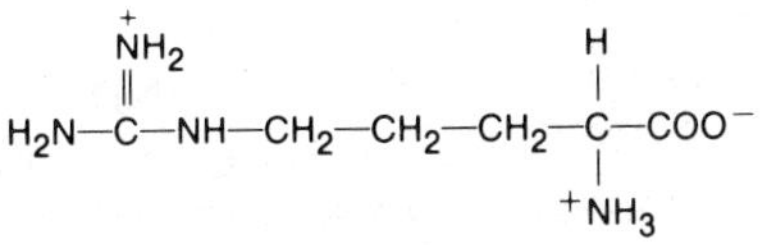

$$
\begin{array}{c}
\overset{+}{N}H_2 \qquad\qquad\qquad H \\
\parallel \qquad\qquad\qquad\quad | \\
H_2N-C-NH-CH_2-CH_2-CH_2-C-COO^- \\
| \\
{}^+NH_3
\end{array}
$$

Arginine
(Arg)

UREA CYCLE. In the cytosol of liver cells arginine is broken apart into urea, which is excreted, and into ornithine, a urea cycle metabolite. In other reactions of the urea cycle arginine is produced from ornithine.

This synthesis of arginine in the urea cycle is at the heart of the question of arginine's essentiality. Those who classify it as essential explain that the enzyme *arginase* in the urea cycle breaks down arginine to ornithine and urea so fast that there is no net arginine available for protein synthesis. Others maintain that, while arginine must be provided preformed in the diet (is essential) in rapidly growing infants and children, the net amount the body can synthesize is sufficient for adults.

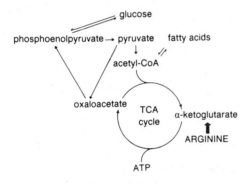

The carbons of arginine
enter metabolic pathways

When surplus arginine is present, or when the demand for energy is great enough to require degradation of amino acids, the carbon skeleton of arginine enters the TCA CYCLE at α-ketoglutarate. The skeleton is first converted to ornithine (in the urea cycle), and then to glutamate γ-semialdehyde, which is oxidized to the amino acid GLUTAMATE. (As shown in the following diagram, the imino acid PROLINE enters the TCA cycle along the same path.) The glutamate formed is oxidatively deaminated by *glutamate*

23

dehydrogenase with NAD^+ as coenzyme to yield α-ketoglutarate and an ammonium ion (NH_4^+). Thus rearranged, 4 carbons of arginine enter the TCA cycle at α-ketoglutarate and the amino group enters the urea cycle. See also: AMINO ACID DEGRADATION; ESSENTIAL AMINO ACIDS; UREA CYCLE.

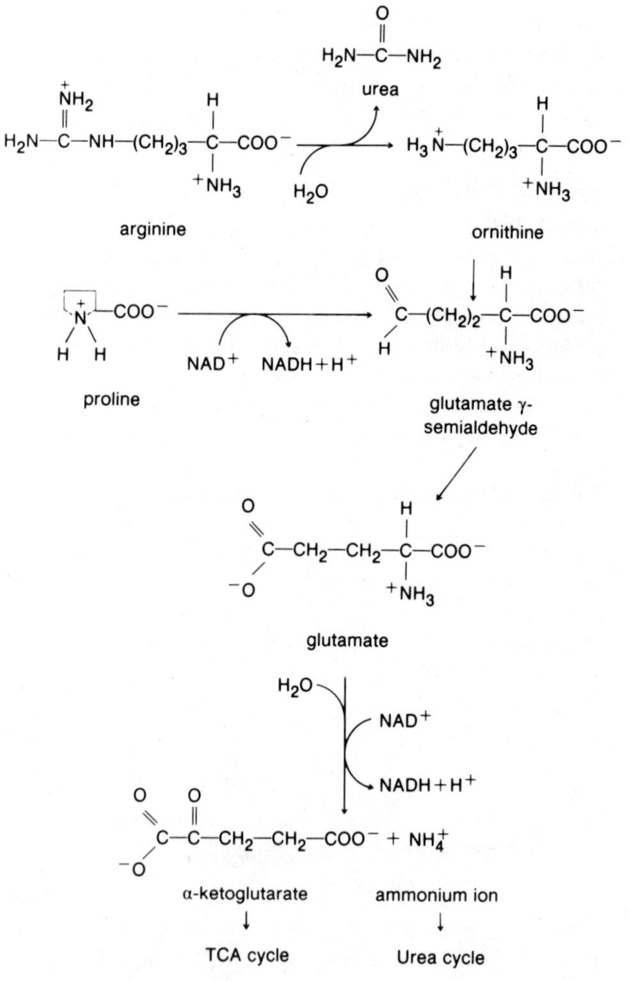

The degradation of arginine and proline

argininemia. High levels of ARGININE in serum owing to a deficiency of the enzyme *arginase*. Symptoms include severe mental retardation.

SUGGESTED READINGS

See suggested readings for INBORN ERRORS OF METABOLISM.

argininosuccinicacidemia. A condition in which argininosuccinate, a UREA CYCLE intermediate, accumulates in the blood and other body fluids. This high level is caused by a deficiency of the enzyme *argininosuccinase* and results in mental retardation, liver disease, and epilepsy.

SUGGESTED READINGS

See suggested readings for INBORN ERRORS OF METABOLISM.

aromatic amino acids. Amino acids whose side chains contain a ring structure. They are PHENYLALANINE, TRYPTO-PHAN, and TYROSINE.

artificial sweeteners. See NONNUTRITIVE SWEETENERS.

ascorbic acid. See VITAMIN C.

asparagine (Asn). A dietarily nonessential, glucogenic (glycogenic), four-carbon, α-amino acid that is an amide of ASPARTATE, another amino acid.

Like GLUTAMINE, asparagine is polar and uncharged due to the amide group on its side chain. It can be hydrolyzed easily to aspartate or synthesized from aspartate in a reaction catalyzed by *asparagine synthetase,* a vitamin B_6-dependent enzyme.

If asparagine is degraded for energy, the enzyme *asparaginase* catalyzes its conversion to aspartate, which is transaminated to oxaloacetate in a vitamin B_6-dependent reaction. Oxaloacetate then either combines with ACETYL-CoA and enters the TCA CYCLE or is converted to phosphoenolpyruvate (PEP) and proceeds toward reforming GLUCOSE (GLUCONEOGENESIS).

$$O \quad\quad H$$
$$\overset{\displaystyle \|}{C}-CH_2-\overset{\displaystyle |}{\underset{\displaystyle |}{C}}-COO^-$$
$$H_2N \quad\quad\quad {}^+NH_3$$

Asparagine
(Asn)

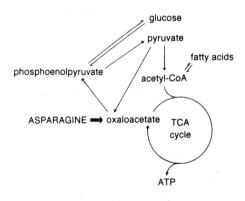

The carbons of asparagine
enter metabolic pathways

$$^-OOC-CH_2-\overset{\overset{\displaystyle H}{|}}{\underset{\underset{\displaystyle {}^+NH_3}{|}}{C}}-COO^-$$

Aspartate
(Asp)

aspartame. A nonnutritive sweetener composed of two AMINO ACIDS, ASPARTATE and PHENYLALANINE. See also: NON-NUTRITIVE SWEETENERS.

aspartate (Asp). A dietarily nonessential, glucogenic (glycogenic), four-carbon α-amino acid that, like GLUTAMATE, has an acidic side chain. Sometimes aspartate is referred to as aspartic acid; however, aspartate is used here to denote its ionized state—a negative charge on the terminal carboxyl group—at the pH of body tissues.

Aspartate plays an important role in transfer of electrons across the membrane between the mitochondria and cytosol of the cells of some tissues. This membrane will not allow NADH to cross from the cytosol into the mitochondrion. However, the complex MALATE-ASPARTATE SHUTTLE can transport the crucial electrons from NADH out of or into the mitochondria for operation of the RESPIRATORY CHAIN.

In the cytosol, electrons (reducing equivalents) are transferred from cytosolic NADH to oxaloacetate (OAA). OAA is then acted on by *malate dehydrogenase* to form malate, which can pass through the membrane. Malate then gives up its reducing equivalents to matrix NAD^+, forming NADH, which can pass them directly to the respiratory chain.

Another important role of aspartate is as the donor of one of the nitrogens in urea and, with fumarate, as a link between the UREA CYCLE and the TCA CYCLE. This nitrogen comes to aspartate from glutamate by transamination and is carried into the cytosol by aspartate. Then aspartate uses an ATP and combines with citrulline (which has entered the cytosol from the mitochondria) to form argininosuccinate. This is the first step of the urea cycle.

Three of aspartate's carbons and a nitrogen are incorporated into the pyrimidine ring of the pyrimidine bases cytosine, thymine, and uracil. Through this action, aspartate becomes vital to the transmission of genetic information because these bases are incorporated into DNA and/or RNA.

The degradation of aspartate by transamination to oxaloacetate permits its carbon skeleton to enter the TCA cycle. In this process α-ketoglutarate is converted to glutamate, which will be oxidatively deaminated by *glutamate dehydrogenase,* yielding an ammonium ion and reforming α-ketoglutarate. The carbons of aspartate can also enter the TCA cycle via fumarate from the urea cycle. See also: AMINO ACID DEGRADATION; MALATE-ASPARTATE SHUTTLE; TCA CYCLE; UREA CYCLE.

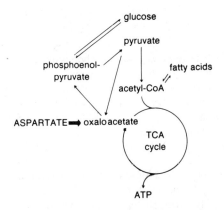

The carbons of aspartate
enter metabolic pathways

aspartic acid. See ASPARTATE.

ATP. See ADENOSINE TRIPHOSPHATE.

**ATP, ADP, AMP (adenosine triphosphate, adenosine di-
phosphate, adenosine monophosphate).** The universal nucleotides by which energy is captured, transferred,
and used in all living organisms, both plant and animal.

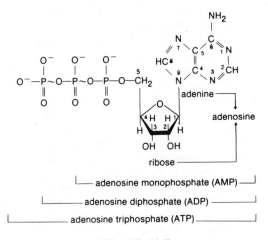

ATP, ADP, AMP

The three compounds are composed of a purine base (adenine) and a five-carbon sugar (ribose) to form the nucleoside (adenosine) portion of their structures. The only differences among the three are the number of phosphate

adenosine—P~P~P = ATP

adenosine—P~P = ADP

adenosine—P = AMP

groups attached at the #5-carbon of the ribose and the amount of standard free energy of hydrolysis available when the bonds between the phosphates are broken.

The two terminal phosphate bonds on ATP and the one on ADP are so-called "high-energy" bonds often denoted by a wavy line in structural formulas. The term "high-energy bonds" may give the impression that they are different from other chemical bonds; however, they are no different. What is unique is the great negativity within the structure of ATP that causes stress as the negatively charged portions attempt to move as far away as possible from each other. This stress drives the reaction toward the breaking of the bonds by hydrolysis. The products, ADP and P_i, also are negatively charged, which makes them repel each other and makes it difficult for them to recombine. This, too, pushes the reaction toward hydrolysis. It takes a great deal of energy (gleaned from the oxidation of energy nutrients) to overcome the repulsion of like charges on ADP and P_i and reform ATP.

The hydrolysis of ATP to ADP and P_i, or to AMP and PP_i (pyrophosphate), usually occurs simultaneously with a reaction that will use the free energy—an action called a "coupled reaction." If a cell requires the assembly of compounds A and B to synthesize compound AB, then A and B will be attracted to the active site of the appropriate enzyme; ATP also will be present. The enzyme will become the avenue by which energy from the hydrolysis of ATP will be transferred to the bonding of A and B. This is an economical use of time and energy and also precludes other reactions taking place inadvertently.

The free energy released upon hydrolysis of these high-energy phosphate bonds generates heat that maintains body temperature and is used to power most cellular reactions, such as synthesis of more complex molecules from simpler ones; muscle contraction; sending signals along a nerve; ACTIVE TRANSPORT of inorganic ions and cellular nutrients across membrane barriers against a concentration gradient; and activation of a molecule so that it can enter into certain reactions, for example, the phosphorylation of GLUCOSE to glucose 6-phosphate so that glucose degradation may proceed toward the release of energy.

SUGGESTED READINGS

Cross, R. L. 1981. The mechanism and regulation of ATP synthesis by F_1-ATPases. *Ann. Rev. Biochem.* 50:681–714.

avidin. A glycoprotein found in raw egg whites that binds biotin in the intestinal tract and inhibits the absorption of biotin. See also: BIOTIN, THE VITAMIN.

b

B-complex vitamins. See B-VITAMIN TERMINOLOGY.

B-vitamin terminology. Many of the vitamins have both names and number. In 1979 the Committee on Nomenclature of the American Institute of Nutrition agreed on the names that would be used and then published their decision in the *Journal of Nutrition* 1979; 198:8–15.

In this text the correct names will be used but the reader should be aware of the other names that may appear in the literature.

Correct names	Other names commonly used
thiamin	vitamin B_1
riboflavin	vitamin B_2
niacin	nicotinic acid, nicotinamide, niacinamide
vitamin B_6	pyridoxine, pyridoxal, pyridoxamine
folacin	folate, folic acid
vitamin B_{12}	cobalamin
pantothenic acid	pantothenate
biotin	none

basal metabolic rate (BMR). The rate at which the body uses oxygen when it is at rest and food has not been ingested for 12 hours. See also: IODIDE.

basic amino acids. Amino acids whose side chains have positively charged amino groups. They are HISTIDINE, LYSINE, and ARGININE.

beriberi. A cluster of symptoms caused by a deficiency of the vitamin THIAMIN. This vitamin is crucial to the gleaning

$$NH_2—CH_2—CH_2—COOH$$

β-alanine

A naturally occurring amino acid
that is not found in proteins

of energy from food, particularly in the metabolism of GLU-COSE, the fuel of choice for the brain. Neural disorders, then, accompany thiamin deficiency. Other deficiency symptoms include cardiovascular problems, anorexia, and painful muscles in the calves. Increased physical activity exacerbates these symptoms. See also: THIAMIN; THIAMIN PYROPHOSPHATE.

beta alanine (β-alanine). A naturally occurring amino acid not found in proteins. It is a part of COENZYME A, PANTO-THENIC ACID, and carnosine.

beta alaninemia (β-alaninemia). A high level of β-alanine in the blood and other body fluids caused by the absence of the enzyme β-*alanine-α-ketoglutarate aminotransferase*.

SUGGESTED READINGS

See suggested readings for INBORN ERRORS OF METABOLISM.

beta carotene (β-carotene). A carotenoid, which is a precursor of VITAMIN A, found in plant foods. β-carotene is responsible for the yellow and orange colors of the vitamin A-rich vegetables, such as carrots. Carotenoids are added as a coloring agent to such foods as cheese and margarine.

beta oxidation (β-oxidation). The enzymatic process that occurs in mitochondria whereby FATTY ACIDS are oxidatively degraded at the second carbon atom (the beta carbon) from the carboxyl group. These two-carbon fragments are successively released as ACETYL-COA while the fatty acid carbon chain is shortened by two carbons with each release. See also: FATTY ACID OXIDATION.

bile pigment. A breakdown product of the HEME portion of hemoglobin, myoglobin, and cytochromes. See also: BILIRUBIN; BILIVERDIN; HEME.

bile salts. Derivatives of CHOLESTEROL that are synthesized in the liver and stored in the gallbladder. Bile salts are released into the small intestine where they act as detergents and emulsify the dietary LIPIDS, that is, they break up lipids into very small globules. After emulsification, a molecule of a digestive ENZYME can get close enough to a molecule of a lipid to hydrolyze its bonds.

An important bile salt is glycocholate, which results from the bonding of cholyl-CoA with GLYCINE. Another is taurocholate, which is formed by cholyl-CoA and taurine. Taurocholate is the principal bile salt formed in infants, whereas glycocholate is formed mainly in adults. See also: ENTEROHEPATIC CIRCULATION.

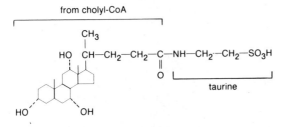

from cholyl-CoA

glycocholic acid

A bile salt derived from cholesterol

from cholyl-CoA

taurocholic acid

A bile salt derived from cholesterol

SUGGESTED READINGS

Gaull, G. E. 1982. Taurine in the nutrition of the human infant. *Acta Paediatr. Scand.* [Suppl.] 296:38–40.

Rassin, D. K., Gaull, G. E., Jarvenpas, A. L., and N. C. R. Raiha. 1983. Feeding the low-birth-weight infant. II. Effects of taurine and cholesterol supplementation on amino acids and cholesterol. *Pediatrics* 71(2):179–186.

bilirubin. A bile pigment resulting from the breakdown of HEME, the nonprotein iron-containing portion of hemoglobin, myoglobin, and cytochromes. Heme in hemoglobin is responsible for carrying oxygen from the lungs and releasing it to the cells. When there is an accelerated breakdown of hemoglobin (hemolysis) or a defect in the liver's ability to dispose of bilirubin, the bilirubin spills into the blood and produces the deep yellow color in the skin and eyes known as jaundice. In adults jaundice indicates a serious but treatable condition; however, in premature babies the increase in bilirubin may cause serious brain damage which can be fatal. See also: BILIVERDIN; HEME; JAUNDICE.

biliverdin.   A product of the first step in the degradation of the HEME portion of hemoglobin, myoglobin, and cytochromes. The enzyme for this reaction is *heme oxygenase* and the reductant is NADPH. Biliverdin is reduced further to bilirubin by *biliverdin reductase* and another molecule of NADPH. The reactions from heme to bilirubin can be seen in the changing colors of bruises.   See also: BILIRUBIN; HEME.

biotin, the coenzyme.   Attached to carboxylases, this coenzyme form of the B-vitamin, biotin, becomes a carrier of activated carbon dioxide (in a carboxyl group) in such important reactions as the biosynthesis of GLUCOSE from non-carbohydrate sources (GLUCONEOGENESIS) and the biosynthesis of FATTY ACIDS. Biotin as a coenzyme of carboxylases also plays a key role in degradations of odd-chain fatty acids and of the amino acids ISOLEUCINE, VALINE, METHIONINE, and LEUCINE.

Carboxylases have a LYSINE in their structure to which biotin is attached. The carboxyl group of biotin reacts with the epsilon-amino group on the end of the specified lysine. The combination of biotin-enzyme (biotinyllysine) is termed "biocytin." The amide link connects the two parts of biocytin making a "long arm" that can swing carbon dioxide, a product of the TCA CYCLE, from one active site of an ENZYME to another site on the same enzyme to complete a series of reactions.

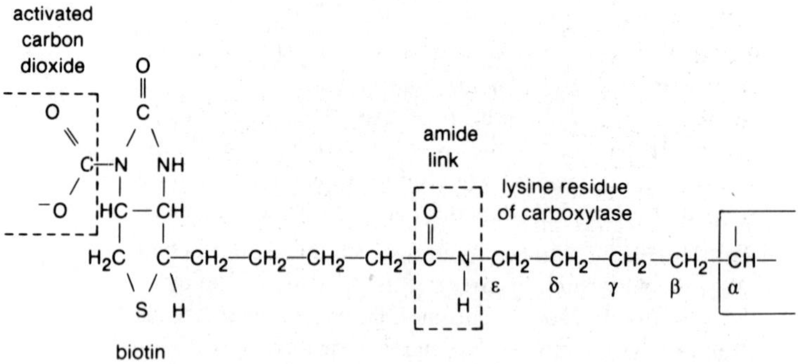

The "long arm" of biotin linked to a lysine residue of a carboxylase picks up the activated carbon dioxide

In gluconeogenesis the long arm provided by the connection of biotin to the lysine residue of *pyruvate carboxylase* is used in the formation of oxaloacetate (a four-carbon compound) from pyruvate (a three-carbon compound). Oxaloacetate can then proceed through phosphoenolpyruvate to the synthesis of glucose. This addition of carbon dioxide to pyruvate takes place in two major steps: carbon dioxide first becomes attached to the biotin-enzyme intermediate and next it becomes attached to pyruvate. The ATP required in the first step activates the carbon dioxide with enough energy for the transfer occurring in the second step. A MAGNESIUM ion is required for the $ATP:Mg^{++}$ complex of the first step, and a MANGANESE ion is required in the second step.

Step 1

$$\text{Biotin}-\text{Enzyme} + HCO_3^- \quad \xrightarrow[Mg^{++}]{ATP \quad ADP+P_i}$$

Carboxy—Biotin—Enzyme

Step 2

$$\text{Carboxy}-\text{Biotin}-\text{Enzyme} + \text{Pyruvate} \xrightarrow{Mn^{++}}$$

Biotin—Enzyme + Oxaloacetate

ACETYL-COA is the positive modulator of the *pyruvate carboxylase* reaction; that is, the enzyme is activated when there is a high level of acetyl-CoA. The rise in acetyl-CoA may be due to a high level of ATP so that the acetyl-CoA is not needed for the production of energy through the TCA CYCLE; or, the acetyl-CoA entry into the TCA cycle may be slowed down by a lack of carbohydrate intermediates, principally oxaloacetate. In either case, the stimulation of the *pyruvate carboxylase* reaction will provide oxaloacetate that (1) can lead through phosphoenolpyruvate to the synthesis of glucose, or (2) can combine with acetyl-CoA to form citrate, bringing acetyl-CoA into the TCA cycle for the production of energy.

Acetyl-CoA carboxylase, another biotin-carboxylase, is the facilitator in the conversion, in the cytosol, of acetyl-CoA (a two-carbon compound) to malonyl-CoA (a three-carbon compound). The carboxylation of acetyl-CoA, the committed step in FATTY ACID SYNTHESIS, occurs similarly to the two-step *pyruvate carboxylase* reaction. In the first step, the biotin-enzyme combination uses the energy from ATP to pick up carbon dioxide in the form of a bicarbonate ion (HCO_3^-). This forms the carbon dioxide-biotin-enzyme group that is activated so that it has the energy to participate in the second step. In the second step, the "long arm" of the complex swings the carbon dioxide over to an acetyl-CoA

33

to form malonyl-CoA. Fatty acid synthesis may now continue.

The positive modulator of *acetyl-CoA carboxylase* is citrate. Citrate is not consumed in fatty acid synthesis; however, it participates by carrying acetyl-CoA out of the mitochondria, where it was formed from pyruvate, and into the cytosol, where fatty acid synthesis takes place.

Propionyl-CoA carboxylase is another biotin-dependent carboxylase with mechanisms similar to the ones already discussed. This carboxylase adds an activated carbon dioxide to propionyl-CoA and forms the D-isomer of methylmalonyl-CoA in the degradative path of odd-carbon fatty acids. These fatty acids are found mostly in plants and marine organisms. The D-isomer is converted to the L-isomer that is then acted upon by a VITAMIN B_{12}-dependent enzyme, *methylmalonyl-CoA mutase*, and forms succinyl-CoA, an intermediate in the TCA cycle. The same reaction occurs in the degradative paths of the amino acids, methionine, threonine, valine, and isoleucine. Leucine is another amino acid that relies on biotin. In one step of leucine's degradation, biotin is required as a coenzyme for the conversion of β-methyl crotonyl-CoA to β-methyl glutaconyl-CoA.   See also: BIOTIN, THE VITAMIN; FATTY ACID OXIDATION; FATTY ACID SYNTHESIS; GLUCONEOGENESIS.

SUGGESTED READINGS

See suggested readings for BIOTIN, THE VITAMIN.

biotin, the vitamin.   A water-soluble B-vitamin widespread in food. Best food sources include liver, kidney, egg yolk, tomatoes, and yeast. Biotin exists in foods either in its free form or bound to a protein. Enzymes located in the brush border of the small intestine cleave the protein-bound biotin; the free biotin that is released is absorbed in the proximal small intestine and the distal colon. Biotin is also synthesized by bacteria in the intestinal tract; however, the extent of the daily requirement met by intestinal synthesis is unknown.

Biotin is actively transported into cells. Within the cell, biotin is converted to biotinyl 5'-adenylate by a kinase, in a reaction that requires the ATP:Mg^{++} complex. The biotinyl moiety is then attached to the apoenzyme (the inactive protein part) of the carboxylase by a synthetase to form the holoenzyme (the complete, active carboxylase).

Biotin's importance stems from its role as a coenzyme in carboxylations during which it carries an activated carbon dioxide molecule (in a carboxyl group) from one active site to another on a carboxylase. These reactions result in an elongation of the substrate through the addition of a carbon

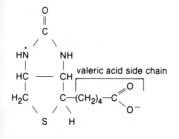

*reactive group

Biotin

dioxide molecule. One such enzyme, the biotin-dependent *acetyl-CoA carboxylase* in the cytosol, makes three-carbon malonyl-CoA from two-carbon acetyl-CoA in the committed step of FATTY ACID SYNTHESIS. Three other biotin-dependent enzymes are found in the mitochondria where they are critical in such processes as the degradation of odd-numbered fatty acids, degradation of certain AMINO ACIDS, as well as in GLUCONEOGENESIS.

Biotin was first discovered in certain foods that were known to protect against symptoms of dermatitis, hair loss, and loss of muscular control which developed in rats fed a diet high in raw egg whites. These symptoms, caused by a carbohydrate-containing protein named avidin found in raw egg white, were alleviated by addition of biotin to the diet. Each of the four polypeptide chains that compose avidin combines with biotin and prevents its absorption from the intestine.

In comparison with the wealth of knowledge about other B-vitamins, little is known about biotin. Definitive research has been hampered by the difficulty in producing a biotin-deficient diet. As stated previously, biotin is widespread in food and is needed in only tiny amounts—about 200 µg a day. As a consequence, spontaneous biotin deficiency has rarely been reported in humans; however, experimental biotin deficiency has been produced in both animals and humans by the consumption of large amounts of raw eggs and/or the use of antibiotics to wipe out the intestinal bacteria that synthesize biotin.

Sydenstricker et al. (1942) reported that they had produced biotin-deficiency symptoms in human subjects with a diet devoid of biotin and including avidin. In about three to four weeks, four subjects developed a scaly dermatitis and in about seven weeks they exhibited a disordered mental state, a grayish pallor and anorexia. Two showed electrocardiographic changes and all had a decrease in hematocrit and number of red blood cells. The symptoms were relieved in only a few days after the subjects received biotin injections.

In the years since Sydenstricker's experiment, research has been limited to isolated case studies. Until 1979 there was no "refined biochemical analysis of the metabolic effects of biotin deficiency" (Roth 1981). In 1979, an 11-year-old child was found who had consumed a diet of raw eggs for six years and had developed hyperuricemia, mental retardation, alopecia (hair loss), and a characteristic dermatitis. Enzymatic assays were carried out and, not surprisingly, these showed a deficiency of two carboxylases. Within six days after oral biotin repletion was begun and only cooked eggs were eaten, the metabolities of the carboxylases returned to normal and most of the overt symptoms disappeared. See also: BIOTIN, THE COENZYME for more about the reactions of the carboxylases.

SUGGESTED READINGS

DeTitta, G. T., et al. 1980. Carboxybiotin translocation mechanisms suggested by diffraction studies of biotin and its vitamers. *Proc. Natl. Acad. Sci.* 77:333–337.

Innis, S. M., and D. B. Allardyce. 1983. Possible biotin deficiency in adults receiving long-term total parenteral nutrition. *Am. J. Clin. Nutr.* 37:185–187.

Mock, D. M. et al. 1985. Biotin deficiency complicating parenteral alimentation: Diagnosis, metabolic repercussions, and treatment. *J. Pediatr.* 106:762–769.

Roth, K. S. 1981. Biotin in clinical medicine—A review. *Am. J. Clin. Nutr.* 34:1967–1974.

Stubble, J., S. Fish, and R. H. Abeles. 1980. Are carboxylations involving biotin concerted or nonconcerted? *J. Biol. Chem.* 255:236–242.

Sweetman, L. 1979. Deficiencies of propionyl-CoA and 3-methylcrotonyl-CoA carboxylases in a patient with a dietary deficiency of biotin. *Clin. Res.* 27:118 (abstract).

Sydenstricker, V. P., et al. 1942. Observations on "egg white injury" in man and its cure with biotin concentrate. *JAMA* 118:1199–1200.

Tanaka, K. 1981. New light on biotin deficiency. *N. Engl. J. Med.* 304:839–840.

Wood, H. G., and R. E. Barden. 1977. Biotin Enzymes. *Ann. Rev. Biochem.* 46:385–413.

blacktongue. A disease seen in dogs that is an animal analog of pellagra, the NIACIN deficiency disease in humans.

blood clotting. See VITAMIN K; GLUTAMINE; CALCIUM.

blood glucose level. The concentration of GLUCOSE in the circulatory system stated in terms of milligrams (mg) of glucose per 100 milliliters (ml) of blood. (Different institutions, disciplines, and texts use different methods of measuring concentrations.) Blood glucose is under homeostatic control, that is, it is maintained at a fairly constant level in spite of wide variations in exercise and carbohydrate intake.

After an overnight fast, the normal concentration may range between 70 mg/100 ml and 90 mg/100 ml. During the day, the level in a healthy person may fluctuate between 80 mg/ml and 120 mg/ml as the person eats and resupplies the blood with glucose or exercises and withdraws glucose.

The liver, which controls the blood glucose level, has an enormous capacity to take up and release large amounts of glucose in response to the principal opposing regulators, insulin and glucagon. After carbohydrate consumption and the consequent rise in blood glucose, glucagon secretion by the pancreas is depressed and insulin secretion is stimulated. These actions enhance the uptake of glucose by the peripheral tissues and the synthesis of GLYCOGEN in both liver and muscle. At the same time, the reactions that lead to GLYCOGENOLYSIS and GLUCONEOGENESIS are depressed.

As the cells of the body take up the glucose to use for fuel and the synthesis of glycogen continues, the blood glucose concentration gradually drops. Any excess glucose is metabolized to ACETYL-CoA and used for energy through the TCA CYCLE or, if the ATP level is high, used to synthesize LIPIDS.

When several hours have elapsed since food intake and activity has caused the cells to draw upon blood glucose for fuel, the consequent drop in glucose concentration below normal stimulates the secretion of glucagon and depresses secretion of insulin. Under the influence of glucagon, glycogen in the liver is degraded to glucose, which is released into the blood to maintain blood glucose levels in the acceptable range. Muscle glycogen may be degraded to glucose 6-phosphate by muscle cells; however, glucose 6-phosphate may not be degraded to glucose and released into the blood for general use owing to the lack of the enzyme *glucose 6-phosphatase*. This enzyme in other tissues dephosphorylates glucose for passage across membranes. Lactate, which is generated by muscle cells, is released into circulation and picked up by the liver for glucose production. Adipose tissues release FATTY ACIDS and glycerol into general circulation. Fatty acids may be used for energy by muscle and liver and glycerol can be converted to glucose in the liver.

If the lack of dietary carbohydrate were to continue, as in STARVATION, fasting, or following major surgery, the adrenal cortex would release glucocorticoid hormones. These hormones stimulate synthesis of gluconeogenic ENZYMES in the liver and enhance protein breakdown in other tissues to provide carbon for gluconeogenesis.

DIABETES MELLITUS is a disease in which there is a disturbance of the blood glucose level because of a relative or complete deficiency of insulin and/or a relative or great excess of glucagon. See also: DIABETES MELLITUS.

BMR. See BASAL METABOLIC RATE.

Changes caused by increased blood glucose concentration

Enhances	Depresses
secretion of insulin by pancreas	secretion of glucagon by pancreas
uptake of glucose by peripheral tissues	gluconeogenesis
synthesis of glycogen in liver and muscle	glycogenolysis in liver
conversion of glucose to fatty acids in liver	release of glucocorticoid hormones
conversion of fatty acids to triglycerides by adipose tissue	

Changes caused by decreased blood glucose concentration

Enhances	Depresses
secretion of glucagon by pancreas	secretion of insulin by pancreas
degradation of glycogen in liver and muscle	uptake of glucose by cells
gluconeogenesis	glycogen synthesis
release of free fatty acids and glycerol from adipose tissue	
release of glucocorticoids from adrenal cortex	
breakdown of proteinaceous tissue, particularly muscle	
shift to use of fatty acids for fuel	

branched-chain amino acids. LEUCINE, ISOLEUCINE, and VALINE. These amino acids are present in large amounts in skeletal muscle. Also present, mainly in muscle, are aminotransferases, which remove the amino ($—NH_2$) group from the amino acid. The amino group may be used to aminate pyruvate and thus form ALANINE. This reaction is valuable when the TCA CYCLE intermediates are in low supply or when GLUCOSE is needed. Alanine can be converted easily to pyruvate, which can replenish oxaloacetate in the TCA cycle. Also, the carbons of alanine, through pyruvate and phosphoenolypruvate (PEP), can be used to rebuild glucose. See also: ALANINE; ISOLEUCINE; LEUCINE; STARVATION; VALINE.

SUGGESTED READINGS

Tanaka, K., and L. E. Rosenberg. 1983. Disorders of branched chain amino acid and organic acid metabolism. In *The metabolic basis of inherited disease*, 5th ed., ed. J. B. Stanbury et al., 440–473. New York: McGraw-Hill.
See suggested readings for INBORN ERRORS OF METABOLISM.

buffer. A substance or a group of substances that resist a change in hydrogen-ion concentration of a solution. In the cells of the body where maintenance of a particular PH is vital, the presence of buffers minimizes shifts in hydrogen ion concentration when acids or bases are introduced into the body.

The normal pH of blood, for example, is 7.40, and in a healthy person would not vary by more than about 0.2. If blood pH were to fall below 7.0 or rise above 7.8, the results could be fatal.

The major buffer in blood plasma is the bicarbonate buffer system, which consists of H_2CO_3 (carbonic acid) and HCO_3^- (bicarbonate ion). Another is the phosphate buffer system, which consists of H_3PO_4 (phosphoric acid) and $HPO_4^=$ (biphosphate ion). In the vicinity of the PK′ of these acids, large amounts of either basic or acidic ions can be added without a major shift in the pH of the blood. The pK′ of an acid is the pH at which the acid is half-ionized. See also: ACID-BASE BALANCE; ACIDOSIS; ALKALOSIS; PH; PK′.

C

calcium (Ca⁺⁺). One of the major minerals of the body. Over 99% of the calcium occurs in the skeleton and teeth in a 2:1 ratio with PHOSPHORUS. The other 1% is no less important since it is critical to many vital functions including muscle contraction, nerve signals, blood clotting, integrity of MEMBRANES, and activation of ENZYMES such as *ATPase* and *succinyl dehydrogenase*. Calcium in the blood is found ionized, complexed with citrate, sulfate, or phosphate, or bound to two blood proteins, albumin and globulin.

Calcium ions play a significant role in the initiation of muscle contraction, where they act as intermediaries between nerves and muscles. When the muscle is at rest, calcium ions are pumped into the sarcoplasmic reticulum, a membrane-bound system of tubules and vesicles in a cell. This leaves the area around the muscle fibers low in calcium. When the cell is stimulated by the nerves, the sarcoplasmic reticulum releases a large amount of calcium ions, thereby stimulating contraction. This transport across membranes is catalyzed by calcium-dependent *ATPase*.

Calcium is also involved in GLYCOGEN metabolism, which is responsible for providing the fuel for muscle contraction. The presence of calcium ions and CYCLIC AMP results in the conversion of the enzyme *phosphorylase b* (inactive) to *phosphorylase a* (active), which catalyzes the catabolism of glycogen to GLUCOSE. At the same time, *glycogen synthase*, which, as its name implies, catalyzes the synthesis of glycogen from glucose, is converted from its active form to its inactive form. These reactions assure the phosphorylation of glucose to glucose 6-phosphate so that it can enter GLYCOLYSIS. Calcium ions, then, stimulate the contraction as well as provide for the release of glucose 6-phosphate to fuel the contractions. When the stimulus ends, calcium is removed, and the phosphorylase and the synthase revert to their original forms.

Some of these actions of calcium are thought to be mediated by calmodulin, a cytoplasmic calcium-binding regulatory protein that acts in smooth muscle. The binding of calcium ions to calmodulin stimulates the activities of some enzymes, such as *phosphodiesterase,* the enzyme which contributes to the relaxation of muscle by destroying the cyclic AMP that remains after the emergency is over.

Another calcium-binding regulatory protein is troponin C, a part of the troponin system of three proteins by which muscle contraction is mediated uniquely in striated muscle. These three proteins are troponin T (TpT), troponin I (TpI), and troponin C (TpC). Troponin C is similar to calmodulin in that each binds four molecules of calcium and each is about the same molecular weight; however, calmodulin acts in smooth muscle while the troponin system acts in striated muscle.

Although it has been known that calcium and VITAMIN K take active roles in the clotting of blood, it took many years to define the roles. The first ten glutamates on the amino end of prothrombin are carboxylated to γ-carboxy-glutamate by a vitamin K-dependent enzyme. It is this arrangement that binds calcium ions and produces the prothrombin that leads to the clotting of blood.

The blood calcium level is kept under homeostatic control in a number of ways. These include:

Hormonal control. These processes are under the direction of parathyroid hormone, which acts to raise blood concentrations back to normal, and calcitonin, which acts to lower blood calcium levels when they are greater than normal.

Bonding to proteins. Calcium in the blood is bound to two blood proteins, albumin and globulin, which release calcium if the blood calcium level drops.

Controlling absorption. The synthesis of a calcium-binding protein in the intestinal cells, aided by VITAMIN D, is increased if the blood calcium level drops. The result is that if more calcium is needed, more will be absorbed from the food eaten.

Storing the excess, then releasing it. If the blood level of calcium rises, more will be stored in the bones; and if the blood level drops, calcium will be resorbed from the bones.

Excretion or reabsorption in the kidneys. More calcium will be excreted in the urine if the plasma concentration of calcium is too high, and more will be returned to the blood stream if the calcium level is too low.

Thus far, it has not been shown that the short-term rise or fall of dietary calcium has any effect on the functions of calcium or on the blood calcium level. However, a consistently low dietary intake of calcium may have serious effects on growth in children and on the brittleness of bones in older persons, especially women.

The best food sources of calcium are milk or milk products and seafoods, especially canned seafoods if the bones are eaten. Other good sources are leafy, dark green vegetables, excepting those such as spinach that have a high oxalate content. Oxalate may combine with calcium and form an insoluble compound that cannot be absorbed.

Dietary protein and phosphorus appear to affect calcium balance in humans. High dietary intakes of protein, with constant dietary intakes of calcium and phosphorus, increase calcium excretion via the kidneys. A high dietary intake of phosphorus (that may occur when a person consumes a large number of soft drinks) accompanied by a constant dietary intake of protein and calcium may decrease calcium excretion by the kidneys. When both protein and phosphorus intakes are high (as might occur in a high meat diet), the urinary excretion of calcium is raised, but calcium balance seems to be unaffected.

Diets that depend largely on seeds and cereal, which have high phytate levels, may decrease calcium absorption because of the formation of insoluble compounds. Undigested fat in the intestine, as may occur in some disease states, forms a soap with the calcium, thus preventing its absorption.

Absorption of calcium may be increased by the presence of lactose (the sugar in milk), vitamin D, and the AMINO ACIDS LYSINE and ARGININE. Calcium may be excreted via the kidneys, feces, or sweat. That which is excreted in the feces may be either from dietary calcium or from calcium that has been absorbed and then secreted into the intestines.

SUGGESTED READINGS

Bikle, D. D., R. L. Morrissey, and D. T. Zolock. 1979. The mechanism of action of Vitamin D in the intestine. *Am. J. Clin. Nutr.* 32:2322–2338.

Cummings, J. H., et al. 1979. The effect of meat protein and dietary fiber on colonic function and metabolism. I. Changes in bowel habit, bile acid excretion, and calcium absorption. *Am. J. Clin. Nutr.* 32:2086–2093.

DeLuca, H. F. 1979. The Vitamin D system in the regulation of calcium and phosphorus metabolism. *Nutr. Rev.* 37:161–193.

Gallagher, J. C., et al. 1982. 1,25-dihydroxyvitamin D₃: Short- and long-term effects on bone and calcium metabolism in patients with postmenopausal osteoporosis. *Proc. Natl. Acad. Sci.* 79:3325–3329.

Halloran, B. P., and H. F. DeLuca. 1980. Calcium transport in small intestine during pregnancy and lactation. *Am. J. Physiol.* 239:E64–E68.

Hegsted, M., et al. 1981. Urinary calcium and calcium balance in young men as affected by level of protein and phosphorus intake. *J. Nutr.* 111:553–562.

Jackson, C. M., and Y. Nemerson. 1980. Blood coagulation. *Ann. Rev. Biochem.* 49:765–811.

Klee, C. B., T. H. Crouch, and P. G. Richman. 1980. Calmodulin. *Ann. Rev. Biochem.* 49:489–515.

Prenen, J. A. C., P. Boer, and E. J. D. Mees. 1984. Absorption kinetics of oxalate from oxalate-rich food in man. *Am. J. Clin. Nutr.* 40:1007–1010.

Schuette, S. A., and H. M. Linkswiler. 1982. Effects of Ca and P metabolism in humans by adding meat, meat plus milk, or purified proteins plus Ca and P to a low protein diet. *J. Nutr.* 112:338–349.

Spencer, H., L. Kramer, M. DeBartolo, et al. 1983. Further studies of the effect of a high protein diet as meat on calcium metabolism. *Am. J. Clin. Nutr.* 37:924–929.

Spencer, H., L. Kramer, D. Osis, and C. Norris. 1978. Effect of a high protein (meat) intake on calcium metabolism in man. *Am. J. Clin. Nutr.* 31:2167–2180.

Spencer, H., L. Kramer, N. Rubio, and D. Osis. 1986. The effect of phosphorus on endogenous fecal calcium excretion in man. *Am. J. Clin. Nutr.* 43:844–851.

calmodulin. A calcium-binding regulatory protein residing in the cytoplasm and affecting certain enzymes. Calmodulin, with practically the same amino acid sequence, is found in all animal species. See also: CALCIUM.

SUGGESTED READINGS

Klee, C. B., T. H. Crouch, and P. G. Richman. 1980. Calmodulin. *Ann. Rev. Biochem.* 49:489–515.

calorie. A unit in which heat energy is measured. A calorie (lowercase c) is the amount of heat necessary to raise 1 gram (gm) of water 1°C (Celsius) at standard conditions of temperature and pressure.

The energy derived from foods when they are oxidized in the body is measured in kilocalories (thousands of calories). A kilocalorie is the amount of energy required to raise 1000 gm. of water 1°C. Kilocalorie is written Calorie (capital C) or it may be abbreviated to "Kcalorie" or "Kcal." Thus, whenever the word calorie is used in connection with food or nutrition, the meaning is always kilocalorie or Calorie.

cAMP. See CYCLIC AMP.

carbohydrate digestion. The chemical separation of polysaccharide and disaccharide molecules of starch- and sugar-containing foods into monosaccharides, their building units. Carbohydrates principally contribute fuel for the work of the body, especially GLUCOSE for the neural tissues; and they contribute carbons for synthesis of a wide variety of biomolecules.

Carbohydrate-rich foods are plant foods that, in addition to fuel, supply the body with vitamins, minerals, and fiber. Before they can be useful to the body, these substances, with the exception of fiber, must be separated from each other through digestion and absorbed into the bloodstream.

Digestion begins with the mechanical act of chewing, or mastication. During mastication food is mixed with saliva which moistens and dissolves some of the constituents. More importantly, saliva contains the enzyme *amylase,* which randomly hydrolyzes the α-1,4 bonds between the glucose units of the starch molecules, yielding maltose, some glucose, and dextrins (small starchlike molecules). When the bolus of food reaches the stomach, digestion of starch ceases as *amylase* is inactivated by the lower PH of the gastric juices. However, if a large meal is eaten, *salivary amylase* may continue to work in the interior of the bolus. Digestion of remaining starch resumes when the material enters the duodenum.

Starch is comprised of two kinds of polysaccharides, amylose and amylopectin. Amylose consists of long, unbranched chains of glucose units bound by α-1,4 bonds; amylopectin, in addition to α-1,4 bonds between glucose units, is highly branched, the branches arising from an α-1,6 bond about every twelfth glucose residue. The enzymes *amylase* and *glucosidase* are present in the alkaline pancreatic juice that is secreted into the duodenum. *Pancreatic amylase* resumes hydrolyzing the α-1,4 bonds while *glycosidase,* also called "debranching enzyme," hydrolyzes the α-1,6 bonds, resulting in the complete degradation of amylose and amylopectin into glucose and maltose.

The small intestine now contains a mixture of disaccharides and monosaccharides. Maltose and other disaccharides are hydrolyzed to their constituent monosaccharides by enzymes present in the brush border membranes of the intestinal wall. *Maltase* hydrolyzes maltose yielding two molecules of glucose; *lactase* acts on lactose yielding galactose and glucose; and *sucrase (invertase)* acts on sucrose yielding glucose and fructose. Glucose and galactose, both monosaccharides, have a common transport mechanism by which they enter the epithelial cells of the intestinal lining. The energy for this transport comes from hydrolysis of ATP which is dependent on SODIUM ions (Na^+) being expelled from the cell as glucose is transported in. The absorption of fructose is by diffusion, a much slower process. These monosaccharides are then transported into the bloodstream where they are available to the cells.

GLYCOGEN and cellulose, both complex carbohydrates, are not dietary sources of monosaccharides for humans. Glycogen, a starchlike polysaccharide stored in the liver, is intended to be a source of quick energy for an animal. However, very little is present in meat intended for human consumption because glycogen stores usually have been depleted by the time death of the animal occurs. Cellulose is made up of unbranched strings of glucose molecules bound by β-1,4 bonds. Because humans do not have enzymes to break these bonds, the glucose residues are not available for energy production. However, cellulose in plants is valuable in human diets as a source of indigestible fiber against which the muscles of the digestive tract can exercise and be strengthened.

After absorption from the gut into the bloodstream and entry into the portal vein, the monosaccharides are routed to the liver and redirected. Fructose and galactose are converted to glucose. If the BLOOD GLUCOSE LEVEL has dropped, glucose will enter the general circulation. If the blood glucose level is normal and there is no need for energy (i.e., ATP level is high), then glucose will be stored as glycogen in the liver; if glycogen stores are full, glucose will be diverted through GLYCOLYSIS to ACETYL-COA. If there is no need for energy (i.e., ATP level is high), the acetyl-CoA will be used to synthesize various LIPIDS—mostly TRIACYLGLYCEROLS—and will be stored as fat in adipose tissues.

Some groups of humans are intolerant of milk because they lack *lactase*, the enzyme that cleaves the bond between galactose and glucose of the milk sugar, lactose. The absence of lactase seems to be an inherited trait for it appears in some racial groups. The resulting accumulation of lactose in the intestinal tract attracts water from the lining. Action on lactose by intestinal bacteria may result in flatulence, nausea, and diarrhea. This reaction should not be confused with an allergic reaction to the protein in milk or to an inability to tolerate fat. See also: CARBOHYDRATE STRUCTURES, for descriptions of various carbohydrates discussed; GLYCOGEN, for special characteristics of glycogen stored in muscle rather than in liver; GLYCOLYSIS; PENTOSE

PHOSPHATE PATHWAY; RESPIRATORY CHAIN; TCA CYCLE, for an understanding of glucose metabolism.

carbohydrate structures. Carbohydrates originate with the photosynthetic reactions in green plants whereby solar energy causes carbon dioxide and water to combine into the basic unit of animals' food chain, GLUCOSE.

Carbohydrates comprise three classes: monosaccharides, oligosaccharides, and polysaccharides. The word "saccharide" means sugar and the carbohydrates are made of sugars, either singly, as in the monosaccharide glucose, or in short chains of sugars, as in the oligosaccharide sucrose (also a disaccharide), or in long chains, as in the polysaccharide starch.

The name carbohydrate dates from early chemical analyses when it was observed that most carbohydrates have a ratio of one carbon (carbo-) molecule to one water (-hydrate) molecule—in other words, a hydrated carbon, $(CH_2O)_n$. It is now known that all carbohydrates do not have this exact empirical formula and carbohydrate derivatives may contain other elements, such as SULFUR, PHOSPHORUS, and NITROGEN.

Nutritionally, carbohydrates are classified as "simple" (the sugars) or "complex" (dietarily, the starches). The most abundant simple sugar is glucose, a hexose, $C_6H_{12}O_6$,

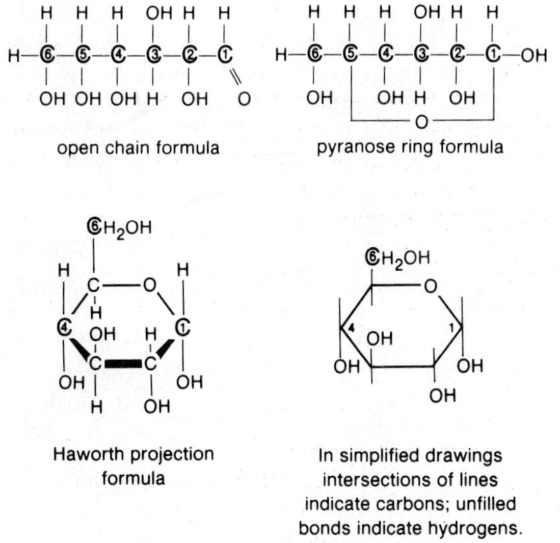

open chain formula

pyranose ring formula

Haworth projection formula

In simplified drawings intersections of lines indicate carbons; unfilled bonds indicate hydrogens.

Structural formulas for α-D-glucose

shown structurally in several ways. In the Haworth projection formula the bold lines indicate the part of the molecule that extends out from the page toward the reader.

Galactose and fructose, other hexoses, differ from each other, not in the chemical composition, but in the arrangement of their atoms.

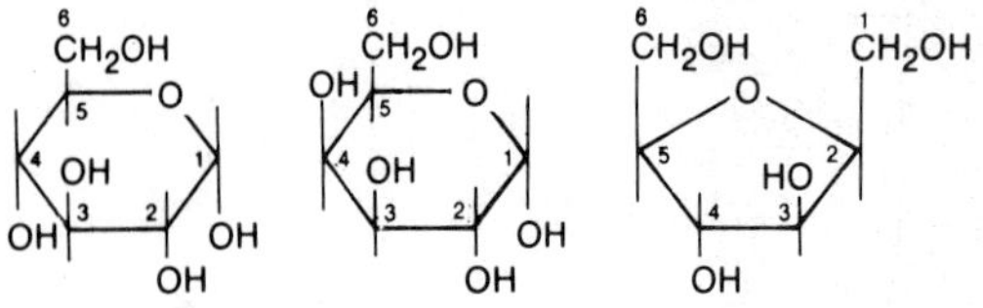

α-glucose   α-galactose   α-fructose   α-D-ribose   α-D-2-deoxyribose

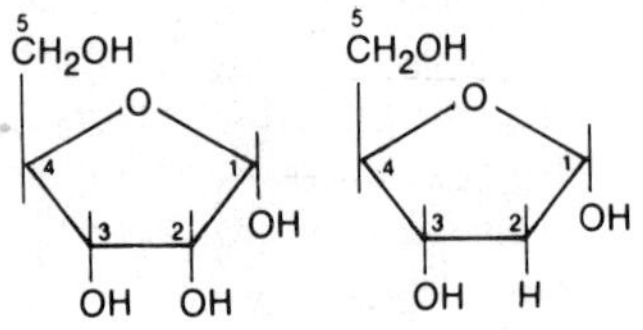

Hexoses   Pentoses

Examples of five-carbon sugars, the pentoses, are ribose and deoxyribose, which are important in the structures of DNA and RNA. Other sugars with different numbers of carbons are less abundant in the body and, while important, will not be discussed here.

Two monosaccharides united chemically comprise a disaccharide. These also are considered simple because there is only one bond to be broken before the two monosaccharides can be absorbed from the gut. The best-known disaccharide is sucrose, or table sugar, which is composed of one molecule of glucose joined in a glycosidic linkage to one molecule of fructose. The glycosidic bond is formed by a condensation reaction when the alpha hydroxyl group on the first sugar reacts with the anomeric carbon of the second sugar and water is released.

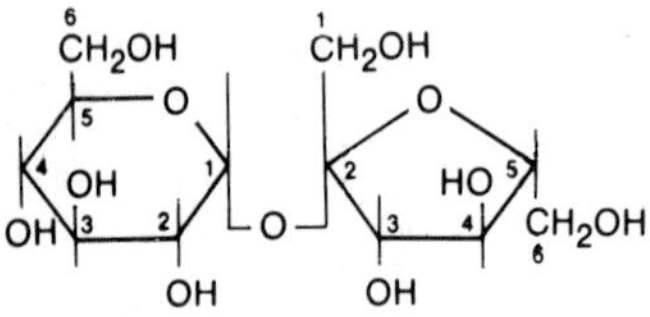

α-glucose   β-fructose

Sucrose

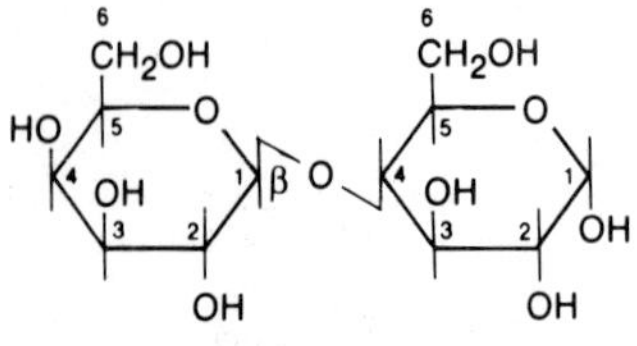

Lactose, the disaccharide found in milk, is composed of glucose and galactose. Maltose, composed of two glucose molecules, is the disaccharide that results from the hydrolysis of starch.

The complex carbohydrates, consisting only of glucose units, are starch, GLYCOGEN, and cellulose. They are classed as complex because they are large molecules with many bonds that must be broken so that monosaccharides can be released and absorbed.

β-galactose   α-glucose

Lactose

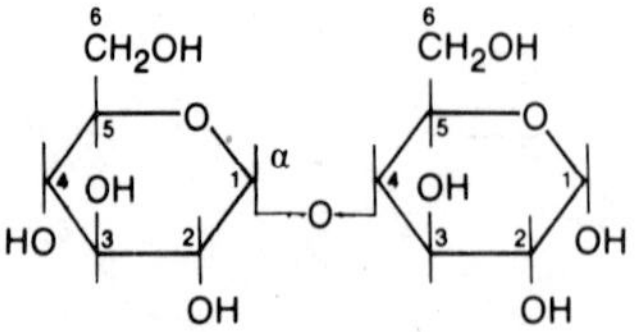

Both starch and glycogen are storage forms of glucose. Starch is stored in plant seeds, fruits, stems, and roots to supply glucose for future growth. Both unbranched starch, amylose, and branched starch, amylopectin, exist. Glycogen, stored in animal liver and muscle, is used as a source of

Maltose

energy between feedings or during an emergency. It is more highly branched than amylopectin. Both starch and glyco- gen are made of chains of glucose units joined in α-1,4 gly- cosidic bonds with branches made by α-1,6 bonds. Cellu- lose differs from starch and glycogen in that its glucose units are bonded by β-1,4 linkages. "Beta" (β) refers to the position of the hydroxyl group on carbon 1 of glucose. Hu- mans lack the enzyme that breaks the β-1,4 linkage, there- fore they cannot utilize the bond's energy. Cellulose is the main structural component of plant cell walls and provides support for the plant body.

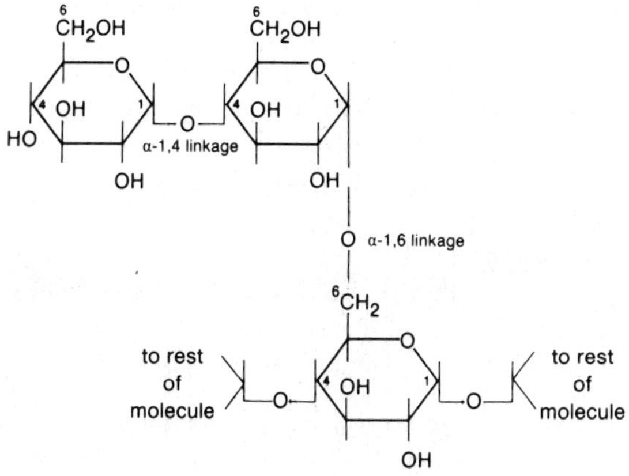

Branch point for glycogen or amylopectin

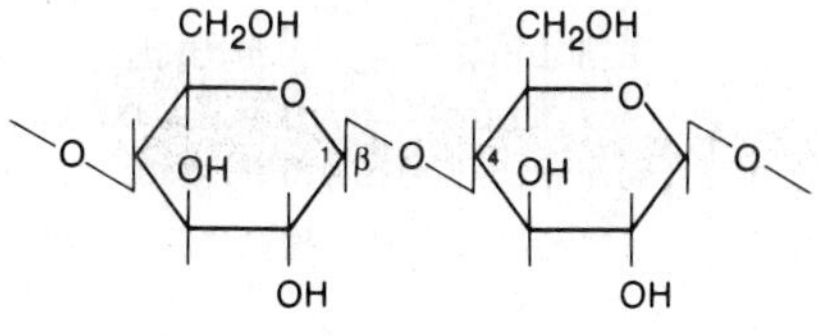

Cellulose

Although cellulose is commonly referred to as "fiber," other polysaccharides also considered as "fibers" include hemicellulose, pectin, mucilages, and guar gum. Hemicellu- lose, known for its water-holding capacity, is found in fruits and vegetables; pectin and guar gum act as thickening agents in foods and when ingested help to lower serum cholesterol. See also: GLYCOGEN, for information about glycosidic bonds; CARBOHYDRATE DIGESTION, GLYCOLYSIS, TCA CYCLE, for catabolism of carbohydrates; GLUCONEOGENESIS; GLUCOSE; GLYCOGENESIS; GLYCOGENOLYSIS; PENTOSE.

carbonyl group.   See ACETALDEHYDE; KETONE BODIES.

carboxylase.   A class of ENZYMES that catalyzes the addition of a carboxyl group to a substrate.

carboxylation.   The addition of a carboxyl group to a substrate. An example is the addition of CO_2 to ACETYL-CoA to form malonyl-CoA in the first step of FATTY ACID SYNTHESIS.

Carnitine

carnitine.   A hydroxy-carboxylic acid related to CHOLINE and found in high concentrations in muscle. Some lower organisms lack the ability to synthesize carnitine, but mammals make it from LYSINE. Carnitine, when associated with the enzyme *carnitine palmitoyl transferase,* plays a role in transporting long-chain fatty acyl groups into the inner mitochondrial membrane where oxidation will take place.

SUGGESTED READINGS

Borum, P. R. 1983. Carnitine. *Ann. Rev. Nutr.* 3:233–259.

Khan-Siddiqui, L., and M. S. Bamji. 1983. Lysine-carnitine conversion in normal and undernourished adult men— suggestion of nonpeptidyl pathway. *Am. J. Clin. Nutr.* 37:93–98.

Mitchell, M. E. 1978. Carnitine metabolism in human subjects. *Am. J. Clin. Nutr.* 31:293–306.

Vacha, G. M., et al. 1983. Favorable effects of L-carnitine treatment on hyper-triglyceridemia in hemodialysis patients. *Am. J. Clin. Nutr.* 38:532–540.

Carnosine

carnosine.   A dipeptide synthesized from β-alanine and HISTIDINE in an ATP-requiring reaction catalyzed by the enzyme *carnosine synthetase.* Carnosine is concentrated in muscle where it activates myosin *ATPase* activity. Although its physiologic functions are not well understood, it is thought that it buffers the pH of contracting muscle. The enzyme *carnosinase,* two forms of which exist in human tissue, degrades carnosine into β-alanine and histidine. The kidney and intestinal enterocytes also take up and degrade carnosine.

carrier.   A substance, common to all life forms, that can pick up a group of atoms and transfer it to another compound. A list of some of these follows:

Acyl carrier protein (ACP) carries intermediates in FATTY ACID SYNTHESIS.

ATP carries activated phosphoryl groups.

BIOTIN carries activated CO_2 groups.

COENZYME A carries activated acyl groups.

$FADH_2$ carries electrons (hydrogens).

Lipoamide carries activated acyl groups.

NADH, NADPH carry electrons (hydrogens).

S-adenosylmethionine carries activated methyl groups.

Tetrahydrofolate (FH_4) carries activated one-carbon units.

THIAMIN PYROPHOSPHATE (TPP) carries activated aldehyde groups.

Uridine diphosphate glucose (UDP-glucose) carries activated GLUCOSE.

catabolism. Degradative reactions. See also: METABOLISM.

catecholamines. A group of amines composed of epinephrine (also called adrenalin), norepinephrine (also called noradrenalin), and dopamine. These amines are synthesized from the amino acid TYROSINE and are secreted by the adrenal medulla, which is closely associated with the nervous system.

Catecholamines generally stimulate the sympathetic nervous system. One of their most widely known effects is that of the "fight-or-flight" cluster of actions—protective actions in response to a life-altering event or danger. The response is to a judgment made in the brain to sensory stimuli that the brain has received. The alarm the brain sends to the adrenal medulla increases the blood adrenalin level one thousandfold in a few seconds.

The "fight-or-flight" reactions include withdrawal of blood from the peripheral tissues and its concentration deep in the body where life-sustaining organs reside, slowdown of digestive processes, increase of respiration rate and heart beat, widening of the pupils, breakdown of GLYCOGEN to GLUCOSE in liver and in skeletal muscle, and lipolysis of fat in fat stores, to name a few.

In the synthesis of epinephrine, dopa is produced from tyrosine by the action of *tyrosine hydroxylase*. A VITAMIN B_6-dependent decarboxylase then produces dopamine, the compound important in controlling the tremor of Parkinson's disease. Norepinephrine is made by the action of a hydroxylase on dopamine and a transferase catalyzes the transfer of a methyl group from S-adenosylmethionine to the norepinephrine to form epinephrine.

Epinephrine exerts its actions by binding to receptors on the surface of cells and by "transmitting a signal" to activate *adenylate cyclase,* which converts ATP to CYCLIC AMP (cAMP). Once produced, cAMP activates various kinases and thereby affects phosphorylation and dephosphorylation.

By such a roundabout path, epinephrine stimulates GLYCOGENOLYSIS in skeletal muscle and inhibits glycogen synthesis. Normally, skeletal muscles rely on FATTY ACIDS and KETONE BODIES for fuel, but use glucose for spurts of physical activity such as a person in danger might need. At the same time, in the liver glycogenolysis and GLUCONEOGENESIS are enhanced while glycogen synthesis is inhibited.

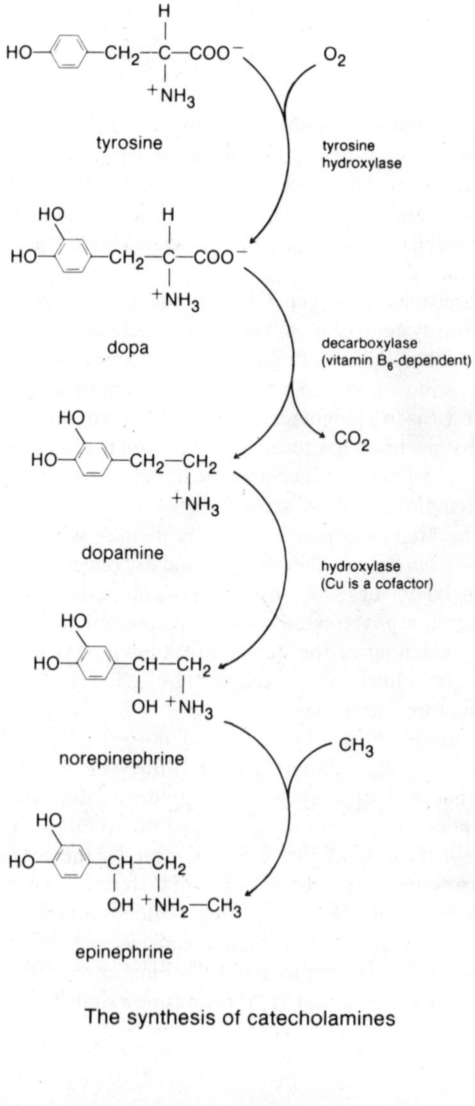

The synthesis of catecholamines

In addition, catecholamines inhibit the use of glucose in the peripheral tissues by the shutdown of insulin secretion from the pancreas. Their effect on fat metabolism is to increase hydrolysis of triglycerides by, again, the stimulation of *adenylate cyclase* to produce cAMP.

After the catecholamines have effected the desired changes, they are inactivated and their catabolites are excreted in the urine. *Monoamine oxidase,* an important enzyme present in the mitochondria, is responsible for much of the degradation of epinephrine. A group of drugs known as monoamine oxidase inhibitors (MAOIs), which elevate the level of epinephrine in the brain, are often prescribed as antidepressants. Physicians and pharmacists warn patients who are taking these drugs of the dangers of self-medicating with over-the-counter cold or reducing medications while taking the prescribed MAOIs. They also warn against eating foods that are high in tyramine, a bacterial breakdown product of the amino acid tyrosine. These foods include aged cheese, such as Camembert and cheddar; fermented sausages, such as bologna and salami; pickled herring; beer; ale; red wine, especially Chianti; figs; raisins; soy sauce; meat that is treated with tenderizer; and others. The combination of MAOIs with these "wine and cheese party" foods may produce dangerous levels of catecholamines in the brain.

CDP. See CYTIDINE DIPHOSPHATE.

cellulose. A structural polysaccharide found primarily in plants and composed of glucose units bonded together by β-1,4 linkages. See also: CARBOHYDRATE DIGESTION; CARBOHYDRATE STRUCTURE; FIBER.

cephalin. A phospholipid, similar to lecithin, present in the brain of mammals. See also: LIPIDS.

cerebroside. A lipid or fatty substance present in nerves and other tissues. A cerebroside is a sphingolipid.

chelation. A combination of metallic ions with certain heterocyclic ring structures so that the ion is held by chemical bonds from each of the participating rings. For example, hemoglobin is a heterocyclic ring that holds, or chelates, the IRON ions. When this structure is diagrammed, it appears that the metallic ion is being held by a claw.

chloride (Cl⁻). The major anion in the extracellular fluid. Small amounts of chloride are found intracellularly in, for example, erythrocytes (red blood cells) and gastric mucosa cells (lining of stomach). The most common dietary source of chloride is table salt. Chloride deficiencies are usually secondary to vomiting, diarrhea, and certain disease states.

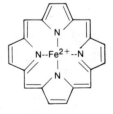

The heme portion of hemoglobin showing the chelation of iron

The chloride ion is important in the formation of gastric hydrochloric acid. Chloride ions are also important in maintaining the ACID-BASE BALANCE of blood by shifting between the plasma and erythrocyte portions. The exchange between the chloride and bicarbonate ions across the erythrocyte membrane has been referred to as the "chloride shift."

The normal concentration of chloride ions in plasma is around 100 mEq/l; usually this is without wide variation. Changes in concentration generally follow those of sodium or of loss of fluid from the upper intestinal tract, as in vomiting.

cholesterol. A high-molecular-weight cyclic alcohol contained in foods of animal origin and synthesized in the body from ACETYL-CoA. Cholesterol is a structural component of cell MEMBRANES and plasma LIPOPROTEINS, which transport LIPIDS in the blood. Its derivatives, including BILE SALTS, steroid hormones, and VITAMIN D, are of great importance in maintaining healthy tissues.

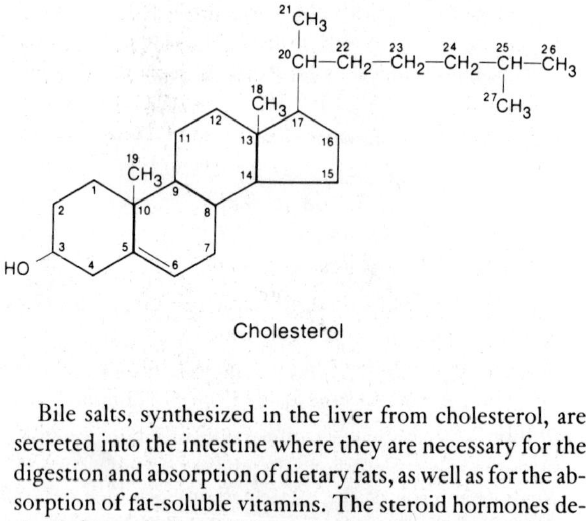

Cholesterol

Bile salts, synthesized in the liver from cholesterol, are secreted into the intestine where they are necessary for the digestion and absorption of dietary fats, as well as for the absorption of fat-soluble vitamins. The steroid hormones derived from cholesterol include the adrenal cortical hormones, such as cortisone, and the reproductive hormones. Vitamin D is made from 7-dehydrocholesterol in the skin after exposure of the skin to sunlight. Membranes that surround the cell and control the entry and exit of vital compounds require cholesterol in their structure.

Cholesterol occurs in foods in both free and esterified forms. During digestion, the ester bond can be broken to release free cholesterol. Free cholesterol, absorbed in the intestinal mucosa, mixes with other lipids, free cholesterols, and protein to form chylomicrons (one type of lipoprotein). From the intestinal cells, the chylomicrons enter the lymph and, ultimately, the blood circulatory system.

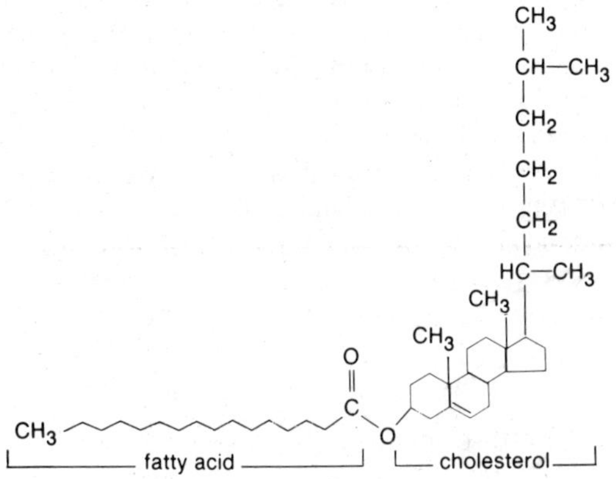

Cholesterol ester

The role of dietary cholesterol in the formation of the plaques of atherosclerosis is the subject of much research. High serum cholesterol levels long have been implicated in the development of atherosclerosis but there is still no consensus as to the extent to which control of dietary cholesterol intake protects a person from coronary heart disease. Epidemiologic evidence points to a high incidence of atherosclerosis among meat-eating cultures. However, there is no consensus whether this occurrence is caused by a diet high in cholesterol, saturated fat, or both. Risk factors, other than dietary cholesterol, include obesity, sedentary lifestyle, and cigarette smoking.

The cholesterol from both dietary intake and endogenous synthesis is carried in the blood as part of lipoproteins: chylomicrons, low-density lipoproteins (LDL), very low-density lipoproteins (VLDL), or high-density lipoproteins (HDL). A high level of LDL-cholesterol in the serum is considered a high-risk factor for coronary heart disease. Conversely, a high level of HDL-cholesterol is an indication of a lower risk of coronary heart disease.

Cholesterol is synthesized in the liver from acetyl-CoA, a degradative product of the oxidation of GLUCOSE, FATTY ACIDS, and AMINO ACIDS. Therefore, higher serum cholesterol levels may result from eating carbohydrate, fat, and protein foods in excess of need, not merely from eating cholesterol-rich foods.

In normal, healthy persons, the rate of cholesterol synthesis is modified by the dietary intake so that the concentration of cholesterol remains fairly constant in various tissues: an increase in dietary intake of cholesterol will lower the amount that the body synthesizes. An exception to this general rule occurs where a person has inherited the genetic condition, familial hypercholesterolemia. Dietary manipulation cannot significantly alter the blood cholesterol level in these patients who are at high risk of coronary heart disease at an early age.

The complex pathway of cholesterol synthesis is simplified here in order to highlight the stages involved. In the first step, two acetyl-CoA molecules react to form acetoacetyl-CoA. Next acetyl-CoA and acetoacetyl-CoA condense to form hydroxymethylglutaryl-CoA (HMG-

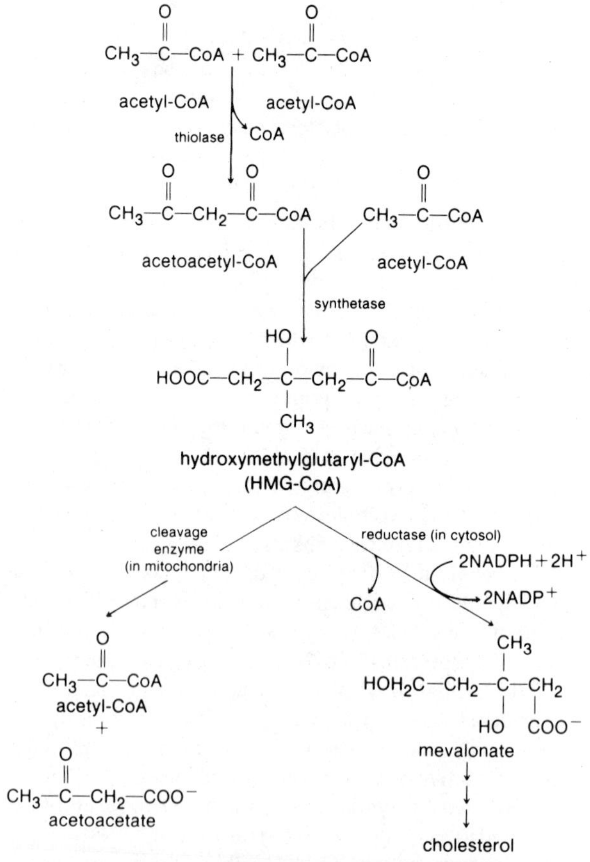

The action of reductase is the committed step
in cholesterol synthesis

CoA), a six-carbon compound. There are two pathways open for this substance. In one, an enzyme in the mitochondria can cleave it back to acetyl-CoA and acetoacetate. In the other, *HMG-CoA reductase*, an enzyme in the cytosol that uses NADPH as its coenzyme, can use HMG-CoA to form mevalonate. The action of the reductase is the committed step in cholesterol synthesis.

Three phosphorylations and a decarboxylation yield the five-carbon compound, isopentenyl pyrophosphate. Condensation of six isopentenyl pyrophosphates produces squalene, a straight-chain thirty-carbon compound. Cholesterol is made from squalene by cyclization, addition of

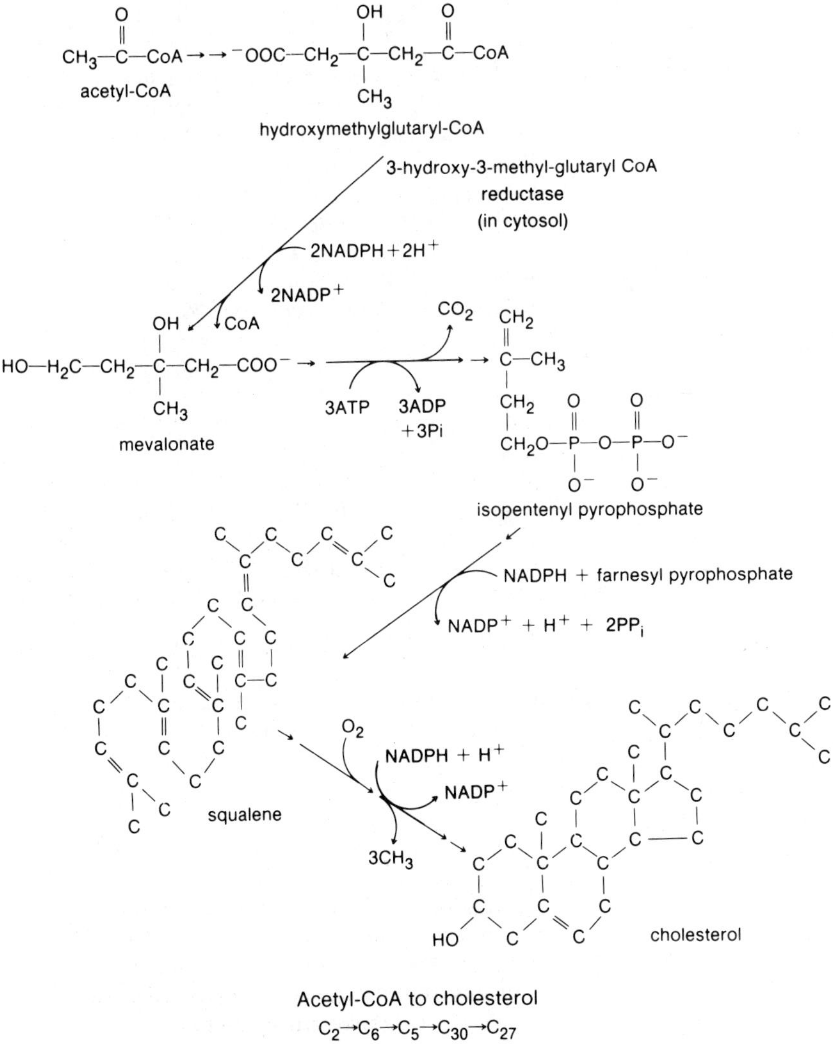

Acetyl-CoA to cholesterol

$$C_2 \rightarrow C_6 \rightarrow C_5 \rightarrow C_{30} \rightarrow C_{27}$$

molecular oxygen, removal of three methyl groups, and the shifting of several bonds. NADPH is used in two steps of this rearrangement. See also: BILE SALTS; FIBER; LIPOPROTEINS; MEMBRANES.

SUGGESTED READINGS

Brown, M. S., and J. L. Goldstein. 1986. A receptor mediated pathway for cholesterol homeostasis. *Science* 232:34–37.

Brown, M. S., and J. L. Goldstein. 1983. Lipoprotein metabolism in the macrophage: Implications for cholesterol deposition in atherosclerosis. *Ann. Rev. Biochem.* 52:223–261.

Council for Agricultural Science and Technology. 1986. Diet and coronary disease, a verbatim report. *Nutrition Today* 21:26–33.

Gallo, L. L. 1983. Cholesterol and other sterols: Absorption, metabolism, roles in atherogenesis. In *Nutrition and heart disease,* ed. E. B. Feldman, 83–110. New York: Churchill Livingstone.

Goldstein, J. L., and M. S. Brown. 1983. Familial hypercholesterolemia. In *The metabolic basis of inherited disease,* 5th ed., ed. J. B. Stanbury et al. New York: McGraw-Hill.

Grundy, S. M. 1983. Absorption and metabolism of dietary cholesterol. *Ann. Rev. Nutr.* 3:71–96.

Hillman, L. C., et al. 1985. The effect of the fiber components pectin, cellulose and lignin on serum cholesterol levels. *Am. J. Clin. Nutr.* 42:207–213.

Lipid Research Clinics Program. 1984. The lipids research clinics coronary primary prevention trial results. *JAMA* 251:351–371.

Schroepfer, G. J., Jr. 1981. Sterol biosynthesis. *Ann. Rev. Biochem.* 50:585–621.

Siperstein, M. D. 1984. Role of cholesterogenesis and isoprenoid synthesis in DNA replication and cell growth. *J. Lipid Res.* 25:1462–1468.

$$H_3C-\overset{+}{\underset{H_3C}{\overset{H_3C}{N}}}-CH_2-CH_2OH$$

Choline

choline. A critical part of lecithin (a phospholipid) and sphingomyelin, both of which are constituents of cell MEMBRANES. Choline is also needed for the synthesis of acetylcholine, a neurotransmitter.

Choline is synthesized by the carboxylation of the amino acid SERINE to ethanolamine in a VITAMIN B_6-dependent reaction. Choline is widespread in food: muscle meats, organ meats, and legumes are good dietary sources; fruits and vegetables are poor sources.

Dietary choline may spare the amino acid METHIONINE in biosyntheses requiring the transfer of methyl groups. Choline is oxidized to betaine which then can provide a methyl group to homocysteine to produce methionine. The conversion to methionine step requires VITAMIN B_{12} and FOLACIN.

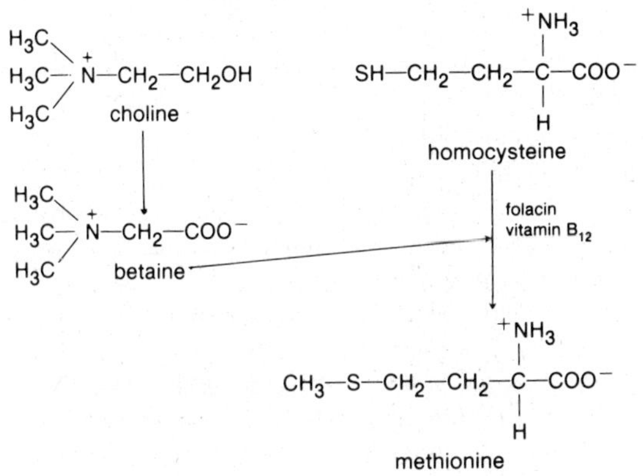

$$H_3C \diagdown \atop H_3C - \overset{+}{N} - CH_2 - CH_2OH \atop H_3C \diagup \quad \text{choline}$$

$$\overset{+NH_3}{\underset{H}{SH - CH_2 - CH_2 - \overset{|}{\underset{|}{C}} - COO^-}}$$
homocysteine

$$H_3C \diagdown \atop H_3C - \overset{+}{N} - CH_2 - COO^- \atop H_3C \diagup \quad \text{betaine}$$

folacin
vitamin B_{12}

$$\overset{+NH_3}{\underset{H}{CH_3 - S - CH_2 - CH_2 - \overset{|}{\underset{|}{C}} - COO^-}}$$
methionine

Betaine, an oxidation product of choline, donates a methyl group to convert homocysteine to methionine. Vitamins B_{12} and folacin are required.

SUGGESTED READINGS

Childs, M. T., et al. 1981. The contrasting effects of dietary soya lecithin and corn oil on lipoprotein lipids in normolipidemic and familial hypercholesterolemic subjects. *Atherosclerosis* 38:217–228.

Kuksis, A. and S. Mookerjea. 1984. Choline. In *Present knowledge in nutrition*, 5th ed., 383–399. Washington, D.C.: The Nutrition Foundation, Inc.

Zeisel, S. H. 1981. Dietary choline: Biochemistry, physiology and pharmacology. *Ann. Rev. Nutr.* 1:95–122.

chromium (Cr^{+++}). A trace metal which is thought to function as part of glucose tolerance factor. See also: INSULIN.

SUGGESTED READINGS

Anderson, R. A., et al. 1982. Urinary chromium excretion of human subjects: Effect of chromium supplementation and glucose loading. *Am. J. Clin. Nutr.* 36:1184–1193.

Evans, G. W., E. E. Roginski, and W. Mertz. 1973. Interaction of the glucose tolerance factor (GTF) with insulin. *Biochem. Biophys. Res. Commun.* 50:718–722.

Liu, V. S. K., and R. P. Abernathy. 1982. Chromium and insulin in young subjects with normal glucose tolerance. *Am. J. Clin. Nutr.* 35:661–667.

Riales, R., and M. J. Albrink. 1981. Effect of chromium chloride supplementation on glucose tolerance and serum lipids including high-density lipoprotein of adult men. *Am. J. Clin. Nutr.* 34:2670–2678.

chromosome. The slender, threadlike structures found in the nucleus of cells that contain the genetic information (DNA) which ultimately controls the processes of the cell. Chromosomes are long because they contain millions of complementary base pairs. See also: DNA; PURINE, PYRIMIDINE BASES; RNA.

chylomicron. A small lipid droplet composed mainly of dietary TRIACYLGLYCEROLS, fat-soluble vitamins, small amounts of CHOLESTEROL and phospholipids, and a thin coating of protein. Chylomicrons are synthesized in the intestinal mucosa cells from products of lipid digestion, given a coating of phospholipids and protein, and released into the lymphatic vessels. From there the chylomicrons are carried via the thoracic duct to the bloodstream for distribution to the tissues. See also: LIPOPROTEINS.

cis-, trans-bonds. Cis and trans describe the position of the substituent groups at each side of a double bond. In the cis-configuration the groups appear on the same side of the double bond; in the trans-configuration the substituent groups are on opposite sides of the double bond.

Two compounds that differ only in the configuration about the double bond are said to be "geometric isomers" of each other, for example, fumaric and maleic acids. Each compound is unique and not interchangeable in biological reactions even though both are identical in their chemical composition. Fumaric acid has a trans-double bond and is active in cells, especially in the TCA CYCLE. Fumaric acid's cis-isomer, maleic acid, exhibits no biological activity.

This difference of position causes two chemically identical compounds to be distinctly different owing to the restriction of rotation about a double bond. Rotation is free about a single carbon-carbon bond so that a compound containing only single bonds can assume many shapes. Palmitic acid, a sixteen-carbon saturated fatty acid with only single bonds, is often incorrectly shown in structural formulas as a long, straight chain. Because there is freedom of rotation about each bond, palmitic acid is more accurately viewed as having a long, flexible, floppy tail. The flexibility about each single carbon-to-carbon bond accounts for the ability of triacylglycerols (such as lard) containing saturated fatty acid molecules to pack together densely so that they are solid at room temperature.

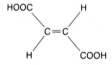

fumaric acid (trans-)

maleic acid (cis-)

Cis-trans isomerism

On the other hand, palmitoleic acid, which is a sixteen-carbon, unsaturated fatty acid with a double bond between carbons 9 and 10, has a rigid bend, or kink, at the point of its double bond. Whether the configuration (the bend) is cis or trans determines the shape of the molecule.

The chains on either side of the double bond will continue to be flexible and will assume many shapes. The kink in the unsaturated fatty acid molecules prohibits them from packing closely together with the result that oils, such as safflower, that contain unsaturated fatty acids are liquid at ordinary temperatures.

In most naturally occurring unsaturated fatty acids in plants and animals the configuration at the double bond is cis rather than trans. The cis-arrangement in fat foods can be altered to trans by processing methods.

SUGGESTED READINGS

Enig, M.G., Munn, R.J., and M. Keeney. 1978. Dietary fat and cancer trends. Fed. Proc. 37:2215–2220.

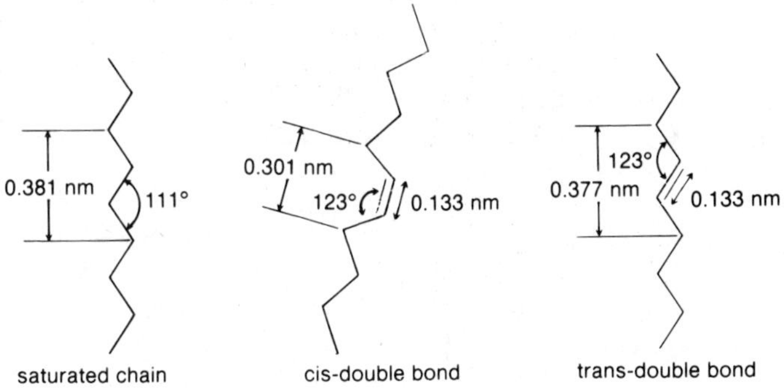

| saturated chain | cis-double bond | trans-double bond |

Configurations of fatty acids

citric acid. An intermediate in the TCA CYCLE. See also: TCA CYCLE.

citric acid cycle. See TCA CYCLE.

citrullinemia. The accumulation of citrulline, a UREA CYCLE intermediate, in the blood and other body fluids resulting from a deficiency of the enzyme *argininosuccinic acid synthetase.*

SUGGESTED READINGS

See suggested readings for INBORN ERRORS OF METABOLISM.

CMP. See CYTIDINE MONOPHOSPHATE.

CoA. See COENZYME A.

cobalamin. See VITAMIN B_{12}.

cobalt. See VITAMIN B_{12}.

codon. A sequence of three bases (triplet) in messenger RNA that specifies the ordering of a particular AMINO ACID. See also: GENETIC CODE; PROTEIN BIOSYNTHESIS; RNA.

coenzyme A (CoA). The coenzyme derived from the vitamin PANTOTHENIC ACID. CoA's function is central to the METABOLISM of nutrients because it carries activated acyl groups. Coenzyme A is synthesized from the vitamin pantothenic acid and the amino acid CYSTEINE, which donates SULFUR. The sulfhydryl group is the active site and is often noted in the naming of compounds containing CoA, for example, acetyl-S-CoA.

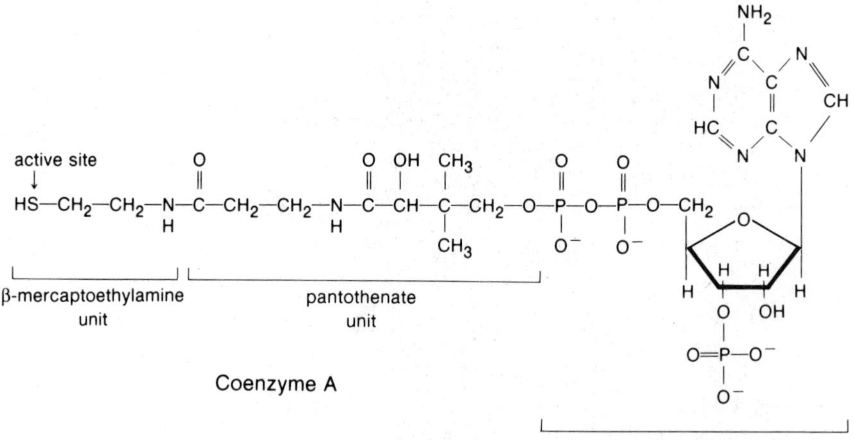

Coenzyme A

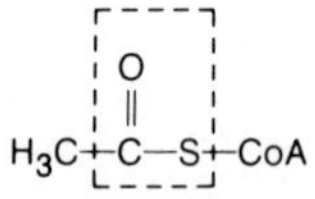

adenine ribose 3′-phosphate

Acetyl-CoA with the thioester functional group encircled

CoA forms a thioester (sulfur-containing) bond with groups such as the two-carbon compound acetate, which is the common degradative product of the metabolism of carbohydrates, FATTY ACIDS, and some AMINO ACIDS. As ACETYL-CoA, the carbons from these fuel nutrients can be oxidized through the TCA CYCLE and RESPIRATORY CHAIN to CO_2, H_2O, and ATP. The thioesters formed with CoA are highly reactive. They include: malonyl-CoA, propionyl-CoA, succinyl-CoA, and methylmalonyl-CoA.

coenzyme B_{12}. When VITAMIN B_{12} (cobalamin) is used as a coenzyme in the cytosol, its cyanide group is replaced with a methyl group forming methylcobalamin. In the mitochondria the cyanide group is reduced and cobalamin joins with 5'-deoxyadenosine to form 5'-deoxyadenosylcobalamin.

Vitamin B_{12} acts as a coenzyme for only two types of reactions: (1) rearrangements, especially intramolecular ones in which a group is transferred from one carbon to an adjacent carbon as in the case of *methylmalonyl mutase* that converts L-methylmalonyl-CoA to succinyl-CoA; and (2) methylations, as in the synthesis of METHIONINE from homocysteine by *homocysteine transmethylase*. See also: VALINE, METHIONINE, ISOLEUCINE, for reactions involving coenzyme B_{12}; CHOLINE; FATTY ACID OXIDATION; VITAMIN B_{12}.

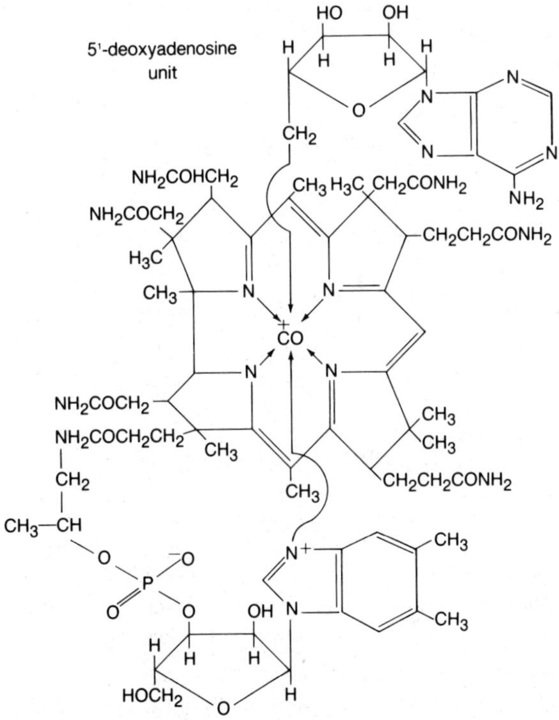

Coenzyme B_{12}
(5'-deoxyadenosyl cobalamin)

coenzyme Q (CoQ). A quinone derivative with a long, isoprenoid tail the length of which varies according to the species. For example, mammalian CoQ is referred to as Q_{10} because the tail contains ten isoprene units. CoQ is also known as ubiquitone because it is ubiquitous in biological systems.

CoQ plays a key role in the RESPIRATORY CHAIN as an electron carrier between flavoproteins and cytochromes. As CoQ accepts and donates electrons it becomes reduced or oxidized. Because of the nonpolar nature of its tail, it can diffuse rapidly through the inner mitochondrial membrane. In fact, CoQ is the only electron carrier that is not tightly bound to this membrane. See also: RESPIRATORY CHAIN.

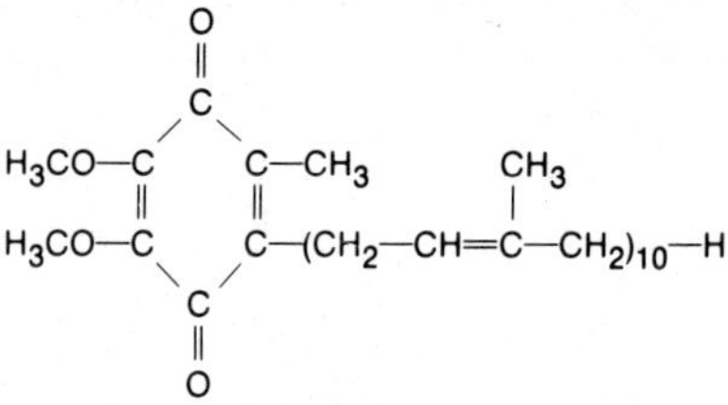

oxidized form of coenzyme Q

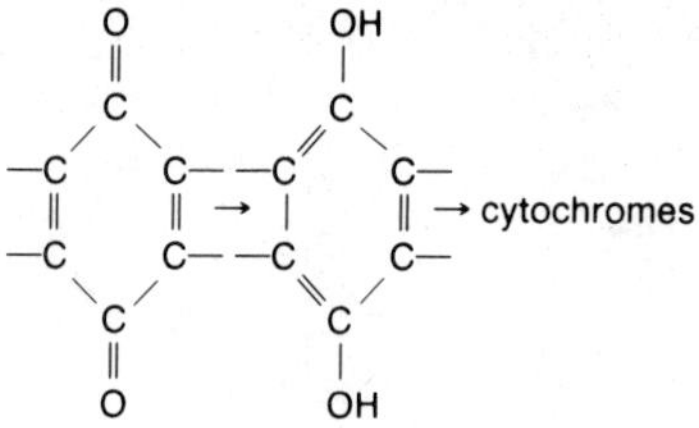

oxidized form → reduced form

Coenzyme Q

cofactor. A small, inorganic or organic substance that is required for the activity of an ENZYME. See also: ENZYME.

collagen. The principal structural protein of bones, teeth, skin, cartilage, tendons, cornea, and blood vessels. As a fibrous protein its length far exceeds its diameter and it possesses a high tensile strength.

Tropocollagen, the precursor of collagen, is a triple helix with chains of about 1000 AMINO ACIDS each. The cross-links that strengthen the conformation of collagen become established after its synthesis and their number increases with a person's age. Therefore collagen of a young person is more soluble; with maturity it becomes stronger. This increasing rigidity of collagen accounts for the cornea's becoming less transparent with a person's advancing age.

The amino acid sequence of collagen is unusual in several ways. It contains two amino acids not ordinarily found in proteins—hydroxyproline and hydroxylysine. Also, collagen contains a high concentration of one amino acid, GLY-CINE, which appears at about every third position along the major portion of its chains. Because of the small size of glycine, the longer side chains of the other amino acids fit within the inner part of the collagen molecule. Another rarity is the number of repetitions of a sequence; in collagen, the repetitions may number 300. The sequence is glycine —X—Y where X is usually proline and Y is usually hydroxyproline.

The synthesis of collagen occurs in several stages similar to those in the formation of fibrin of coagulating blood. First, long polypeptide chains are formed with abundant PROLINE and LYSINE. After the chain is complete, in a reaction catalyzed by *prolyl hydroxylase* and *lysyl hydroxylase,* proline and lysine become hydroxylated to hydroxyproline and hydroxylysine, respectively.

Both reduced (ferrous) IRON and VITAMIN C are required by these hydroxylases. Vitamin C acts as the reducing agent to maintain the ferrous state. Some symptoms of scurvy, a vitamin C-deficiency disease, can be explained by this need for vitamin C during collagen formation. Ill-formed collagen results in swelling of lower extremities, bleeding gums, loss of teeth, inability to stand, and capillaries that leak blood just under the skin.

The strength of collagen relates to many factors. The rigid imino acids, proline and hydroxyproline, limit the rotation around the bonds of collagen and thus stabilize the helix. Both hydroxyproline and glycine residues form intramolecular hydrogen bonds. Van der Waal interactions and hydrogen bonds between residues on different strands also stabilize the triple helix. The establishment of cross-links by rare, covalent bonds between two lysine molecules adds further stability to collagen, a bonding catalyzed by *lysyl oxidase* with COPPER as a cofactor. Whether a bond forms seems to depend on the previous bonds. The ultimate tensile strength of a collagen fiber is determined by the addition of many fairly weak bonds which collectively interact to produce great tensile strength.

When collagen is boiled in water, some of the triple helixes unfold and it becomes more soluble. By this action meat becomes tender and gelatin is formed. This gelatin is a poor source of dietary protein because collagen primarily is made of nonessential amino acids.   See also: IRON; VITAMIN C; COPPER.

SUGGESTED READINGS

Eyre, D. R., M. A. Paz, and P. M. Gallop, 1984. Cross-linking in collagen and elastin. *Ann. Rev. Biochem.* 53:717–748.

Prockop, D. J., and K. I. Kivirikko. 1984. Heritable diseases of collagen. *N. Engl. J. Med.* 311:376–388.

Prockop, D. J., et al. 1979. The biosynthesis of collagen and its disorders. Part 1. *N. Engl. J. Med.* 301:13–23.

Prockop, D. J., et al. 1979. The biosynthesis of collagen and its disorders. Part 2. *N. Engl. J. Med.* 301:77–85.

Scriver, C. R., R. J. Smith, and J. M. Phang. 1983. Disorders of proline and hydroxyproline metabolism. In *The metabolic basis of inherited disease,* 5th ed., ed. J. B. Stanbury et al., 360–381. New York: McGraw-Hill.

competitive inhibition.   The action of an inhibitor which so closely resembles the substrate that it competes with it for a binding site at the enzyme's active center. For example, oxaloacetate in the TCA CYCLE is a competitive inhibitor of *succinate dehydrogenase.* Owing to the similarity of the structure of oxaloacetate and succinate, oxaloacetate is able to fit into the active site of the enzyme, thus blocking succinate's entry; however, oxaloacetate is not acted upon by the *enzyme.*

$$
\begin{array}{cc}
COO^- & COO^- \\
| & | \\
C{=}O & CH_2 \\
| & | \\
CH_2 & CH_2 \\
| & | \\
COO^- & COO^- \\
\text{oxaloacetate} & \text{succinate}
\end{array}
$$

Competitive inhibitors have similar structures

complementary base pairs.   The pairing of the bases adenine (A) with thymine (T) and cytosine (C) with guanine (G). These pairs form the cross bars of the double strands of DNA. If adenine is on one strand, it will be linked to a thymine on the other strand; similarly, cytosine and guanine will be linked. When the double strands are "unzipped" during DNA replication, this complementary pairing assures the exact copying of the DNA. In the case of RNA, adenine (A) pairs with uracil (U).   See also: DNA; PROTEIN BIOSYNTHESIS; RNA.

complete protein.   A protein food that contains all the ESSENTIAL AMINO ACIDS in relatively the same proportions as humans require. Generally, animal flesh and products, except collagen, are considered complete protein foods, whereas plant foods are considered incomplete. Two plant foods, each containing the amino acid that the other lacks, can make an acceptable complete protein. Eggs, the most complete protein food, are the standard against which other protein foods are judged.

copper (Cu$^+$ cuprous, Cu^{++} cupric).   An important trace element that participates as a cofactor in a number of EN-

ZYMES and as a part of ceruloplasmin, a glycoprotein of the α_2-globulin fraction of plasma.

Copper serves as a cofactor for *tyrosinase* (in TYROSINE degradation to melanin), *cytochrome c oxidase* (the last enzyme in the RESPIRATORY CHAIN), *dopamine beta hydroxylase* (which oxidizes the CATECHOLAMINES), *lysyl oxidase* (which is crucial to the formation of the cross-links of COLLAGEN and elastin, two important connective tissues within the body), and as a part of *superoxide dismutase* (which catalyzes the formation of hydrogen peroxide and oxygen).

Copper is stored primarily in the liver where it may be used to synthesize ceruloplasmin (sometimes called ferroxidase I). Ceruloplasmin functions to oxidize ferrous IRON to ferric, thus allowing the transfer of iron from its ferritin stores to transferrin for transport in the blood.

The best sources of copper are organ meats, seafood, vegetables, and nuts. Copper deficiency has been seen in malnourished Peruvian children, in premature infants, and in adults who have received large doses of ZINC for wound healing or for SICKLE CELL ANEMIA. Symptoms of copper deficiency include hypochromic, microcytic anemia, low plasma ceruloplasmin, and abnormalities of connective tissue and the central nervous system.

Copper is absorbed from the stomach and proximal small intestine. It is transported in the blood attached to albumin or to plasma AMINO ACIDS. Copper is excreted along with bile in the feces; only trace amounts are excreted in the urine. See also: COLLAGEN; ELASTIN; PHENYLALANINE; TRYPTOPHAN; TYROSINE.

SUGGESTED READINGS

Danks, D. M. 1983. Hereditary disorders of copper metabolism in Wilson's Disease and Menkes' disease. In *The metabolic basis of inherited disease,* 5th ed., ed. J. B. Stanbury et al., 1251–1268. New York: McGraw-Hill.

Finley, E. B., and F. L. Cerklewski. 1983. Influence of ascorbic acid supplementation on copper status in young adult men. *Am. J. Clin. Nutr.* 37:553–556.

Fischer, P. W. F., A. Giroux, and M. R. L'Abbe. 1984. Effect of zinc supplementation on copper status in adult men. *Am. J. Clin. Nutr.* 40:743–746.

Frieden, E., 1986. Perspectives on copper biochemistry. *Clin. Physiol. Biochem.* 4:11–19.

Klevay, L. M. 1980. Interactions on copper and zinc in cardiovascular disease. *Ann. N.Y. Acad. Sci.* 355:140–151.

Klevay, L. M., et al. 1980. The human requirement for copper. I. Healthy men fed conventional, American diets. *Am. J. Clin. Nutr.* 33:45–50.

Mason, K. E. 1979. A conspectus of research on copper metabolism and requirements of man. *J. Nutr.* 109:1979–2066.

Prasad, A. S., et al. 1978. Hypocupremia induced by zinc therapy in adults. *JAMA* 240:2166–2168.

Rayton, J. K., and E. D. Harris. 1979. Induction of lysyl oxidase with copper. *J. Biol. Chem.* 254:621–626.

Cori cycle.   The process by which lactate produced in skeletal muscles during contraction is recycled in the liver to GLUCOSE.

Two molecules of ATP are made available when glucose is converted to lactate in contracting muscle. The lactate cannot be recycled to glucose in muscle tissue because GLUCONEOGENESIS is blocked by the absence of *glucose 6-phosphatase*. Instead, the lactate diffuses into the bloodstream. When it reaches the liver, it will be reconverted to glucose at a cost of six molecules of ATP.

The Cori cycle is an energetically costly process; nevertheless, it serves the muscles well. When skeletal muscles are at rest, ATP is provided from free FATTY ACIDS and KETONE BODIES that are both oxidized to ACETYL-CoA, which then proceeds through the TCA CYCLE and the RESPIRATORY CHAIN. When extreme demands are placed on the skeletal muscles, however, these fuels are augmented with glucose from stored muscle GLYCOGEN. Throughout the activity there is a large supply of creatine phosphate available to phosphorylate the ADP produced from the use of ATP for contraction.

As the muscles continue to contract, muscle glycogen is depleted. Lactate builds up as the oxygen debt diverts pyruvate from aerobic paths. The decreased NAD^+ and increased NADH encourage the pyruvate-to-lactate reaction. Both pyruvate and lactate will diffuse into the bloodstream and will be carried to the liver. In the liver, gluconeogenesis will produce glucose that will be carried back to the site of muscle contraction. In the muscles, the glucose will again undergo GLYCOLYSIS forming lactate; thus the cycle is repeated.

Some of the oxygen debt will remain after the muscular activity ceases. During the recovery period, the continuing increased action of the heart and lungs will bring additional oxygen to the muscles so that all the fuels can be oxidized by aerobic paths.

Cori's disease (glycogen storage disease: type III).   A disorder inherited recessively and caused by an absence of the ENZYME that debranches GLYCOGEN. It is characterized by increased deposits of glycogen with short outer branches in the liver, muscle, and heart.

SUGGESTED READINGS

Howell, R. R., and J. C. Williams. 1983. The glycogen storage diseases. In *The metabolic basis of inherited disease*, 5th ed., ed. J. B. Stanbury, et al., 141–166. New York: McGraw-Hill.

coupled reaction. Two chemical reactions that have a common intermediate which acts as a vehicle by which energy can be transferred from one set of reactants to the other. An example of a coupled reaction is the production of creatine from creatine phosphate and the production of ATP from ADP.

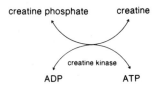

A coupled reaction

creatine phosphate (phosphocreatine). A high energy phosphate compound that has a higher phosphate group transfer potential than ATP. As a phosphagen creatine phosphate acts as a reservoir of phosphate energy for the maintenance of a steady supply of ATP for nerve impulses and muscle contraction. The enzyme *creatine kinase* catalyzes the reversible transfer of phosphate between ATP and creatine phosphate.

In the case of neural tissue, even when at rest, there must be a constant expenditure of ATP to maintain the outward-directed SODIUM ion level and the inward-directed POTASSIUM ion level. When a neuron is excited, it becomes more permeable to sodium ions, so sodium ions flow in while potassium ions flow out. This depolarization carries the message down the neuron; then, when the message has been "delivered," the cell cannot deliver another message until its normal potassium ion and sodium ion levels inside and out of the cell have been restored. This restoration of charge requires ATP, and the ATP that is used must be replenished, in other words, ADP must be phosphorylated. ATP is replenished from the reservoir of creatine phosphate.

In the case of skeletal muscle tissue, creatine phosphate provides the energy for short bursts of activity. When muscles are at rest, phosphates are transferred from ATP to creatine, thus producing creatine phosphate, a reversal of the process as it occurs during muscular activity.

Creatine phosphate

SUGGESTED READINGS

Bessman, S. P., and C. L. Carpenter. 1985. The creatine-creatine phosphate energy shuttle. *Ann. Rev. Biochem.* 54:831–862.

creatinine. A metabolite, along with creatine, that is produced in muscle cells from the breakdown of creatine phosphate. While creatine can be reconverted to creatine phosphate, creatinine production from creatine is irreversible. It is excreted in the urine. The amount of creatinine excreted

Creatinine

for a given person in a given time is fairly constant and is often used to note fluctuations of other metabolites in the urine.

CTP. See CYTIDINE TRIPHOSPHATE.

Cushing's syndrome. A syndrome exhibiting protein loss, fatigue, osteoporosis, excess hair growth, and discoloration of the skin resulting from hypersecretion of glucocorticoids by the adrenal cortex.

cyanocobalamin. See VITAMIN B_{12}.

cyclamate (sodium cyclamate). See NONNUTRITIVE SWEETENERS.

cyclic AMP (cAMP, cyclic adenosine monophosphate). A mediator inside the cell formed in response to such hormones as epinephrine and glucagon. The hormone combines with a specific receptor in the plasma membrane of the target cell and this reaction stimulates *adenylate*

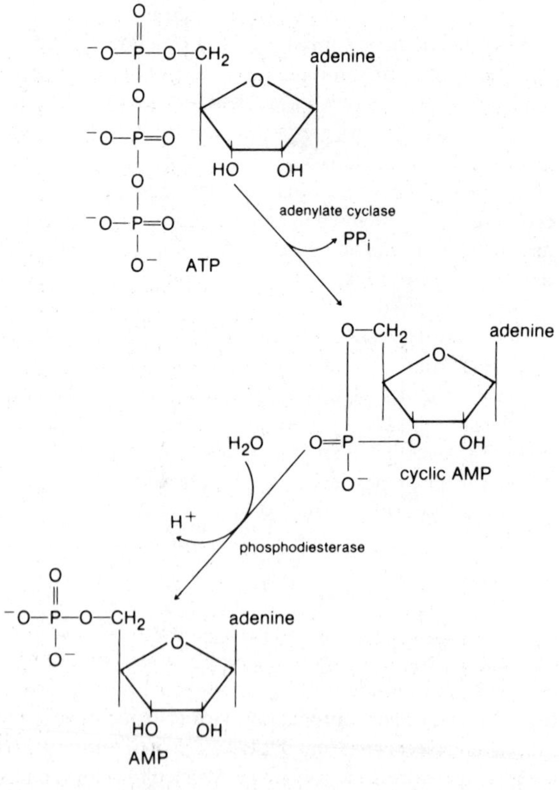

The synthesis and degradation of cyclic AMP

cyclase, also located in the plasma membrane. The hormone itself does not enter the cell but exerts its effect through *adenylate cyclase. Adenylate cyclase* increases the amount of cyclic AMP inside the cell, and cyclic AMP then stimulates the specific process. Cyclic AMP is "turned on" (synthesized) by *adenylate cyclase* and "turned off" (inactivated) by *phosphodiesterase,* which hydrolyzes the bond between the phosphate and the oxygen on carbon-3 of the ribose, forming AMP. See also: CATECHOLAMINES; HORMONE; MEMBRANES; NUCLEOSIDES, NUCLEOTIDES.

cystathioninuria. A high level of cystathionine in the urine caused by an absence of the enzyme *cystathionase,* which converts cystathionine to CYSTEINE during the synthesis of cysteine from METHIONINE.

SUGGESTED READINGS

See suggested readings for INBORN ERRORS OF METABOLISM.

cysteine (Cys). A nonessential, glucogenic (glycogenic), three-carbon α-amino acid that, like METHIONINE, has a SULFUR atom in its side chain.

Cysteine is an important amino acid in the protein of hair, hoofs, and the keratin of the skin, as well as in many ENZYMES and other proteins. Cysteine functions to stabilize the conformation of protein structure. The sulfur of a cysteine side chain joins readily with the sulfur of another cysteine molecule forming cystine which is a disulfide bridge. The two cysteines may be on the same chain, causing the chain to fold back on itself, or on adjacent chains holding them together. The union of the two cysteines becomes a disulfide bridge, the predominant covalent cross-link of proteins.

$$HS-CH_2-\overset{\overset{\displaystyle H}{|}}{\underset{\underset{\displaystyle ^+NH_3}{|}}{C}}-COO^-$$

Cysteine
(Cys)

$$^-OOC-\overset{\overset{\displaystyle H}{|}}{\underset{\underset{\displaystyle ^+NH_3}{|}}{C}}-CH_2-\overset{\text{disulfide bridge}}{S-S}-CH_2-\overset{\overset{\displaystyle H}{|}}{\underset{\underset{\displaystyle ^+NH_3}{|}}{C}}-COO^-$$

Cystine

The formation of a disulfide bridge, when DNA calls for only sulfhydryl groups, can be undesirable. For example, denaturation of proteins often comes about through oxidation of the sulfhydryl groups and subsequent formation of a disulfide bridge, resulting in a loss of protein activity. Frequently, activity can be restored by the addition of reduced sulfhydryl compounds such as the amino acid cysteine or the compound glutathione. Glutathione is essential for maintaining normal red cell structure and for keeping hemoglobin IRON in the ferrous ($+2$) state.

Cysteine is synthesized from methionine, an essential amino acid, which contributes the sulfur, and from SERINE, a NON-ESSENTIAL AMINO ACID, which contributes the carbon skeleton. Methionine is activated by the lysis of ATP into pyrophosphate and inorganic phosphate. Adenosine is attached to the methionine at its sulfur atom, then after a methyl group is transferred to an acceptor, the adenosine is released, yielding homocysteine. Homocysteine, carrying the sulfhydryl group from methionine, then combines with

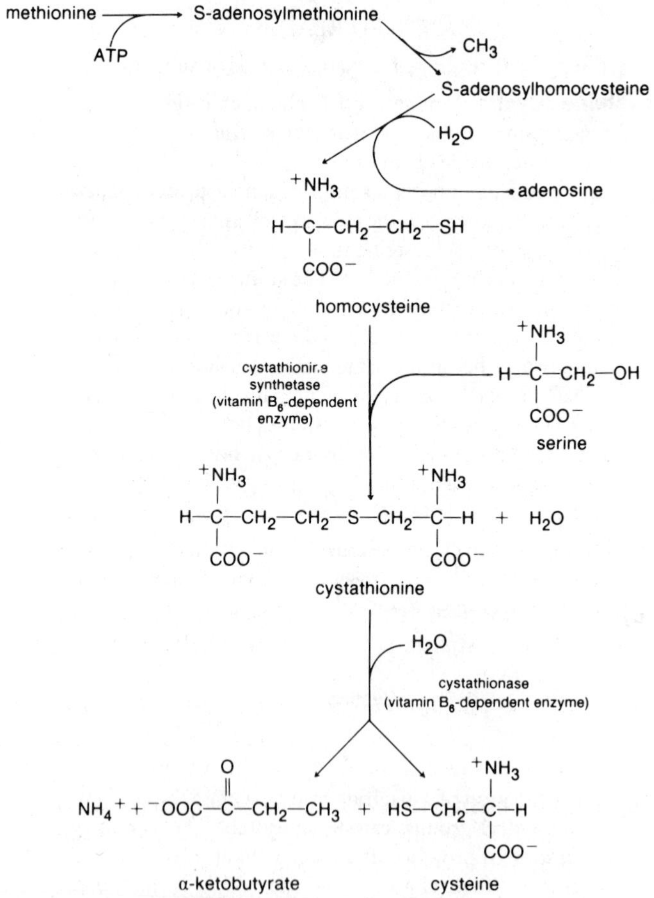

The synthesis of cysteine from methionine and serine

serine under the influence of a VITAMIN B_6-dependent enzyme, *cystathionine synthetase*. The resulting compound is cleaved to cysteine and α-ketobutyrate (and NH_4^+) by another vitamin B_6-dependent enzyme, *cystathionase*.

When a protein containing a disulfide bridge is degraded, cystine is broken into two cysteine molecules by the action of an NADH-dependent oxidoreductase; then the cysteines are degraded to pyruvate by several reactions involving transaminases, desulfinases, or sulfhydrases. Through pyruvate, the carbon skeletons of cysteine can enter the TCA CYCLE and be used for energy, or, through phosphoenolpyruvate, can re-form GLUCOSE and replenish the blood glucose supply.

SUGGESTED READINGS

Cooper, A. J. L. 1983. Biochemistry of sulfur-containing amino acids. *Ann. Rev. Biochem.* 52:187–222.

cystine. A molecule resulting from two CYSTEINE molecules joined at their SULFUR atoms. See also: CYSTEINE.

SUGGESTED READINGS

Cooper, A. J. L. 1983. Biochemistry of sulfur-containing amino acids. *Ann. Rev. Biochem.* 52:187–222.

cystinuria. An inherited amino-aciduria that, due to renal carrier deficiencies, prevents the renal tubules from reabsorbing cystine, LYSINE, ARGININE, and ornithine. There is a tendency to form kidney stones composed of the insoluble cystine.

SUGGESTED READINGS

Segal, S., and S. O. Thier. 1983. Cystinuria. In *The metabolic basis of inherited disease*, 5th ed., ed. J. B. Stanbury et al., 1774–1791. New York: McGraw-Hill.

cytidine. A nucleoside composed of cytosine (a pyrimidine) and ribose. See also: NUCLEOSIDES, NUCLEOTIDES.

cytidine diphosphate (CDP). A nucleotide composed of cytosine (a pyrimidine), ribose, and two phosphates. See also: NUCLEOSIDES, NUCLEOTIDES.

cytidine monophosphate (CMP, cytidylate). A nucleotide composed of cytosine (a pyrimidine), ribose, and one phosphate. See also: NUCLEOSIDES, NUCLEOTIDES.

cytidine triphosphate (CTP). A nucleotide composed of cytosine (a pyrimidine), ribose, and three phosphates. See also: NUCLEOSIDES, NUCLEOTIDES.

cytochromes. Electron carriers that act sequentially. For example, in the RESPIRATORY CHAIN cytochromes pick up electrons from reduced COENZYME Q and deliver them to oxygen. All cytochromes contain a HEME prosthetic group. The IRON in the heme group alternates between the reduced, ferrous ($+2$), state and the oxidized, ferric ($+3$), state. This shift in valence enables cytochromes to pick up and deliver one electron (as opposed to NADH, $FADH_2$, and CoQ, which handle two electrons).

Coenzyme Q/cytochrome *c*
reductase complex:

CoQ (reduced) $\rightarrow$ cyt *b* $\rightarrow$ FeS $\rightarrow$ cyt C_1

Cytochrome *c*
oxidase complex:

cyt *c* $\rightarrow$ cyt *a* $\rightarrow$ cyt a_3 $\rightarrow$ O_2

Cytochrome *b*, cytochrome c_1, and the iron-sulfur protein (FeS) are a part of the coenzyme Q/cytochrome *c* reductase complex; cytochrome *a* and cytochrome a_3 are a part of the cytochrome *c* oxidase complex. See also: HEME, for cytochrome structure; RESPIRATORY CHAIN, for cytochromes as electron carriers.

cytosine. A pyrimidine base. See also: PURINE, PYRIMIDINE BASES.

d

D. A small, capital D preceding the name of a compound signifies that the compound is a stereoisomer and has an absolute configuration like that of D-glyceraldehyde. See also: AMINO ACIDS, for a more complete discussion of stereoisomers.

dAMP. See DEOXYADENYLATE.

dCMP. See DEOXYCYTIDYLATE.

deaminase. A class of ENZYMES that catalyze the removal of an amino group ($-NH_2$) from an amino acid.

deamination. The removal of an amino group ($-NH_2$) from an amino acid. See also: VITAMIN B_6.

decarboxylase. A class of ENZYMES that catalyze the removal of a carboxyl group ($-COOH$) from a substrate.

decarboxylation. The removal of a carboxyl group ($-COOH$) from a compound. For example, pyruvate, the three-carbon compound that is the end product of GLYCOLYSIS, is converted to ACETYL-COA, the two-carbon compound that enters the TCA CYCLE, by the process of decarboxylation. In this step, the hydrogens and electrons are carried in $NADH + H^+$, which will be converted to ATP by the RESPIRATORY CHAIN; thus, another name for this process is oxidative decarboxylation.

degrade. To breakdown large molecules to simpler ones.

dehydratases. VITAMIN B_6-dependent ENZYMES that catalyze the removal of water. During the direct deamination of the amino acids SERINE and THREONINE, dehydration precedes deamination.

dehydrogenase. A class of ENZYMES that catalyze the removal of a pair of hydrogens from a substrate.

delta G (ΔG). Free energy that is available to do work.

delta G° (ΔG°). Standard free energy in chemical reactions.

delta G°′ (ΔG°′). Standard free energy of biochemical reactions. See also: ENERGETICS.

denaturation. The partial or complete unfolding of the native configuration of the polypeptide chain of proteins. Acid and high temperature promote protein denaturation.

deoxyadenosine. A nucleoside containing adenine (a purine) and deoxyribose. See also: NUCLEOSIDES, NUCLEOTIDES.

deoxyadenylate (deoxyadenosine monophosphate, dAMP). A nucleotide containing adenine (a purine), deoxyribose, and one phosphate. See also: NUCLEOSIDES, NUCLEOTIDES.

deoxycytidine. A nucleoside containing cytosine (a pyrimidine) and deoxyribose. See also: NUCLEOSIDES, NUCLEOTIDES.

deoxycytidylate (deoxycytidine monophosphate, dCMP). A nucleotide containing cytosine (a pyrimidine), deoxyribose, and one phosphate. See also: NUCLEOSIDES, NUCLEOTIDES.

deoxyguanosine. A nucleoside containing guanine (a purine) and deoxyribose. See also: NUCLEOSIDES, NUCLEOTIDES.

deoxyguanylate (deoxyguanosine monophosphate, dGMP). A nucleotide containing guanine (a purine), deoxyribose, and one phosphate. See also: NUCLEOSIDES, NUCLEOTIDES.

deoxyribonucleic acid. See DNA.

deoxyribose. A five-carbon sugar. See also: PENTOSE.

deoxythymidine. A nucleoside containing thymine (a pyrimidine) and deoxyribose. See also: NUCLEOSIDES, NUCLEOTIDES.

deoxythymidylate (deoxythymidine monophosphate, dTMP). A nucleotide containing thymine (a pyrimidine), deoxyribose, and one phosphate. See also: NUCLEOSIDES, NUCLEOTIDES.

dGMP. See DEOXYGUANYLATE.

diabetes mellitus. A disease in which the blood GLUCOSE concentration is unstable due to a relative or complete deficiency of insulin and a relative or great excess of glucagon. The dominant presenting symptom is hyperglycemia caused by an overproduction of glucose and an inefficient clearance of glucose in the peripheral tissues. This condition may be the expression of a genetic defect, follow a viral infection, or both.

There are two types of diabetes mellitus. Type 1 diabetes, insulin-dependent diabetes (IDD), seems to have a permissive genetic background but usually follows another event, perhaps a chemical or viral assault. Results from studies of hereditary factors have been inconclusive—the studies have been hampered by imprecise diagnoses that have included many persons without the disease. Formerly, Type 1 was called by various names, including "juvenile-onset" diabetes and "brittle" diabetes. In Type 1, ketogenesis is present, which results from the mobilization of free FATTY ACIDS from the adipose tissues and, at the same time, the increased activity of the liver's FATTY ACID OXIDATION system.

Type 2 diabetes, non-insulin-dependent diabetes (NIDD), seems to be determined completely by genetic factors. Formerly, Type 2 was known as "maturity-onset" diabetes. Diet and weight reduction may control Type 2 diabetes in obese people. Obesity, however, is not the sole factor responsible for the insulin resistance because persons with normal weight can develop Type 2 diabetes. Oral antidiabetic drugs and even insulin occasionally are required in its treatment. Persons with Type 2 diabetes usually are insulin resistant, that is, the effectiveness of insulin in disposing of a glucose load is impaired whether the insulin level is high, medium, or low.

The National Diabetes Data Group recommends that the age classifications of Type 1 and Type 2 diabetes be dropped since age of onset in both types is not a clear diagnostic guide. This group also recommends procedures for diagnosis of diabetes. Traditionally, diagnosis of diabetes has been based on elevated blood glucose concentrations following an overnight fast and consumption of a glucose load. This standard oral glucose tolerance test has resulted in overdiagnosis of diabetes, especially in patients with an elevated blood glucose level that is caused by the presence of another disease, for example, pancreatitis, or by an increase of stress-related hormones.

SUGGESTED READINGS

Bantle, J. P., et al. 1983. Postprandial glucose and insulin responses to meals containing different carbohydrates in normal and diabetic subjects. *N. Engl. J. Med.* 309:7–12.

Brownlee, M., and A. Cerami. 1981. The biochemistry of the complications of diabetes mellitus. *Ann. Rev. Biochem.* 50:385–432.

Foster, D. W. 1983. Diabetes mellitus. In *The metabolic basis of inherited disease,* 5th ed., ed. J. B. Stanbury et al., 99–117. New York: McGraw-Hill.

Heller, A., and L. Jovanovic. 1985. Artificial sweeteners: Safety and utility in the treatment of diabetes mellitus. In *Nutrition and diabetes,* ed. L. Jovanovic and C. M. Peterson, 37–50. New York: Alan R. Liss.

Menendez, C. E., and B. J. Stoecker. 1985. The role of the diet in improving glycemic control. In *Nutrition and diabetes,* ed. L. Jovanovic and C. M. Peterson, 15–36. New York: Alan R. Liss.

National Diabetes Data Group. 1979. Classification and diagnosis of diabetes mellitus and other categories of glucose intolerance. *Diabetes* 28:1039–1057.

diacylglycerol. A compound resulting from the esterification of two fatty acids to a glycerol molecule.

dicoumarol. An antagonist of vitamin K. See also: VITAMIN K.

digestion. The enzymatic hydrolysis of food that occurs in the gastrointestinal tract. See also: CARBOHYDRATE DIGESTION; LIPID DIGESTION; PROTEIN DIGESTION.

diglyceride. See DIACYLGLYCEROL; LIPIDS.

disulfide bridge. See CYSTEINE; CYSTINE.

DNA (deoxyribonucleic acid). The molecule that carries, in the sequence of its bases, the genetic language of a species or an individual. DNA, which makes up the genes and, thus, the chromosomes, is found almost exclusively in the nucleus of eukaryotic cells. The biochemistry of these molecules explains the way heredity is copied faithfully during the lifetime of a person or from generation to generation within families and species. (The reader may wish to review GENETIC CODE; NUCLEOSIDES, NUCLEOTIDES; PURINE, PYRIMIDINE BASES; REPLICATION; RNA; TRANSLATION, before continuing.)

DNA is composed of two "vertical" chains of alternating phosphate and deoxyribose (sugar) molecules that can be envisioned as the uprights of a ladder. The structure of this "backbone" is constant throughout the molecules. The crosspieces of the "ladder" are composed of hydrogen-bonded purine and pyrimidine bases. In every species that has been studied, the ratio of purine to pyrimidine bases is nearly 1.0. This is due to the complementary base pairing of a single purine with a single pyrimidine—i.e., adenine is paired to thymine and guanine is paired to cytosine.

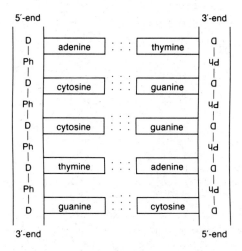

5'-end   3'-end

5'-end   3'-end

3'-end   5'-end

The "ladder" of deoxyribonucleic acid (DNA)

The "rungs" of the ladder are formed by purine
and pyrimidine pairs — guanine ⋮ cytosine and
adenine ⋮ thymine. The purines are adenine
and guanine. The pyrimidines are thymine
and cytosine.

D - deoxyribose sugar
Ph - phosphate

⋮ 3 hydrogen bonds

⋮ 2 hydrogen bonds

The external backbone of the double helix consists of phosphate-deoxyribose (phosphate-sugar) chains strongly bound by covalent bonds. The 5'-hydroxyl of one pentose in bonded by a phosphodiester bond to the 3'-hydroxyl of the adjacent pentose.

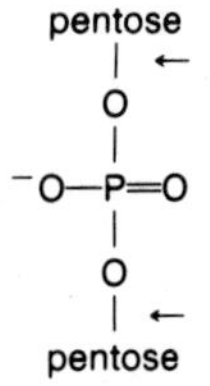

In contrast to the strength of the phosphodiester bonds of the backbone, the bases in the interior of the double helix are bonded with weak hydrogen bonds—two hydrogen bonds between adenine and thymine, and three hydrogen bonds between guanine and cytosine. These weak hydrogen bonds make the crosspieces easy to break.

The ladder of DNA is twisted around an axis to form a double helix. In this configuration the plane of the bases is perpendicular to the axis and to the planes of the sugars. Interestingly, the space within the helix is just the correct size for one purine and one pyrimidine; distortion of the helix

pentose
| ←
O
|
⁻O—P=O
|
O
| ←
pentose

Phosphodiester bond

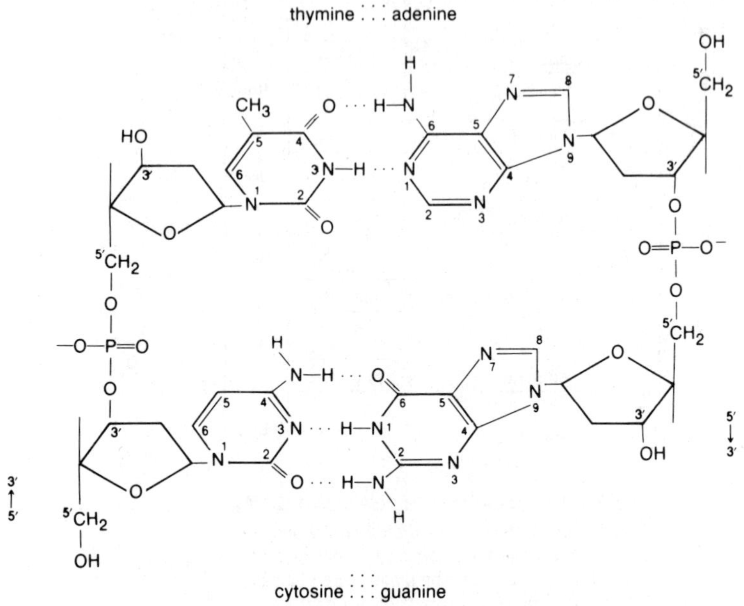

thymine ⋮⋮ adenine

cytosine ⋮⋮⋮ guanine

Deoxyribonucleic acid (DNA) showing hydrogen bonds between bases
and the direction of phosphate-deoxyribose backbones.

results if two pyrimidines or two purines form hydrogen
bonds between them.

The double helix of DNA shows remarkable integrity: in
the same individual, every diploid cell contains identical
DNA material. Within a species, the base composition, that
is, the amount of adenine, cytosine, guanine, and thymine,
does not vary with age, nutritional status, or shift in environment. Species that are close to each other in evolution-
ary history have similar DNA base composition, while
those that are evolutionarily divergent have dissimilar DNA
composition.

The genetic language is written in the sequence of the
complementary base pairs that compose the crosspieces, or
ladder rungs. Because there are no physical restrictions on
the sequence of bases, each purine-pyrimidine pair may be
identical to or different from the adjacent pair, thus making
possible the infinite number of unique DNA molecules—
hence, proteins—found throughout all life forms.

Through the complementarity of base pairs, DNA is rep-
licated in a dividing cell so that each daughter cell receives
the complete store of genetic knowledge. In each new cell

there will be one strand of the original DNA from the parent cell and a freshly duplicated strand. During replication the hydrogen bonds holding the base pairs together in the parent cell are broken and the two chains come apart (become "unzipped") leaving the single bases exposed. Each base is now ready to attach to its complement, which is in its activated form of deoxyribonucleoside 5'-triphosphate.

As each matching of base pairs occurs, the two extra phosphates are released as pyrophosphate, whose hydrolysis provides the energy for the next matching of base pairs. Each new nucleotide is added to the 3'-hydroxyl end of the already existing nucleotide, thus the direction of elongation is $5' \longrightarrow 3'$ and the direction of the two phosphate-deoxyribose chains of completed DNA is antiparallel. Each DNA chain has one end that has the 5'-OH group of the sugar and the other end that has the 3'-OH group, which is not attached to another nucleotide. The notation of a sequence of bases is stated from the 5'-end to the 3'-end in the same manner as the sequence of AMINO ACIDS in protein is read from the amino end of the "first" amino acid to the carboxyl end of the "last" amino acid.

Also, because of the complementarity of base pairs, the information carried in DNA can be transferred to single-stranded messenger RNA, which will carry the information out of the nucleus into the cytosol, a process known as transcription. Messenger RNA becomes the template for aligning amino acids in the proper sequence to make the prescribed protein. Certain molecules that must be present in the cell for replication and transcription to occur include *DNA-polymerase*, which will direct the addition of deoxyribonucleotides to the developing DNA chain; Mg^{++}; all four of the triphosphates of the deoxyribonucleosides (dATP, dTTP, dGTP, dCTP); DNA that will be the template; and a primer fragment of DNA with an exposed 3'-hydroxyl group for the nucleotide to attach to since the *polymerase* will not begin a new strand.

Less than 0.1 percent of DNA is present in mitochondria. This extra-nuclear DNA has a slightly different base composition and is much smaller than the DNA found in the nucleus. There is much speculation about the origins of mitochondrial DNA: one such explanation holds that mitochondria are vestigial chromosomes of ancient bacteria that entered the cytoplasm of eukaryotic cells and continued to reproduce there. The percentage of mitochondrial DNA (mDNA) is greater in fertilized and dividing cells because of the greater number of mitochondria in these cells. See also: GENETIC CODE; NUCLEOSIDES, NUCLEOTIDES; PURINE, PYRIMIDINE BASES; RNA.

SUGGESTED READINGS

Klobutcher, L. A., and F. H. Ruddle. 1981. Chromosome mediated gene transfer. *Ann. Rev. Biochem.* 50:533–554.

Record, M. T., Jr., et al. 1981. Double helical DNA: Conformations, physical properties, and interactions with ligands. *Ann. Rev. Biochem.* 50:997–1024.

Waring, M. J. 1981. DNA modification and cancer. *Ann. Rev. Biochem.* 50:159–192.

dopamine. See CATECHOLAMINES.

D-ribose. A five-carbon sugar. See also: DNA; PENTOSE; PENTOSE PHOSPHATE SHUNT; RNA.

dTMP. See THYMIDYLATE.

dynamic state. A condition within a cell, tissue, or organ in which a structure is constantly being produced and destroyed in such a way that there is no net gain or loss. To outward appearance, the tissue, once made, is completed and there is no more coming and going of nutrients across its threshold. Close study, however, reveals a high level of metabolic activity.

Bone is an excellent example of a tissue in a dynamic state. It may appear that once full growth has been achieved, no more activity occurs within bone unless there is healing following a break; however, bone tissue is being broken down continuously by cells called osteoclasts and the minerals are being resorbed into the bloodstream. At the same time, osteoblasts are using minerals from the blood supply to rebuild bone tissue.

eicosanoids. A group of compounds known as PROSTAG-
LANDINS that are derived from the C-20 fatty acids. See
also: ESSENTIAL FATTY ACIDS; FATTY ACIDS; PROSTAGLANDINS.

elastin. The substance in major connective tissues found in
ligaments and arterial walls. Elastin is similar to COLLAGEN in
that both are rich in GLYCINE and LYSINE, but, unlike collagen,
elastin has few PROLINES. COPPER is required for the formation of cross-links in elastin. Elastin is characterized by
being elastic, that is, it will stretch when a force is applied
and will return to its original length when the force is released. This quality is especially valuable in arterial walls,
which must withstand expansion when the heartbeat pushes
a surge of blood through the arteries. Then, to maintain
blood pressure, the walls must contract after the surge has
passed.

SUGGESTED READINGS

Eyre, D. R., M. A. Paz, and P. M. Gallop. 1984. Cross-
linking in collagen and elastin. *Ann. Rev. Biochem.*
53:717–748.

Sandberg, L. B., N. T. Soskel, and J. G. Leslie. 1981. Elastin
structure, biosynthesis, and relation to disease states. *N.
Engl. J. Med.* 304:566–579.

electron acceptor. A member of an oxidation/reduction
pair that can receive electrons from the electron donor; thus
it is an oxidizing agent or oxidant. Oxygen is the ultimate
acceptor in the RESPIRATORY CHAIN.

electron donor. A member of an oxidation/reduction pair
that can donate electrons to an electron acceptor; thus it is
a reducing agent or reductant. Hydrogen is a strong reducing agent whereas water is a weak reducing agent.

electron transport chain. See RESPIRATORY CHAIN.

Embden-Meyerhoff pathway. See GLYCOLYSIS.

emulsion. A mixture of fat in water in which the fat is broken into very small droplets that are dispersed throughout the water. If the emulsion is to be sustained, an emulsifying agent, such as a detergent, must be present. In the case of the emulsion of fats in the watery fluids of the digestive tract, BILE SALTS act as the emulsifying agent. Their hydrophilic ends form an interface between the fat droplets and the water, thereby allowing *lipases* to act on the fat.

enantiomer. A mirror image of a compound that has an asymmetrical carbon atom. Such compounds have optical activity, that is, they rotate the plane of polarized light and are said to be optical isomers, stereoisomers, or enantiomers of each other. Although enantiomers of a compound are similar chemically, their biological properties are different.

endoplasmic reticulum. An interconnected network of flattened tubules in the cytoplasm of cells. Regions with ribosomes attached to the cytoplasmic surfaces of the tubules are called rough endoplasmic reticulum; these regions are involved in the synthesis of proteins for export.

endorphin. A peptide present in the brain that has morphinelike properties. Beta endorphin reacts similarly to morphine, even to the extent that its effects are counteracted by naloxone, an antagonist of morphine.

energetics. The physical laws of energy and energy transformations that operate during every chemical reaction. The principles of energetics explain many of the puzzling questions of biochemistry and nutrition such as why some cellular chemical reactions proceed spontaneously while others do not, or how complex, highly ordered molecules can be built within the cell, an action that seems to defy the law that all reactions go toward increasing disorder.

The principles of energetics of chemical reactions in biological systems are based on the first and second laws of thermodynamics. The first law of thermodynamics, the familiar conservation-of-energy law, states that energy can neither be created nor destroyed but can be converted from one form to another. The second law, which states that all chemical changes move toward less order and more randomness, will be considered below.

Energy occurs as a variety of forms including heat, chemical, light, electrical, or solar energy. Work done by machines is accomplished through successive conversions of energy from one form to another. In the biological world, solar energy is converted to the chemical energy stored in plants that, when eaten by animals, can be converted to the mechanical energy of contracting muscles or can be stored as chemical energy in fat deposits. None of these conversions is very efficient because each involves some loss of energy. Considering this loss, how can the first law of thermodynamics be correct?

The first law of thermodynamics operates in a closed "universe" in which there is a working "system" plus its "surroundings." It is in that universe, not in the system, that total energy remains constant. If the system loses energy, it is lost to the surroundings so that the total energy of the two parts of the universe remains constant. In the cells of the body, GLUCOSE, which contains stored energy, can be oxidatively degraded into carbon dioxide, water, and ATP, the molecule that carries cellular energy. When this reaction occurs, however, not all the energy stored in the bonds of glucose will be conserved in the bonds of ATP, carbon dioxide, and water—some will be lost as heat energy. These three compounds, each containing some of glucose's energy, may be used in other ways; therefore they contain useful energy. Heat energy that was dissipated into the immediate surroundings (the cytosol of the cell) cannot be redirected toward work. Consequently, above the amount of heat needed for warmth, this heat is useless energy. In the meantime, the total energy of the universe remains constant—that is, the energy of the system (the glucose molecule) plus the energy in its surroundings (the cytosol) remains constant. The ultimate surroundings of the glucose molecule is not the cytosol but the universe itself, including outer space. The heat energy moves from the cytosol to the circulatory systems, out of the body via the lungs, kidneys, pores of the skin, and intestinal excreta, and ultimately into the atmosphere.

The energy principle of the first law of thermodynamics is expressed mathematically as

$$\Delta E_{system} \rightarrow E_B - E_A = Q - W$$

where ΔE represents the total energy of the system, E_A is the energy possessed by the system at the beginning of a reaction, and E_B is the energy the system possesses when the reaction ends (has reached equilibrium). Q is the heat the system has absorbed and W is the work accomplished. An important element in energy transformations in biological reactions is missing if we are left with the question "How can highly ordered molecules be structured if all energy reactions lead to disorder?" This equation does not include the changes in orderliness—the entropy (ΔS)—that occur.

The second law of thermodynamics includes the idea of changes in entropy.

The second law of thermodynamics states that any physical or chemical change moves in a direction that leads to an increase in the randomness, the entropy (S), of the universe. What must be brought into the equation being developed here is the idea of work accomplished: Where is the energy that is useful, i.e., that gets work done?

Useful energy can be in two forms, free energy and heat energy. Free energy is that which is available to do work when temperature and atmospheric pressure remain constant. Heat energy can do work only when the system requires a change in temperature, such as burning coal to change the physical state of water from liquid to gas. In biological systems that require maintenance of a particular temperature, heat energy (above that small amount that maintains a viable temperature) is useless energy; it merely contributes to the entropy of the universe.

The second law of thermodynamics is expressed mathematically as

$$\Delta S_{universe} \rightarrow \Delta S_{system} + \Delta S_{surroundings}$$

where $\Delta S_{universe}$ stands for the change in entropy of a universe that is the total of the change in entropy of the system (ΔS_{system}) plus the change in entropy of the surroundings ($\Delta S_{surroundings}$). If the value of $\Delta S_{universe}$ increases, the numerical value will be greater than zero and the reaction will proceed spontaneously.

It is difficult to measure entropy, however. To overcome this difficulty there must be included in the evolving equation an additional function; that of free energy (G). As stated above, free energy can do work at constant temperature and pressure. As a reaction proceeds toward equilibrium, free energy decreases while entropy increases. A combination of the first and second laws of thermodynamics is expressed mathematically as

$$\Delta G = \Delta E - T\Delta S$$

where ΔG is the change in free energy, ΔE is the change in total energy, ΔS is the change in entropy, and T is the absolute temperature.

In the special instances of chemical reactions, the standard free energy change ($\Delta G°$) is a more useful concept than free energy change (ΔG). The value of $\Delta G°$ is derived from the equilibrium constant (K'_{eq}), a term that incorporates the effect of the concentrations of reactants and products on a given reaction.

If the equilibrium constant of a reaction is 1.0, the standard free energy change is 0. If the equilibrium constant is greater than 1.0, the standard free energy change will be negative and the reaction will be exergonic. Only those reactions with a negative standard free energy change will proceed spontaneously in the direction written. Reactions with a positive standard free energy change (an equilibrium constant less than 1.0) will proceed in the reverse direction only with an input of energy.

Another factor that must be incorporated into those special energy equations—the ones that deal with biochemical reactions—is that of pH, because chemical reactions occurring in living organisms take place within a limited pH range. Standard conditions of temperature and pressure include a standard pH of 7.0. The pH factor is included in the special symbol $\Delta G^{\circ\prime}$.

From the discussion of the energetics of biochemical reactions so far, $\Delta G^{\circ\prime}$ incorporates many concepts including the first and second laws of thermodynamics; the values for standard temperature, pressure, and pH; the effects of concentrations of reactants and products (the equilibrium constant K'_{eq}); and the difference between useful and useless energy.

When $\Delta G^{\circ\prime}$ is given for a specific reaction and for its reverse direction, it can be known in which direction the biochemical reaction will proceed spontaneously. The direction with the more negative value for $\Delta G^{\circ\prime}$ will prevail. A reaction that has a positive $\Delta G^{\circ\prime}$ will need to be coupled with a reaction that has a negative value for $\Delta G^{\circ\prime}$. For example, if a reaction is involved in synthesizing a protein and has a positive $\Delta G^{\circ\prime}$, it may be coupled with the hydrolysis of ATP, which will furnish the free energy for the synthesis. The following table shows the standard free energy changes of some typical biochemical reactions.

Standard free energy changes ($\Delta G^{\circ\prime}$) of some common biochemical reactions (at standard conditions of pH, temperature, and pressure)

Reaction	$\Delta G^{\circ\prime}$ (kcal)
glucose + $6O_2 \rightarrow 6CO_2 + 6H_2O$	-686
glucose $1-PO_4 \rightarrow$ glucose $6-PO_4$	-1.7
glutamine + $H_2O \rightarrow$ glutamate + NH_4^+	-3.4
pyrophosphate + $H_2O \rightarrow$ 2 phosphate	-8.0
sucrose + $H_2O \rightarrow$ glucose + fructose	-7.0

enterohepatic circulation. The path of BILE SALTS from liver to bile duct to intestine where 99 percent may be reabsorbed from the ileum and sent back to the liver by way of the portal circulation. Some vitamins and minerals also undergo enterohepatic circulation.

enthalpy. The thermodynamic function of a system equivalent to the internal energy plus the product of the pressure and the volume.

entropy. The randomness or disorder of a system. A measure of the capacity of a system to undergo spontaneous change. All reactions proceed in the direction of greatest stability with the energy distributed in the most unordered way possible, that is, with the greatest entropy. See also: ENERGETICS.

enzyme. A highly specialized protein molecule that serves as a catalyst for a specific chemical reaction and is not consumed or permanently altered by the reaction. Since it is a protein, however, its activity is altered by heat, changes in pH, radiation, or any other environmental condition that affects protein conformation.

The enzyme molecule has an active site to which the reactants are attracted, providing a place where the reaction can occur more quickly and efficiently than it would if it depended on chance encounters of the reactants. The active site of an enzyme is an arrangement of atoms in one small part of the large complex protein that creates a three-dimensional cleft or crevice into which the substrate will fit. In some enzymes, the active site is molded after the substrate has been engaged (induced fit). In most enzymes, however, the active site and the substrate are exact complements of each other, in the same manner as a lock and key. An inhibitor, a substance that keeps the enzyme from being active, functions because it fits into the active site and prevents the substrate and enzyme from engaging. Some poisons work this way. On the other hand, it is often beneficial for the active site to be unusable until it is in the presence of its substrate; such a form of the enzyme is called a ZYMOGEN.

Many enzymes can be active only if they are combined with other substances. These additions, called cofactors, may include metallic ions such as IRON, MAGNESIUM, MANGANESE, or ZINC. For example, cytochromes require iron, *phosphotransferases* require magnesium, *arginase* requires manganese, *alcohol dehydrogenase* requires zinc, and *pyruvate phosphokinase* requires both POTASSIUM and magnesium. Other cofactors may be large organic molecules such as vitamins, in which case they are usually called coenzymes. For example, *carboxylases* require BIOTIN as the coenzyme, and *transaminases* require the coenzyme form of VITAMIN B$_6$.

Some enzymes will act on a broad range of substances while others are highly specific for a substrate and will not act on even closely similar compounds. An example of the latter is *trypsin*, a digestive enzyme that will split a peptide bond only if it is on the carboxyl side of LYSINE or ARGININE. Two features must be present for enzymes to be substrate specific. First, the substrate must have the specific bond that the enzyme is designed to attack; second, there must be a group on the enzyme that positions and holds the substrate and enzyme together. This group, or place, is the binding site.

Enzyme action is influenced by the concentration of the substrate. If the substrate concentration is low, the rate of enzyme action will increase with an increase in the available substrate up to a concentration where an increase in substrate produces no significant rate increase. This point is termed the maximum velocity (V_{max}). Each enzyme has a characteristic concentration of the substrate, the Michaelis-Menten constant (K_m), that produces one-half the maximum velocity ($\frac{1}{2}V_{max}$).

Enzymes are also affected by the PH of the surrounding medium. At an optimum pH, where enzyme action is at its peak, the proton acceptors and proton donors in the active site are fully ionized. This characteristic of enzymes allows them to be activated ("turned on") or deactivated ("turned off") by a change in pH. The devastating effect that small changes in pH have on the body is due to the effect of pH changes on the action of enzymes.

An "enzyme complex" is composed of a group of enzymes that alter the starting compound in sequential, small stages until the desired end product is obtained. These enzymes are often attached, in the proper sequence, to a membrane, or they are confined within an organelle so that the series of changes can take place in the least amount of time and with a minimum of opportunity for engaging in other chance encounters. The enzymes of the RESPIRATORY CHAIN form such a complex: they are attached to the inner membrane of the mitochondria where they act like a "bucket brigade" handing the electrons from one compound to the next.

The compartmentalization of enzymes allows incompatible reactions to take place simultaneously. An example of this is the oxidation of FATTY ACIDS taking place inside the barrier of the mitochondrial membrane, while the synthesis of fatty acids occurs on the other side of the membrane in the cytoplasm of the cell.

In the early years of biochemical investigation and enzyme identification, enzymes were often named by addition of the suffix "ase" to the name of the substrate on which they acted. For example, *arginase* acts on ARGININE, *lactase* acts on lactose, and so forth. Some of the early names, however, did not follow this system, for example, *trypsin* and *chymotrypsin*. After the isolation of many enzymes, the Committee on Enzyme Nomenclature of the International Union of Biochemistry established a system of classification and nomenclature that allows scientists to identify each one accurately. In the enzyme catalog published by this committee, there are six classifications of enzymes based on the kind of work they do:

1. oxido-reductases   electron transfer
2. transferases   transfer of groups
3. hydrolases   hydrolysis
4. lyases   addition at a double bond
5. isomerases   isomerization
6. ligases   formation of bond with ATP cleavage

See also: ACIDOSIS; ALKALOSIS; THIAMIN PYROPHOSPHATE, for a discussion of one enzyme at work.

enzyme inhibitor. A substance that interacts to modify the conformation of the active center or the substrate-binding site of an ENZYME, slowing or preventing its catalytic action.

epinephrine (adrenalin). A hormone, produced mainly by the adrenal medulla, that produces effects on target tissues by raising CYCLIC AMP concentrations in the cells. It promotes GLYCOGENOLYSIS in muscle and liver, activates lipolysis in adipose tissue, and raises blood glucose concentrations and fatty acid levels. Epinephrine and norepinephrine are also known as CATECHOLAMINES and are both synthesized from the amino acid TYROSINE. See also: CATECHOLAMINES.

equilibrium constant (K'_{eq}). The point of equilibrium of any chemical reaction, that is, the point at which the forward and the reverse reactions of molar concentrations of the reactants and products will be equal. This point is unique for every chemical reaction and allows many useful calculations. The equilibrium constant (K'_{eq}) is calculated from

$$K'_{eq} = \frac{[C][D]}{[A][B]}$$

where [A] and [B] are molar concentrations of the reactants and [C] and [D] are molar concentrations of the products of a reaction. These terms are commonly used in the generalized equation A + B → C + D. The brackets denote molar concentrations.

erythropoietic porphyria. A mild form of a genetic disorder in which porphyrins are excreted in urine.

essential amino acids (EAA). Those AMINO ACIDS that a species cannot synthesize in sufficient quantity and that the species obtains preformed in its food. There is no implication of "necessary" as opposed to "unnecessary" in this designation except in the sense that it is necessary to eat foods daily which contain these amino acids. All amino acids, essential and nonessential, are necessary for the construction of body proteins. Scientists generally concur that eight amino acids, ISOLEUCINE, LEUCINE, LYSINE, METHIONINE, PHENYLALANINE, THREONINE, TRYPTOPHAN, and VALINE, are essential for human beings.

There is some disagreement, however, over the essentiality of ARGININE and HISTIDINE. Some scientists consider histidine as being essential for infants but not for children or adults; others consider the amount of arginine that is reformed by the UREA CYCLE to be sufficient for adults. Yet others explain that not enough net arginine is synthesized in the urea cycle to provide for the amino acid needs during rapid growth. McMurray (1983) states that "low arginine diets, though adequate to sustain growth and body maintenance, may lead to defective spermatogenesis; low histidine diets promote eczema and reduced growth in infants and interfere with hemoglobin synthesis." Jones, Kopple, and Swendseid (1982) reported that "these observations [on adult men] indicate a need for exogenous histidine." Jackson (1983) suggested that essentiality may depend on the carbon skeleton structure and the body's ability to aminate it. Though this disagreement has not been resolved, newer techniques now in use may clarify human dietary amino acid needs.

Sometimes special conditions cause an amino acid to be essential in that situation. For example, two amino acids, CYSTEINE and TRYOSINE can be synthesized from methionine and phenylalanine, respectively, and are considered nonessential. However, cysteine and tyrosine become essential if there is any interference in their conversion, such as a defective enzyme or immature development as found in premature infants. See also: ARGININE; PHENYLALANINE.

SUGGESTED READINGS

Gaull, G. E., J. Sturman, and N. C. R. Raiha. 1972. Development of mammalian sulfur metabolism: Absence of cystathionase in human fetal tissues. *Pediatr. Res.* 6:538–547.

Jackson, A. A. 1983. Amino acid: Essential and nonessential? Lancet 2:1034–1037.

Jones, M. R., J. D. Kopple, and M. E. Swendseid. 1982. $^{14}CO_2$ expiration after ^{14}C-histidine administration in normal and uremic men ingesting two levels of histidine. *Am. J. Clin. Nutr.* 35:15–23.

Kopple, J. D., and M. E. Swendseid. 1975. Evidence that histidine is an essential amino acid in normal and chronically uremic man. *J. Clin. Invest.* 55:881–891.

McMurray, W. C. 1983. Essentials of human metabolism. Philadelphia: Harper & Row, pp. 208–211.

Wixom, R. L., et al. 1977. Total parenteral nutrition with selective histidine depletion in man. *Am. J. Clin. Nutr.* 30:887–899.

essential fatty acids (EFA). The polyunsaturated FATTY ACIDS, linoleic acid ($18:2\Delta^{9,12}$ or $18:2\omega6$) and linolenic acid ($18:3\Delta^{9,12,15}$ or $18:3\omega3$). Because mammals lack the enzymes to insert double bonds beyond carbon number 9, these two essential fatty acids must be included in the diet. Plant foods, such as peanuts, corn, and safflower, provide ample amounts of essential fatty acids in the diet.

Linoleic and linolenic acids are important precursors of the regulatory compounds PROSTAGLANDINS, leukotrienes, and thromboxanes. They are also important in maintaining normal fluidity of cell MEMBRANES and in lowering plasma CHOLESTEROL concentrations.

Linoleic acid ($18:2\omega6$) is converted to γ-linolenic acid ($18:3\omega6$) by Δ^6 *desaturase*. Another enzyme, an *elongase*, catalyzes the next reaction to yield dihomo γ-linolenic acid ($20:3\omega6$). This compound is usually incorporated into phospholipids in cell membranes, used to synthesize prostaglandins (series 1) and/or converted to arachidonic acid ($20:4\omega6$) by a Δ^5 *desaturase*. Arachidonic acid may also be incorporated into the phospholipids of cell membranes or be used to synthesize protaglandins (series 2), thromboxanes, and leukotrienes.

A similar series of reactions, utilizing the same enzymes, may convert α-linolenic acid ($18:3\omega3$) to eicosapentaenoic acid ($20:5\omega3$). This compound, which can be obtained by consuming marine animals, is also a precursor of prostaglandins (series 3) and thromboxanes, or it may provide fluidity to membranes as part of phospholipids. Arachidonic

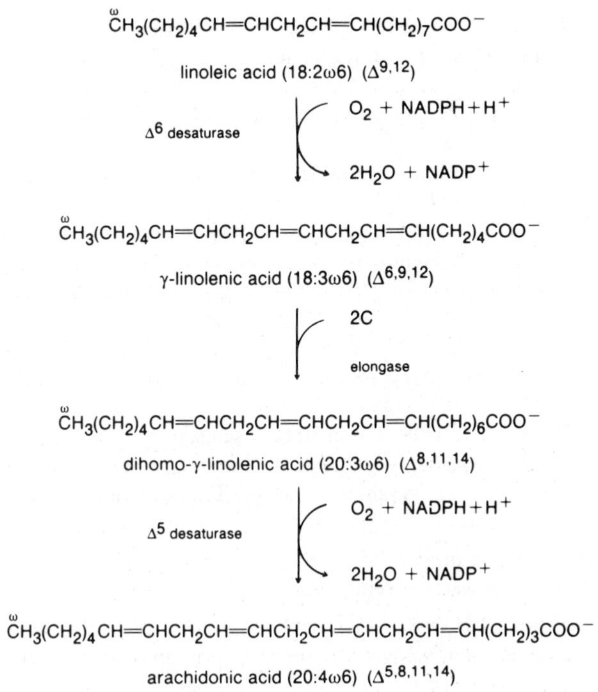

$$\overset{\omega}{C}H_3(CH_2)_4CH{=}CHCH_2CH{=}CH(CH_2)_7COO^-$$

linoleic acid (18:2ω6) ($\Delta^{9,12}$)

Δ^6 desaturase $\qquad O_2 + NADPH + H^+$

$2H_2O + NADP^+$

$$\overset{\omega}{C}H_3(CH_2)_4CH{=}CHCH_2CH{=}CHCH_2CH{=}CH(CH_2)_4COO^-$$

γ-linolenic acid (18:3ω6) ($\Delta^{6,9,12}$)

$\qquad 2C$

elongase

$$\overset{\omega}{C}H_3(CH_2)_4CH{=}CHCH_2CH{=}CHCH_2CH{=}CH(CH_2)_6COO^-$$

dihomo-γ-linolenic acid (20:3ω6) ($\Delta^{8,11,14}$)

Δ^5 desaturase $\qquad O_2 + NADPH + H^+$

$2H_2O + NADP^+$

$$\overset{\omega}{C}H_3(CH_2)_4CH{=}CHCH_2CH{=}CHCH_2CH{=}CHCH_2CH{=}CH(CH_2)_3COO^-$$

arachidonic acid (20:4ω6) ($\Delta^{5,8,11,14}$)

The conversion of linoleic acid to arachidonic acid

acid and eicosapentaenoic acid compete with each other for the activity of *cyclooxygenase*, the enzyme that acts on both of these unsaturated fatty acids to produce prostaglandins and thromboxanes.

In general, the prostaglandins, thromboxanes, and leukotrienes affect smooth muscle contraction and relaxation and/or vascular and bronchial constriction and dilation. In addition, these compounds are thought to affect leukocyte chemotaxis—in other words, either enhance or retard white blood cells' reaction to chemical substances. Leukotrienes are also thought to be involved in hypersensitivity (allergic) reactions.   See also: FATTY ACIDS; FATTY ACID NOMENCLATURE; FATTY ACID OXIDATION; PROSTAGLANDINS.

SUGGESTED READINGS

Adam, O., and G. Wolfram. 1984. Effect of different linoleic acid intakes on prostaglandin biosynthesis and kidney function in man. *Am. J. Clin. Nutr.* 40:763–770.

Crawford, M. A. 1983. Background to essential fatty acids and their prostanoid derivatives. *Br. Med. Bull.* 39:210–213.

Friedman, Z. 1980. Essential fatty acids revisited. *Am. J. Dis. Child* 134:397–408.

Hammarstrom, S. 1983. Leukotrienes. *Ann. Rev. Biochem.* 52:355–377.

Lewis, R. A., and K. F. Austen. 1984. The biologically active leukotrienes: Biosynthesis, metabolism, receptors, functions, and pharmacology. *J. Clin. Invest.* 73:889–897.

Meng, H. C. 1983. A case of human linolenic acid deficiency involving neurological abnormalities. *Am. J. Clin. Nutr.* 37:157–159.

Willis, A. L. 1984. Essential fatty acids, prostaglandins and related eicosanoids. In *Present knowledge in nutrition,* 5th ed., 90–115. Washington, D. C.: The Nutrition Foundation, Inc.

ester. The product of a reaction of an acid with an alcohol in which water is removed.

ethanol (C_2H_5OH). The alcohol resulting from the alcoholic fermentation of GLUCOSE. The principal alcohol in alcoholic beverages. See also: ACETALDEHYDE.

eukaryotes (eucaryotes). Organisms whose cells contain a membrane-bounded nucleus. With the exception of the bacteria and blue-green algae (the prokaryotes), all living organisms are eukaryotes.

FAD. See FAD, FMN.

FAD, FMN (flavin adenine dinucleotide, flavin mono-nucleotide). Two important coenzymes that are carriers of hydrogens (with their electrons) during oxidation and reduction reactions in the METABOLISM of energy nutrients as well as in the degradation of a number of other compounds. Even though these coenzymes' chemical names are incorrect, they are commonly accepted. FAD and FMN are also known as the "flavin coenzymes."

A critical portion of FAD's and FMN's structures is RIBO-FLAVIN, one of the B-vitamins. In the figure, the reactive region in riboflavin's isoalloxazine ring is encircled with a dashed line.

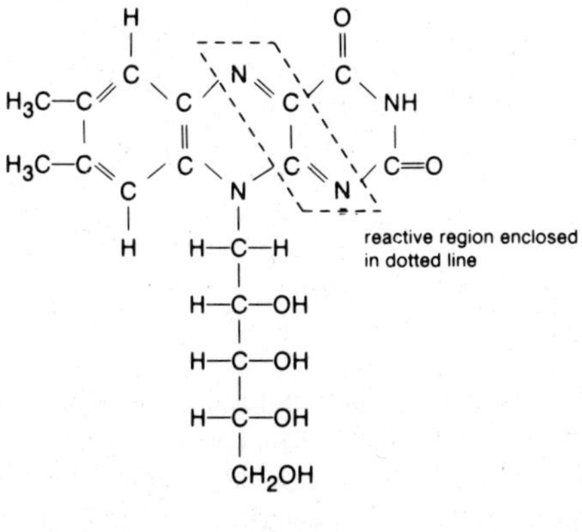

Riboflavin

FAD and FMN alternate between the oxidized and reduced states with a change in the number of hydrogens and
a shift in the placement of double bonds in the riboflavin
portion of their structures. See figures.

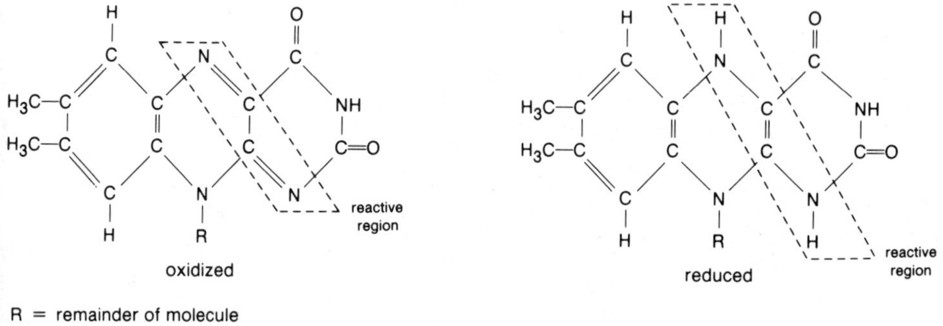

R = remainder of molecule

Oxidized and reduced forms of FAD

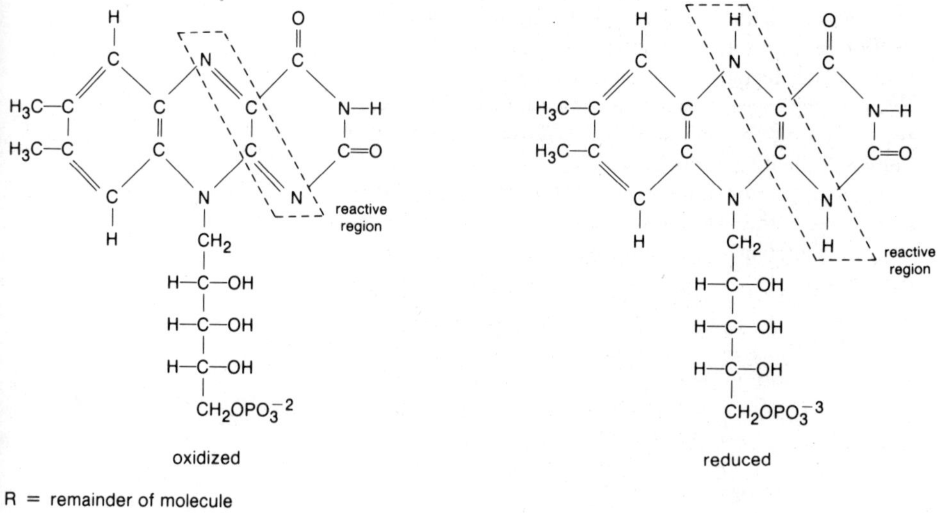

R = remainder of molecule

Oxidized and reduced forms of FMN

In the oxidation/reduction reactions by which the energy
nutrients are oxidized, FAD, like NAD^+, is a two-hydrogen
carrier but, unlike NAD^+, FAD accepts both hydrogens
given up by the substrates and becomes $FADH_2$. The original donors of the hydrogens are GLUCOSE, FATTY ACIDS, GLYC-
EROL, and AMINO ACIDS which derive from the digestion of

carbohydrate, fat, and protein foods. The ultimate acceptor molecule is oxygen. However, the transfer of hydrogens (and their electrons) from original donor to ultimate acceptor is accomplished by successive, small, oxidative and reductive steps using carrier molecules such as the flavin coenzymes.

FAD and FMN participate in oxidations and reductions by first being tightly bound to an enzyme (E^1) that has a specific task to perform. The substrate (S^1—H—H) enters the active site of the enzyme and forms a substrate-enzyme complex. Within the substrate-enyzme complex, hydrogens are removed from the substrate and picked up by FAD. This removal of two hydrogens from the substrate causes the bonds within the substrate to shift so that a new substance (S) is formed. The new substance is then separated from the complex. Succeeding reactions will separate the enzyme from its coenzyme and contribute the hydrogens to a carrier molecule in the RESPIRATORY CHAIN. The enzyme and FAD are then prepared to participate in another reaction.

a. $E^1 + FAD \rightarrow E^1{-}FAD$

b. $S^1\big\langle{\,^H_H} + E^1{-}FAD \rightarrow S^1{-}H_2{-}E^1{-}FAD$

c. $S^1{-}H_2{-}E^1{-}FAD \rightarrow S{-}E^1{-}FADH_2$

d. $S{-}E^1{-}FADH_2 \rightarrow S + E^1{-}FADH_2$

These structural alterations by enzyme-FAD combinations are found in a variety of important reactions in the reclaiming of energy from the bonds of fuel nutrients, as in the following five illustrations.

In the TCA CYCLE, FAD joins with the enzyme *succinate dehydrogenase* to alter succinate so that it becomes fumarate.

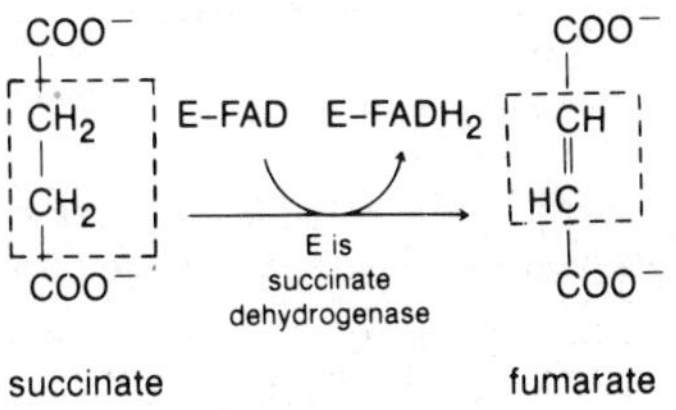

The conversion of succinate to
fumarate in the TCA cycle

Note that fumarate has a carbon-carbon double bond in the place where succinate had a carbon-carbon single bond.

In the first step of FATTY ACID OXIDATION, FAD joins with *acyl-CoA dehydrogenases,* which act on fatty acids of different lengths, to remove two hydrogens from carbons #2 and #3, an action that will lead to a fatty acid two carbons shorter. As in the synthesis of fumarate, the removal of two hydrogens has produced a double bond where there had been a single bond.

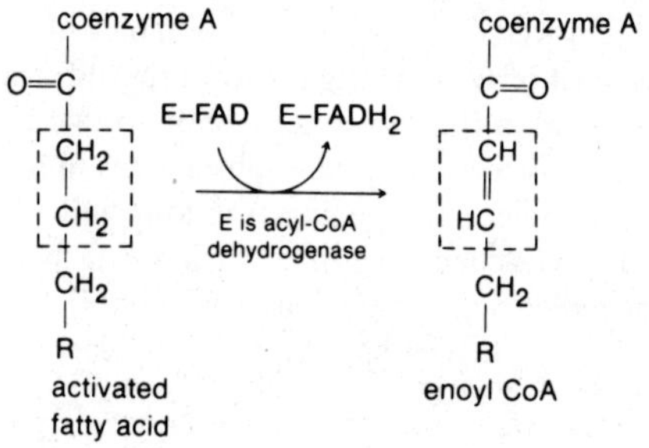

Removal of hydrogens during
fatty acid oxidation

In a pathway necessary to the continuation of glycolysis—the GLYCEROL PHOSPHATE SHUTTLE—FAD links with a mitochondrial enzyme *glycerol dehydrogenase* to produce dihydroxyacetone phosphate. The enzyme-FAD removes two hydrogens and forms a double bond to oxygen to produce a molecule (dihydroxyacetone phosphate) that is able to migrate out of the mitochondria.

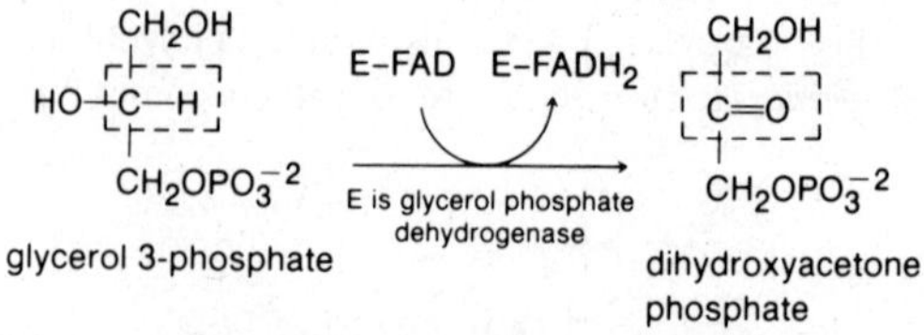

The glycerol phosphate shuttle conversion of glycerol
3-phosphate to dihydroxyacetone phosphate

In the first step of releasing methyl groups from dietary CHOLINE for the building of biomolecules, FAD joins with the enzyme *choline dehydrogenase* to produce betaine aldehyde.

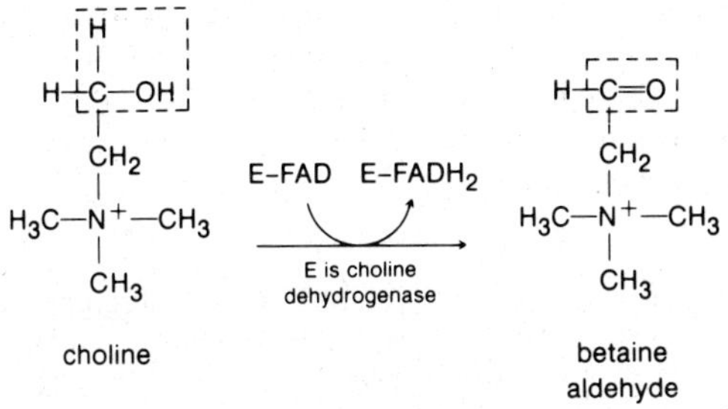

The conversion of choline to
betaine aldehyde

In the pyruvate dehydrogenase complex that converts pyruvate to acetyl-CoA, FAD joins with the enzyme *dihydrolipoyl dehydrogenase* to regenerate lipoic acid so that more pyruvate can be converted to acetyl-CoA. In this action, the removal of two hydrogens creates a sulfur-sulfur bond.

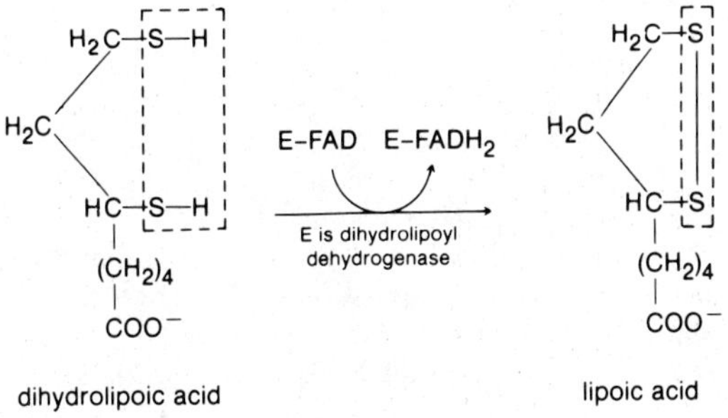

The regeneration of lipoic acid

After release of the new substance formed by the action of an enzyme-FAD combination on a substrate, the enzyme will be "set free" from its coenzyme. Also, the coenzyme will donate its hydrogens to acceptor molecules such as iron-sulfur proteins, coenzyme Q, or, in one case, another coenzyme, NAD^+. The transfer of the hydrogens to acceptor molecules sets off the complex series of events of the respiratory chain in which the final acceptor molecule is oxygen. Each $FADH_2$ generates 2 ATP after passage through the respiratory chain. See also: TCA CYCLE; RESPIRATORY CHAIN.

Fanconi's syndrome. A recessive, inherited disease associated with cystinosis. The syndrome is characterized by abnormalities of renal proximal tubular function and includes glycosuria, phosphaturia, aminoaciduria, and bicarbonate wasting.

SUGGESTED READINGS

Morris, R. C., and A. Sebastian. 1983. Renal tubular acidosis and Fanconi syndrome. In *The metabolic basis of inherited disease*, 5th ed., ed. J. B. Stanbury et al., 1808–1844. New York: McGraw-Hill.

fat. See LIPIDS.

fat-soluble vitamins. Vitamins A, D, E, and K are brought into the body mostly in fat-rich foods. Additionally, VITAMIN D can be made by the action of ultra violet light on 7-dehydrocholesterol in the skin. Excess intake is stored in fatty tissues and the liver. Vitamins A and D can reach toxic levels. See also: VITAMIN A; VITAMIN D; VITAMIN E; VITAMIN K.

fatty acid nomenclature. The naming of FATTY ACIDS is based on the name of the hydrocarbon in the alkane series from which a particular fatty acid is derived. Alkanes are given the Latin name for the total number of carbons in the longest straight chain. Exceptions to this convention include the 1- to 4-carbon alkanes whose common names are too firmly established to change. The final "e" on the hydrocarbon's name is replaced with "oic" to denote the saturated fatty acid form. Thus saturated fatty acid names end in "anoic." If there is one double bond in the chain, the unsaturated fatty acid's name ends in "enoic;" if there are two double bonds, the fatty acid's name ends in "dienoic."

Notational systems have been devised to designate the number of carbon atoms and the location of double bonds within the fatty acid chain. In one such system, for example,

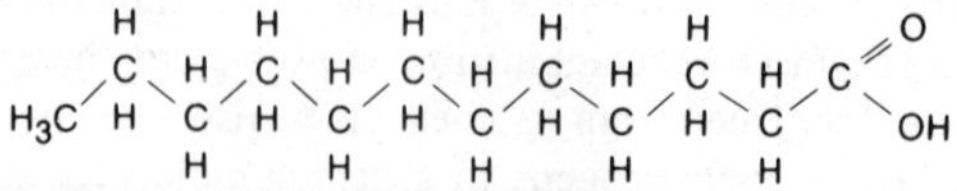

Dodecanoic acids (lauric acid),
a saturated fatty acid, $C_{12}H_{24}O_2$

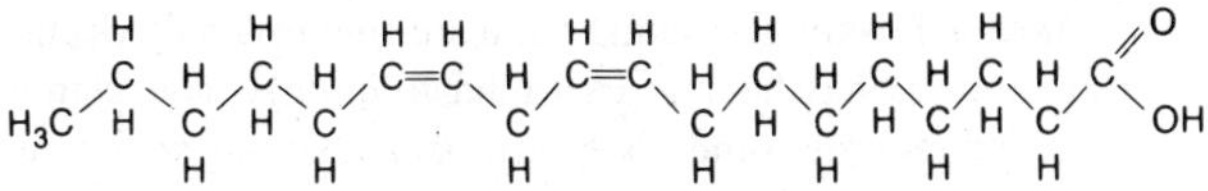

Octadecadieonic acid (linoleic acid),
an unsaturated fatty acid, $C_{18}H_{32}O_2$

beginning with the carboxyl carbon as carbon 1, if the fatty acid has 18 carbons and no double bonds (stearic acid), the notation is 18:0. If another 18-carbon fatty acid has one double bond between carbons 9 and 10 (oleic acid), the notation is 18:1;9. The notation for linoleic acid, an 18-carbon chain with two double bonds between carbons 9 and 10 and between carbons 12 and 13, is 18:2;9,12. When special significance is placed on the configuration about the double bond, cis or trans is designated in the notation.

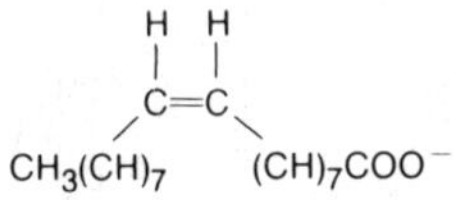

18:1;9 or 18:1ω9
Octadecanoic acid (oleic acid or oleate)

In another system of notation, the omega (ω) system, the methyl carbon (ω carbon) is carbon 1 and the position of the double bond nearest the methyl end is noted. Thus, linolenic acid would be noted as 18:3ω3. The chemist would recognize that there are three repeats of the structure —CH=CH—CH— and that the other double bonds are at carbon 6 and carbon 9. Linoleic acid is shown below under the two systems of notation.

$$\overset{18}{C}H_3(CH_2)_4\overset{13}{C}H=\overset{12}{C}HCH_2\overset{10}{C}H=\overset{9}{C}H(CH_2)_7\overset{1}{C}OO^-$$

18:2;9,12

$$\overset{\omega}{C}H_3\overset{2}{C}H_2\overset{3}{C}H_2\overset{4}{C}H_2\overset{5}{C}H_2\overset{6}{C}H=CHCH_2\overset{9}{C}H=CH(CH_2)_7COO^-$$

18:2ω6

Linoleic acid

Included in the following table are five naturally occurring unsaturated fatty acids found in animals and plants, with their common and systematic names, structural formulas, and notational symbols.

SOME NATURALLY OCCURRING UNSATURATED FATTY ACIDS

Common name	palmitoleic	oleic	linoleic	linolenic	arachidonic
Systematic name	Δ^9-hexa-decanoic	Δ^9-octa-decanoic	$\Delta^{9,12}$-octa-decadienoic	$\Delta^{9,12,15}$-octa-decatrienoic	$\Delta^{5,8,11,14}$-eicosa-tetraenoic
Symbol ω Series	16:1;9 16:1ω7	18:1;9 18:1ω9	18:2;9,12 18:2ω6	18:3;9,12,15 18:3ω3	20:4;5,8,11,14 20:4ω6

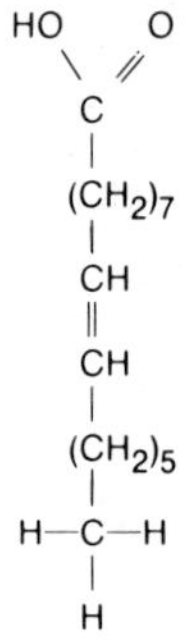

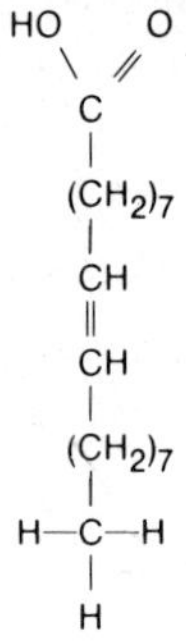

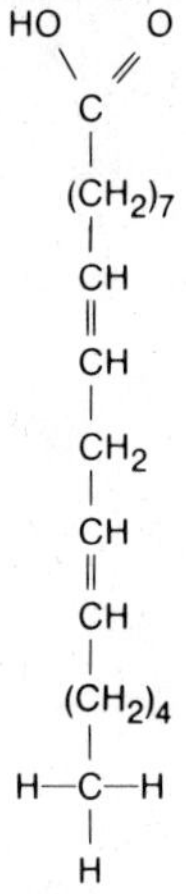

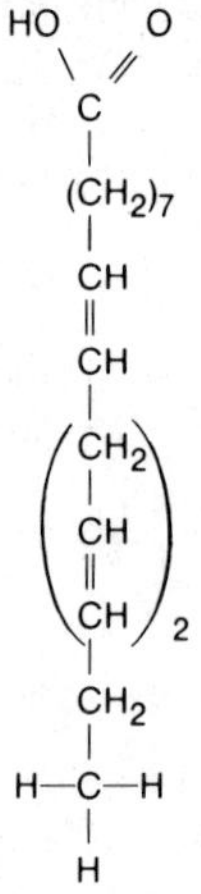

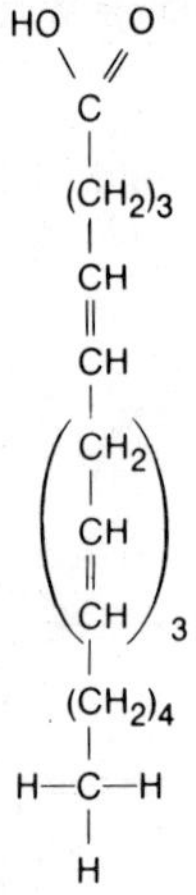

palmitoleic:
$$HO\!-\!C(\!=\!O)\!-\!(CH_2)_7\!-\!CH\!=\!CH\!-\!(CH_2)_5\!-\!CH_2\!-\!CH_3$$

oleic:
$$HO\!-\!C(\!=\!O)\!-\!(CH_2)_7\!-\!CH\!=\!CH\!-\!(CH_2)_7\!-\!CH_2\!-\!CH_3$$

linoleic:
$$HO\!-\!C(\!=\!O)\!-\!(CH_2)_7\!-\!CH\!=\!CH\!-\!CH_2\!-\!CH\!=\!CH\!-\!(CH_2)_4\!-\!CH_2\!-\!CH_3$$

linolenic:
$$HO\!-\!C(\!=\!O)\!-\!(CH_2)_7\!-\!CH\!=\!CH\!-\!(CH_2\!-\!CH\!=\!CH)_2\!-\!CH_2\!-\!CH_2\!-\!CH_3$$

arachidonic:
$$HO\!-\!C(\!=\!O)\!-\!(CH_2)_3\!-\!CH\!=\!CH\!-\!(CH_2\!-\!CH\!=\!CH)_3\!-\!(CH_2)_4\!-\!CH_2\!-\!CH_3$$

Examples of some saturated fatty acids are noted in the following table. See also: CIS, TRANS BONDS; FATTY ACIDS.

Examples of Some Saturated Fatty Acids

Common name	Systematic name	Number of carton atoms
butyric acid	tetranoic acid	4
caproic acid	hexanoic acid	6
caprylic acid	octanoic acid	8
capric acid	decanoic acid	10
lauric acid	dodecanoic acid	12
myristic acid	tetradecanoic acid	14
palmitic acid	hexadecanoic acid	16
stearic acid	octadecanoic acid	18
arachidic acid	eicosanoic acid	20

fatty acid oxidation. The degradation of a fatty acid. This process yields more Calories per gram, and thus more energy (ATP) than carbohydrate or protein oxidation. The more hydrogen atoms contained in a fuel nutrient, the more ATP will be produced per molecule oxidized. For example, one molecule of glucose with 12 hydrogen atoms yields 38 ATP while one molecule of palmitic acid with 32 hydrogen atoms yields 129 ATP.

Oxidation of FATTY ACIDS occurs in the mitochondria in three stages. In stage one, which takes place on the outer mitochondrial membrane, fatty acid activation is accomplished by joining COENZYME A at its sulfur atom to the carboxyl carbon of the fatty acid, a reaction that converts 1 ATP to AMP and PP_i (pyrophosphate).

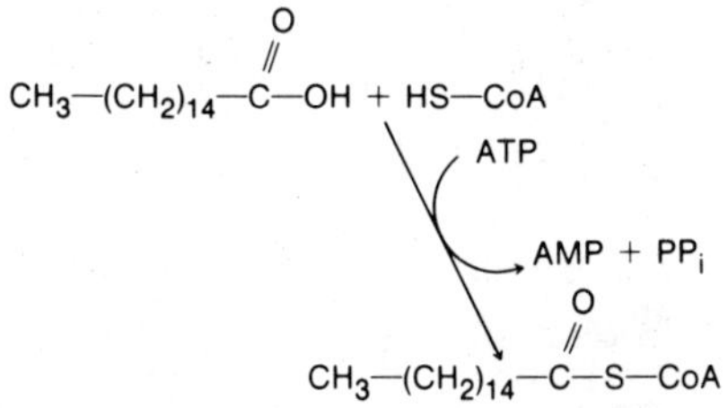

$$CH_3\!-\!(CH_2)_{14}\!-\!\overset{\overset{\textstyle O}{\|}}{C}\!-\!OH \;+\; HS\!-\!CoA$$

ATP

AMP + PP_i

$$CH_3\!-\!(CH_2)_{14}\!-\!\overset{\overset{\textstyle O}{\|}}{C}\!-\!S\!-\!CoA$$

Fatty acid oxidation, stage one: activation of palmitic acid

In stage two, which takes place in the mitochondrial matrix, after transport of long-chain fatty acids across the mitochondrial membrane by carnitine, two-carbon increments are removed from the hydrocarbon chain by beta oxidation. This series of reactions is known as "beta oxidation" because the β carbon, carbon 3, is the most highly oxidized during the oxidations and reductions of the series. In this process, when coenzyme A joins the carboxyl carbon at the end of the chain, the bond between the α and β carbons is weakened, and ACETYL-COA splits off, leaving behind an activated fatty acid that is two carbons shorter.

Because the shorter fatty acid that remains is activated, it returns to the first step of beta oxidation, saving the expenditure of another ATP for activation. The hydrogens that are released are picked up by FAD and NAD^+ forming $FADH_2$ and NADH, while one hydrogen ion is released to the surrounding fluid. $FADH_2$ yields 2 ATP and NADH yields 3 ATP when these molecules unload their hydrogens onto the carriers of the RESPIRATORY CHAIN—each repetition

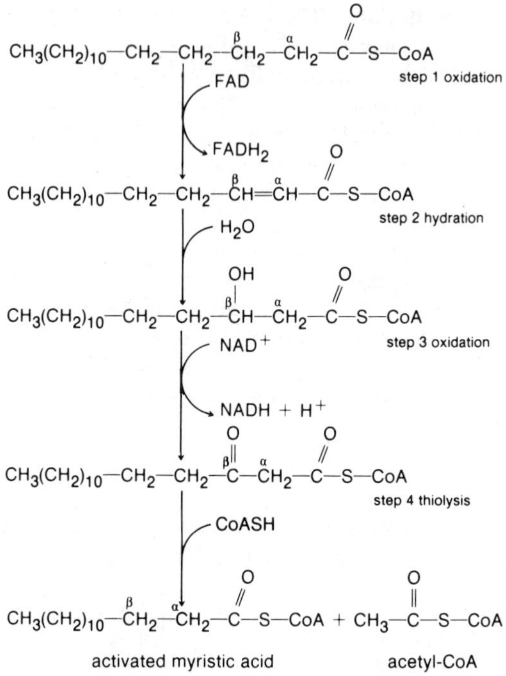

Fatty acid oxidation, stage two: β-oxidation of palmitic acid (16:0) to myristic acid (14:0)

thus yields 5 ATP. Palmitic acid, with its 16 carbons, will undergo 7 rounds for total production of 35 ATP and 8 acetyl-CoAs.

In stage three, each acetyl-CoA that is split off enters the TCA CYCLE in the same manner as acetyl-CoA from any other fuel nutrient. When the 8 acetyl-CoAs go through the TCA cycle and the respiratory chain, they will yield 12 ATP for each turn for a total of 96 molecules of ATP. Thus the total yield from the oxidation of one molecule of palmitic acid is 96 plus 35, or 131 ATP. The net yield, after subtracting for the 2 high-energy phosphate bonds used in the activation step, is 129 ATP.

If entry into the TCA cycle is blocked due to a high level of ATP, then the acetyl-CoAs from the breakdown of dietary fat will go into LIPID synthesis in the same way as acetyl-CoA produced from excess carbohydrate or protein foods. If the TCA cycle carbohydrate intermediates are not maintained, the acetyl-CoAs may be converted into KETONE BODIES, which may be used for energy by the peripheral tissues, or, if they are overproduced, KETOSIS may result.

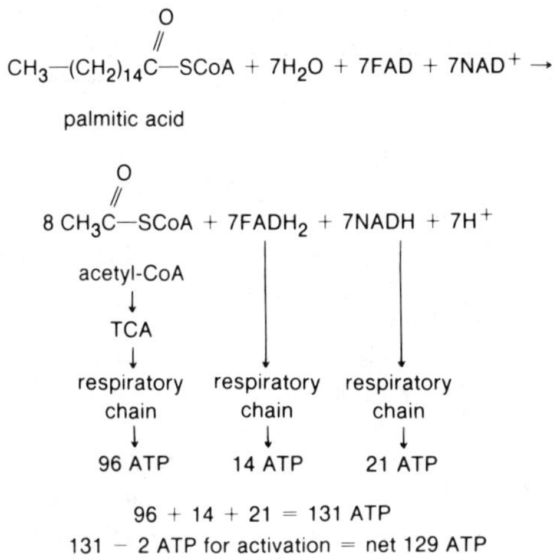

$$CH_3-(CH_2)_{14}C\overset{\overset{\displaystyle O}{\|}}{}-SCoA + 7H_2O + 7FAD + 7NAD^+ \rightarrow$$

palmitic acid

$$8\ CH_3C\overset{\overset{\displaystyle O}{\|}}{}-SCoA + 7FADH_2 + 7NADH + 7H^+$$

acetyl-CoA
↓
TCA
↓
respiratory   respiratory   respiratory
chain   chain   chain
↓   ↓   ↓
96 ATP   14 ATP   21 ATP

96 + 14 + 21 = 131 ATP
131 − 2 ATP for activation = net 129 ATP

Production of 129 ATP from oxidation of one molecule of palmitic acid (16:0)

The oxidation of unsaturated fatty acids is basically identical to that described above for the saturated fatty acids. In this case, the cis double bond is converted to a trans double bond by an isomerase, yielding the D-isomer of 3-hydroxy-acyl-CoA, which must be inverted by an epimerase. Oxidation then continues as for saturated fatty acids.

The oxidation of the odd-numbered fatty acids is similar to that of the even-numbered fatty acids except that in the final round, one molecule each of propionyl-CoA and acetyl-CoA are produced instead of two molecules of acetyl-CoA. Propionyl-CoA is converted to succinyl-CoA in several steps. One step from propionyl-CoA to D-methylmalonyl-CoA requires the vitamin BIOTIN, and another step from L-methylmalonyl-CoA to succinyl-CoA requires VITAMIN B_{12}. Acetyl-CoA and succinyl-CoA then can enter the TCA cycle.

SUGGESTED READINGS

Jones, P. J. H., P. B. Pencharz, and M. T. Clandinin. 1985. Whole body oxidation of dietary fatty acids: Implications for energy utilization. *Am. J. Clin. Nutr.* 42:769–777.

McGarry, J. D., and D. W. Foster. 1980. Regulation of hepatic fatty acid oxidation and ketone body production. *Ann. Rev. Biochem.* 49:395–420.

fatty acids. Highly concentrated energy nutrients that are stored in the body mostly as TRIACYLGLYCEROLS (also called triglycerides). Fatty acids are also building blocks of phospholipids and glycolipids. Structurally, fatty acids occur as either saturated or unsaturated hydrocarbon chains of variable length with a carboxyl group at one end.

Saturated fatty acids are so called because hydrogen fills (or saturates) all the remaining bonds on the singly bonded internal carbons. In unsaturated fatty acids, there are at least two carbons sharing a double bond, therefore each can hold only one hydrogen. Monounsaturated fatty acids have only one double bond whereas polyunsaturated fatty acids have several double bonds along the chain of carbons. The configuration about the double bonds in naturally occurring unsaturated fatty acids is CIS.

The degree of saturation has an effect on the fluidity of the fatty acids: the more saturated a fatty acid, the more firm it will be at a particular temperature. This difference is due to the rotation that is possible around a single bond. Since all the bonds in a saturated fatty acid are single, the chain is highly flexible and the molecules can pack closely together. Because there is no rotation about the double bond of an unsaturated fatty acid, a rigid kink in the chain at the double bond, makes it difficult for these molecules to fit into a compact space. Oils such as safflower or corn oil contain a predominance of polyunsaturated fatty acids. Hard fats such as suet or lard contain a predominance of saturated fatty acids.

Most fatty acids have an even number of carbon atoms, between 14 and 22, with the most common having 16 or 18 carbon atoms. Examples include palmitic acid with 16 carbons and oleic acid with 18 carbons. Fatty acids with odd-numbered chains are most abundant in marine animals. See also: CIS-, TRANS-BONDS; ESSENTIAL FATTY ACIDS; FATTY ACID NOMENCLATURE; FATTY ACID OXIDATION; FATTY ACID SYNTHESIS; LIPIDS; TRIACYLGLYCEROLS.

fatty acid synthesis. Occurs in the cytosol from excess ACETYL-CoA, the degradative product from the oxidation of the fuel nutrients. ACETYL-CoA is successively attached in two carbon increments until the long fatty acid chain is completed.

The first order of business for fatty acid synthesis is to get acetyl-CoA out of the mitochondria where it was synthesized and into the cytosol. To accomplish this, acetyl-CoA bonds to oxaloacetate to form citric acid (the first step of the TCA CYCLE). Citric acid is able to leave the mitochondria. Once citric acid is in the cytosol, it can be cleaved by an ATP-dependent enzyme to acetyl-CoA and oxaloacetate. NADPH, generated from the PENTOSE PHOSPHATE PATHWAY, is the reducing agent. Now, fatty acid synthesis can begin; acetyl-CoA is in the cytosol and the reducing power of NADPH is present.

The ENZYMES of synthesis are organized in the fatty acid synthetase complex so that transfer from the active site of one enzyme to the active site of the next is accomplished in an orderly fashion. The first, and the committed, step of fatty acid synthesis is the carboxylation of acetyl-CoA to malonyl-CoA by *acetyl-CoA carboxylase,* a BIOTIN-dependent enzyme. The energy for the carboxylation of acetyl-CoA is obtained from the hydrolysis of ATP to ADP and P_i. The reaction is stimulated by the presence of citrate and inhibited by the presence of the end product, palmitoyl-CoA.

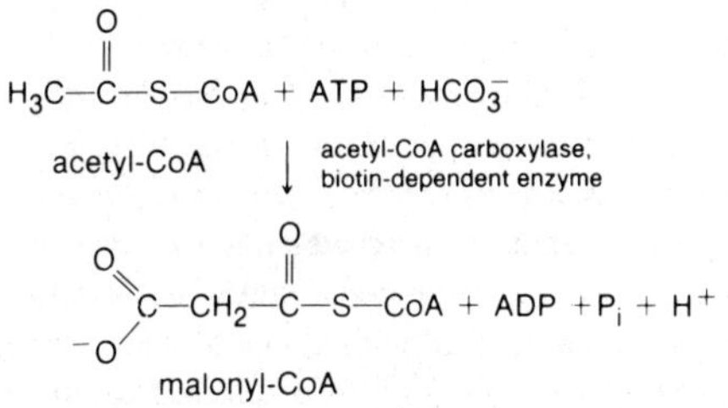

$$H_3C-\overset{\overset{\textstyle O}{\|}}{C}-S-CoA \ + \ ATP \ + \ HCO_3^-$$

acetyl-CoA $\qquad$ acetyl-CoA carboxylase, biotin-dependent enzyme

$$\overset{O}{\underset{-O}{\diagup}}\!\!\diagdown C-CH_2-\overset{\overset{\textstyle O}{\|}}{C}-S-CoA \ + \ ADP \ +P_i \ + \ H^+$$

malonyl-CoA

The conversion of acetyl-CoA to malonyl-CoA

The intermediates of the fatty acid synthesis complex are bound to the sulfhydryl end unit on acyl carrier protein (ACP). Once bound, the acetyl-ACP joins with malonyl-ACP to produce acetoacetyl-ACP, releasing one ACP and CO_2.

$$\text{acetyl-ACP + malonyl-ACP} \xrightarrow{\overset{\text{acyl-malonyl-ACP}}{\text{condensing enzyme}}}$$

$$\text{acetoacetyl-ACP + ACP + CO}_2 \uparrow$$

The production of acetoacetyl-ACP

With each additional round, a malonyl-CoA is formed from the carboxylation of acetyl-CoA in which an ATP is used. In the condensation step, two carbons from the malonyl are used and one goes off as carbon dioxide. Reduction by NADPH is followed by a dehydration and another reduction to complete the addition of two carbons to the chain. This will continue only until palmitoyl-ACP is formed. Palmitoyl-ACP cannot act as the substrate for the condensing enzyme and so is hydrolyzed to ACP and palmitate. For the synthesis of the longer fatty acids and insertion of a double bond between carbons 9 and 10, specific enzymes in the endoplasmic reticulum are needed.

The synthesis of unsaturated fatty acids with double bonds beyond carbon #9 does not take place in humans, only in plants. Therefore, linoleic and linolenic (18:2;9,12 and 18:3;9,12,15) fatty acids are essential nutrients for humans; that is, they must be included in the diet. From these ESSENTIAL FATTY ACIDS a variety of other unsaturated fatty acids as well as PROSTAGLANDINS can be synthesized.

Fatty acid synthesis is not the reverse of FATTY ACID OXIDATION. Synthesis occurs in the cytoplasm of the cell whereas oxidation occurs in the mitochondria. The compartmentalization of these two processes allows the cell to degrade fatty acids to acetyl-CoA for fuel at the same time that it is using excess acetyl-CoAs to make fatty acids. Another difference between the synthesis and oxidation of fatty acids is the use of entirely distinct enzyme systems. Also, the enzymes of synthesis are organized into a complex while those of oxidation are not. Through these safeguards, the two processes do not become an unproductive (futile) cycle. See also: BIOTIN, THE COENZYME.

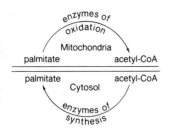

A futile cycle is prevented by compartmentalization and two distinct sets of enzymes

SUGGESTED READINGS

Wakil, S. J., J. K. Stoops, and V. C. Joshi. 1983. Fatty acid synthesis and its regulation. *Ann. Rev. Biochem.* 52:537–579.

favism. A hereditary condition common to persons native to the Mediterranean area resulting in a sensitivity to a species of beans, *Vicia faba.* This condition is aggravated by ingestion of the bean or inhalation of pollen of the plant. Affected persons have an inherited deficiency of the enzyme *glucose 6-phosphate dehydrogenase.* Such persons show similar sensitivity to some drugs. Causative agents in afflicted individuals promote oxidation of erythrocytic glutathione, resulting in hemolytic anemia, vomiting, diarrhea, and may lead to coma.

fiber. Polysaccharides for which humans do not have digestive enzymes; thus fiber contributes no calories to the human diet. Fiber includes cellulose, hemicellulose, pectic substances, gums, and mucilages. Lignin, a nonpolysaccharide, is sometimes included. Fiber is found in fruits, vegetables, whole grains, and legumes.

Hemicellulose has a high water-holding capacity that increases stool bulk. Some of the gel-forming and mucilagenous substances have been shown to reduce serum

CHOLESTEROL by decreasing the absorption of fat and cholesterol. Ingestion of large amounts of dietary fiber may reduce
the absorption of CALCIUM and other divalent metals, forming an insoluble complex.   See also: CARBOHYDRATE STRUC-
TURE; CALCIUM; CHOLESTEROL.

SUGGESTED READINGS

Bell, E. W., et al. 1981. Effects of dietary fiber from wheat,
  corn, and soy hull bran on excretion of fecal bile acids in
  humans. *Am. J. Clin. Nutr.* 34:1071–1076.

Bolton, R. P., K. W. Heaton, and L. F. Burroughs. 1981.
  The role of dietary fiber in satiety, glucose, and insulin:
  Studies with fruit and fruit juice. *Am. J. Clin.
  Nutr.*34:211–217.

Eastwood, M. 1984. Dietary fiber. In *Present knowledge in
  nutrition,* 5th ed., 156–175. Washington, D.C.: The Nutrition Foundation, Inc.

Englyst, H. N., and J. H. Cummings. 1985. Digestion of the
  polysaccharides of some cereal foods in the human small
  intestine. *Am. J. Clin. Nutr.* 42:778–787.

Hillman, L. C., et al. 1985. The effect of the fiber components pectin, cellulose and lignin on serum cholesterol
  levels. *Am. J. Clin. Nutr.* 42:207–213.

Holloway, W. D., C. Tasman-Jones, and K. Maher. 1983.
  Pectin digestion in humans. *Am. J. Clin. Nutr.*
  31:253–255.

Kay, R. M. 1982. Dietary fiber, *J. Lipid Res.* 23:221–242.

Leigh, M. J., and D. D. Miller. 1983. Effects of pH and chelating agents on iron binding by dietary fiber: Implications for iron availability. *Am. J. Clin. Nutr.*
  38:202–213.

Levine, R. A. 1981. An overview of fiber and gastrointestinal disease. In *Nutrition in gastrointestinal disease,* ed. R.
  C. Kurz, 1–16. New York: Churchill Livingstone.

Reinhold, J. G. 1975. Phytate destruction by yeast fermentation in whole wheat meals. *J. Am. Diet. Assoc.*
  66:38–41.

Schwartz, R., B. J. Apgar, and E. M. Wien. 1986. Apparent
  absorption and retention of Ca, Cu, Mg, Mn, and Zn
  from a diet containing bran. *Am. J. Clin. Nutr.*
  43:444–455.

Story, J. A. 1981. The role of dietary fiber in lipid metabolism. *Adv. Lipid Res.* 18:229–246.

fibrin.   A protein synthesized from fibrinogen by the action
of thrombin and required for bloodclotting.   See also: VITA-
MIN K.

fibrinogen.   A blood protein used to synthesize fibrin, a
protein necessary for bloodclotting.   See also: VITAMIN K.

flavin adenine dinucleotide (FAD). One of the coenzyme forms of RIBOFLAVIN. See also: FAD, FMN.

flavin coenzymes. See FAD, FMN.

flavin mononucleotide (FMN). One of the coenzyme forms of RIBOFLAVIN. See also: FAD, FMN.

flavoprotein. A protein that contains the riboflavin-dependent coenzyme FMN or FAD as its prosthetic group. See also: FAD, FMN.

fluoride (F⁻). The ionized form of a mineral that is primarily involved in mineralization of bone and teeth. Its presence in the hydroxyapatite crystal of bone and teeth hardens the crystal. Thus, fluoride is helpful in resistance to tooth decay, and to this end it is often added to municipal drinking water. Fluoride is important, also, in preventing the loss of bone mass.

Fluoride is widely dispersed in foods, but its bioavailability from various foods is still under investigation. Absorption of fluorides is rapid, and excretion is by the urine. In body fluids, it is normally maintained at relatively low levels by skeletal uptake and renal excretion. In the plasma, both ionic and nonionic fluoride is found. Fluoride salts are inhibitors of *enolase*, the enzyme that catalyzes the glycolytic step that produces phosphoenolpyruvate.

SUGGESTED READINGS

Ophaug, R. H., and L. Singer. 1977. Influence of variations in fluoride intake on the ionic and bound fractions of plasma and muscle fluoride. Proc. Soc. Exp. Biol. Med. 155:23–26.

Schamschula, R. G., and D. E. Barmes. 1981. Fluoride and health: Dental caries, osteoporosis and cardiovascular disease. *Ann. Rev. Nutr.* 1:427–436.

Singer, L., R. H. Ophaug, and B. F. Harland. 1980. Fluoride intake of young male adults in the United States. *Am. J. Clin. Nutr.* 33:328–332.

Spencer, H., et al. 1970. Fluoride metabolism in man. *Am. J. Med.* 49:807–813.

FMN. See FAD, FMN.

folacin (folate, folic acid, PGA, pteroylglutamic acid). A B-vitamin that is required for the formation of red blood cells. It is so named because it is found in leafy green vegetables; it is also present in yeast and liver. Structurally, it consists of a pteridine double ring combined with PABA (para-amino benzoic acid) and glutamate.

Most folates occur naturally as polyglutamates whereby additional glutamate residues are bound by peptide linkages

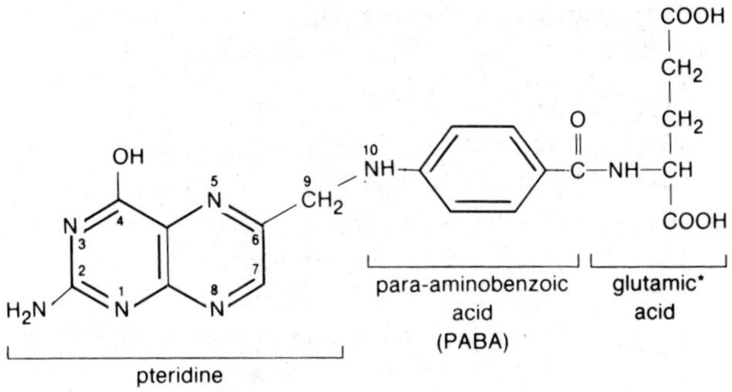

Folacin (pteroylmonoglutamic acid)

(the number of glutamic acids *
may vary from one to eight)

to the gamma carboxyl group of the glutamate. Dietary folacin, as polyglutamate, is hydrolyzed by intestinal conjugases which remove the extra glutamate residues. Folacin as a monoglutamate is then absorbed in the small intestine.

Folacin's biologically active form is tetrahydrofolic acid (FH_4). The conversion into this form requires VITAMIN C and NIACIN and is dependent on VITAMIN B_6 to effect molecular rearrangements that make it suitable for some metabolic purposes.

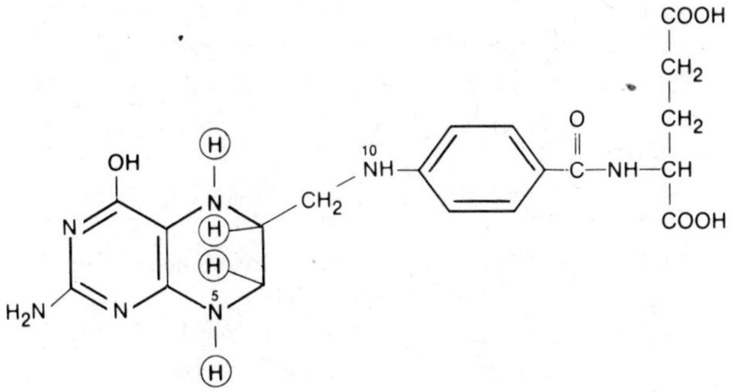

Tetrahydrofolate (FH_4)

The four circled hydrogens are added to folacin when it is reduced to its metabolically active form.

The reactive part of the tetrahydrofolate molecule occurs in the pteridine portion at nitrogens 5 and 10. These nitrogens can receive and transfer carbon units of varying oxidation states. The least oxidized one-carbon unit carried by

methyl	$-CH_3$	least oxidized
methylene	$-\overset{\displaystyle H}{\underset{\displaystyle H}{C}}-$	more oxidized
methenyl	$-C=$	
formyl	$-\overset{}{\underset{\displaystyle O}{C}}-H$	most oxidized
formimino	$-\overset{}{\underset{\displaystyle NH}{C}}-H$	
carbon dioxide	CO_2	

Carbon units carried by folacin

FH_4 is the methyl group, the next most oxidized group is the methylene group, and the most oxidized include the formyl, formimino, and methenyl groups, as well as the compound, carbon dioxide.

Tetrahydrofolate plays a vital role in many biochemical processes due to its ability to accept and release different oxidative states of one-carbon units. For example, METHIONINE is synthesized from homocysteine by the transfer of a methyl group by FH_4 with the help of the vitamin B_6 coenzyme. Purines, a class of base present in DNA, receive some of their carbons from FH_4; another DNA base, thymine, a pyrimidine, receives a methyl group from FH_4. Tetrahydrofolate can also receive one-carbon units as it does in the breakdown of SERINE and HISTIDINE.

Folacin was discovered while scientists were searching for a cure for pernicious anemia, a VITAMIN B_{12}-deficiency disease. They found that vegetables, liver, and yeast relieved some of the symptoms but did nothing to stop the progression of damage to the myelin sheaths of nerves. Today it is known that a high folacin intake coupled with a total absence of animal foods, which would supply vitamin B_{12}, puts the person at risk for the eventual development of undetected megaloblastic anemia. See also: CHOLINE, GLYCINE, SERINE, HISTIDINE, for reactions involving folacin; METHIONINE; PURINE, PYRIMIDINE BASES; VITAMIN B_{12}.

SUGGESTED READINGS

Babu, S., and S. G. Skrikantia. 1976. Availability of folates from some foods. *Am. J. Clin. Nutr.* 29:376–379.

Benkovic, S. J. 1980. On the mechanism of action of folate and biopterin-requiring enzymes. *Am. Rev. Biochem.* 49:227–251.

Colman, N., and V. Herbert. 1980. Folate binding proteins. *Ann. Rev. Med.* 31:433–439.

Erbe, R. W. 1975. Inborn errors of folate metabolism. Part 1. *N. Engl. J. Med.* 293:753–757.

Ghishan, F. K., et al. 1986. Intestinal transport of zinc and folic acid: A mutual inhibitory effect. *Am. J. Clin. Nutr.* 43:258–262.

Lindenbaum, J. 1983. Drug-induced folate deficiency and the hematologic effects of alcohol. In *Nutrition and hematology*, ed. J. Lindenbaum, 33–58. New York: Churchill Livingstone.

Milne, D. B., et al. 1984. Effect of oral folic acid supplements on zinc, copper and iron absorption and excretion. *Am. J. Clin. Nutr.* 39:535–539.

Olinger, E. J., J. R. Bertino, and H. J. Binder. 1973. Intestinal folate absorption. II. Conversion and retention of pteroylmonoglutamate by jejunum. *J. Clin. Invest.* 52:2138–2145.

Rosenberg, I. H. 1975. Folate absorption and malabsorption. *N. Engl. J. Med.* 293:1303–1308.

Shane, B., and E. L. R. Stokstad. 1985. Vitamin B_{12}-folate interrelationships. *Ann. Rev. Nutr.* 5:115–141.

Weir, D. G., and J. M. Scott. 1983. Interrelationships of folates and cobalamins. In *Nutrition and hematology*, ed. J. Lindenbaum, 121–142. New York: Churchill Livingstone.

folate.   See FOLACIN.

folic acid.   See FOLACIN.

free energy.   The energy that is available to perform work as a biochemical system proceeds toward equilibrium. A process will occur spontaneously in nature only if its standard free energy change ($\Delta G°'$) is less than zero.   See also: ENERGETICS.

fructose.   A monosaccharide found principally in fruits. It is metabolized in the body by *hexokinase* to form fructose 6-phosphate or by *fructokinase* to form fructose 1-phosphate. The latter, thought to be the major product of fructose oxidation, is further catabolized by *aldolase B* to glyceraldehyde and dihydroxyacetone phosphate, an intermediate of GLYCOLYSIS. Glyceraldehyde may be converted to glyceraldehyde 3-phosphate, another intermediate in glycolysis, through the action of several ENZYMES.   See also: CARBOHYDRATE STRUCTURE; GLYCOLYSIS.

fumarate.   An intermediate in the TCA CYCLE that connects the TCA and urea cycles.   See also: TCA CYCLE; UREA CYCLE.

g

GABA. See GAMMA AMINOBUTYRATE.

galactose. One of the three principal monosaccharides. When bonded to GLUCOSE, galactose forms the disaccharide lactose, the carbohydrate of milk. Galactose is normally not a large part of the diet unless milk products are the principal source of dietary carbohydrate.

Galactose is readily converted to glucose in the liver where *galactokinase* and ATP phosphorylate it to galactose 1-phosphate. This substance may react with uridine diphosphate glucose (UDP-glucose) to form glucose 1-phosphate and UDP-galactose. Through several steps, UDP-glucose may be converted to glucose. See also: CARBOHYDRATE STRUCTURE.

galactosemia. A metabolic inability, inherited as a recessive trait, to convert galactose to GLUCOSE because of an absence of *galactose 1-phosphate uridyl transferase*. The disease can be detected in utero by amniocentesis. An infant with this condition will fail to thrive within a week after birth.

SUGGESTED READINGS

See suggested readings for INBORN ERRORS OF METABOLISM.

gamma aminobutyrate (γ-aminobutyrate, GABA). A substance produced primarily by decarboxylation of GLUTAMATE by a VITAMIN B_6-dependent enzyme, *glutamate decarboxylase*, in neural tissues. It plays a role as an inhibitory neurotransmitter in quieting the excitability of neurons; in fact, low levels of GABA are associated with convulsions. The synthesis of GABA from glutamate may be viewed as a shunt in the brain whereby the two-step conversion of α-ketoglutarate to succinate via the TCA CYCLE may be bypassed when TCA cycle intermediates are low; then GABA may be catabolized to succinate.

ganglioside. A particular class of glycosphingolipids that are present in the cell membranes of nerve tissue and the spleen.

Gaucher's disease. A familial disorder of lipid metabolism resulting in the accumulation of abnormal glucocerebrosides in the brain and other tissues due to the lack of *glucocerebrosidase* activity. This enzyme normally hydrolyzes glucocerebrosides to GLUCOSE and ceramide.

SUGGESTED READINGS

Brady, R. O., and J. A. Barranger. 1983. Glucosylceramide lipidosis: Gaucher's disease. In *The metabolic basis of inherited disease*, 5th ed., ed. J. B. Stanbury et al., 842–856. New York: McGraw-Hill.

GDP. See GUANOSINE DIPHOSPHATE.

gene. A unit of inheritance. A gene is a segment of a chromosome that carries the information for a single trait, such as eye color, or for a single polypeptide chain, such as the beta chain of hemoglobin. In addition, the gene codes for RNAs and for signal codes that regulate gene activity, such as noting the beginning or the end of transcription.

genetic code. The universal language by which genetic information originating in DNA in the nucleus is carried in the codons of messenger RNA in the cytosol. All the information carried in DNA is expressed in the body through proteins. The code is a set of three nucleotides (a triplet) that is specific for one amino acid. A string of triplets comprises the code for a protein.

As the mystery of genetic information unravelled, it was realized that somehow the four deoxyribonucleotides—deoxyadenylate (A), deoxyguanylate (G), deoxycytidylate (C), and deoxythymidylate (T)—of DNA must form "words" that spell the twenty AMINO ACIDS of protein. Simple arithmetic showed that twenty combinations of letters could not be obtained if one nucleotide coded for only one amino acid. Also, it was obvious that four bases used in groups of two would make only sixteen combinations (4^2); however, four bases combined in groups of three would make sixty-four combinations (4^3). Experimental evidence has shown that, in fact, there are sixty-four triplet combinations, or codons, in the genetic code. The accompanying figure shows all sixty-four codons as they appear in messenger RNAs.

Because of the occurrence of sixty-four codons for the twenty amino acids, most amino acids have more than one codon. Only two amino acids, METHIONINE and TRYPTOPHAN, have one codon, and some have as many as six. An initiating

The Codons in Messenger RNA

Second letter of codons

		U	C	A	G
First letter of codons, 5′ end	**U**	UUU Phe UUC Phe UUA Leu UUG Leu	UCU Ser UCC Ser UCA Ser UCG Ser	UAU Tyr UAC Tyr UAA End UAG End	UGU Cys UGC Cys UGA End UGG Trp
	C	CUU Leu CUC Leu CUA Leu CUG Leu	CCU Pro CCC Pro CCA Pro CCG Pro	CAU His CAC His CAA Gln CAG Gln	CGU Arg CGC Arg CGA Arg CGG Arg
	A	AUU Ile AUC Ile AUA Ile AUG* Met	ACU Thr ACC Thr ACA Thr ACG Thr	AAU Asn AAC Asn AAA Lys AAG Lys	AGU Ser AGC Ser AGA Arg AGG Arg
	G	GUU Val GUC Val GUA Val GUG Val	GCU Ala GCC Ala GCA Ala GCG Ala	GAU Asp GAC Asp GAA Glu GAG Glu	GGU Gly GGC Gly GGA Gly GGG Gly

*AUG is both initiator code and code for methionine.

codon, AUG, also codes for methionine when methionine appears in the interior of a sequence. Three codons, UAA, UAG, and UGA, note when the terminal amino acid (the carboxyl end) on a protein chain has been attached.

When a cell requires a particular protein, a complementary copy of that protein's gene is transcribed into messenger RNA (mRNA). A complementary copy of a portion of a strand of DNA or RNA is one that contains the complementary nucleotide of each nucleotide to be copied. In double-stranded DNA, guanine (G) and cytosine (C) are complements of each other as are thymine (T) and adenine (A). Thus, when G appears in one strand, C appears in the complementary strand and vice versa. When T appears in one strand, A appears opposite on the other strand and vice versa. In RNA, however, thymine is replaced by uracil. Therefore, if adenine were to appear in a DNA segment that is being transcribed into mRNA, uracil, not thymine, would appear in the complementary copy on mRNA; thus adenine is the complement of both uracil and thymine.

Transfer RNA (tRNA) in the cytosol contains a complementary copy of the codon (an anticodon) that is specific for

DNA	T G C
mRNA	A C G
tRNA	U G C

The triplet codes for threonine

one amino acid. It is the function of tRNA to carry the correct amino acid to the mRNA that is attached to the ribosome. At the ribosome the amino acid will be incorporated into the growing protein chain in its proper order. The example at left shows how the codon for THREONINE on DNA would appear on messenger RNA and as the anticodon of transfer RNA.   See also: DNA; NUCLEOSIDES, NUCLEOTIDES; PROTEIN BIOSYNTHESIS; PURINE, PYRIMIDINE BASES; RNA; SICKLE-CELL ANEMIA.

globulin.   A protein in blood plasma that may contain active antibodies against such diseases as measles or diphtheria.

glucagon.   A polypeptide hormone secreted by the α-cells in the pancreas. Glucagon responds to low levels of blood glucose by activating CYCLIC AMP in the liver, thus stimulating GLUCONEOGENESIS and GLYCOGENOLYSIS.

glucogenic amino acids (glycogenic amino acids). Those amino acids whose carbon backbones may be funneled into pyruvate or into the TCA CYCLE at a point where the carbons could be used to rebuild GLUCOSE or GLYCOGEN. Intermediates where the carbons could enter the TCA cycle include α-ketoglutarate, succinyl-CoA, fumarate, and oxaloacetate. The carbons brought in at these points can exit from the cycle in oxaloacetate and proceed through phosphoenolpyruvate to become incorporated into glucose, thus the term "glucogenic." Since excess glucose is converted to glycogen, the term "glycogenic" is also used.

If an amino acid is degraded to ACETYL-CoA or acetoacetyl-CoA, it is classified as a KETOGENIC AMINO ACID. The carbons of these amino acids may be directed to the formation of KETONE BODIES, which cannot be diverted to glucose. It has been generally accepted that carbons of acetoacetate cannot be recovered in glucose, therefore carbons from ketogenic amino acids in humans cannot be converted to glucose. G. F. Cahill (1981), however, showed that this may not be entirely true. He traced the path of carbons from fatty acids through acetoacetate and acetone to glucose and noted that, while this circuitous route may be unimportant in well-fed persons, it may play a crucial role in persons fasting for a prolonged period.

Glucogenic amino acids are vital in maintaining the blood glucose concentration during times when carbohydrate intake is low. During low-carbohydrate dieting, fasting, or STARVATION, body proteins, such as ENZYMES, hormones, antibodies, and muscle tissue, will be disassembled for energy. The glucogenic amino acids released from these proteins will be deaminated and their carbons will be used for synthesizing glucose through the pathway of GLUCONEO-GENESIS.

There is no sharp distinction in the designation of amino acids as glucogenic or ketogenic. Some, notably PHENYLALANINE and TYROSINE, are both. ALANINE, CYSTEINE, and SERINE, which are normally designated as glucogenic, can be degraded to acetyl-CoA, then to acetoacetyl-CoA, and finally to ketone body formation under special circumstances, such as during uncontrolled DIABETES MELLITUS. Generally, the following amino acids are considered glucogenic: alanine ARGININE, ASPARTATE, ASPARAGINE, cysteine, GLUTAMATE, GLUTAMINE, GLYCINE, HISTIDINE, METHIONINE, PROLINE, serine, THREONINE, and VALINE. There is no question about leucine being ketogenic: it is the only amino acid whose carbons lack any possibility of being used to synthesize glucose. Differences of opinion occur, however, regarding the ketogenic properties of other amino acids, such as LYSINE and TRYPTOPHAN. These differences are minor and relate to a judgment of how much glucose or how many ketone bodies are produced by a metabolic path. See also: AMINO ACID DEGRADATION; GLUCONEOGENESIS; KETOGENIC AMINO ACIDS; individual amino acids.

SUGGESTED READINGS

Cahill, G. A. 1981. Jonathon E. Rhoads Lecture. *JPEN* 5(4):281-287.

gluconeogenesis. The synthesis of GLUCOSE from substances such as lactate, some AMINO ACIDS, and glycerol. The gluconeogenic pathway converts pyruvate to glucose. The points of entry into the pathway are pyruvate, oxaloacetate, and dihydroxyacetone phosphate.

Lactate enters the gluconeogenic pathway at pyruvate. Some amino acids enter at pyruvate and oxaloacetate, while others first enter the TCA CYCLE at α-ketoglutarate, succinyl-CoA, or fumarate, are converted to oxaloacetate, and then enter the gluconeogenic pathway. Glycerol enters the pathway at dihydroxyacetone phosphate.

Although many of the individual reactions of gluconeogenesis are reversals of steps in GLYCOLYSIS, the overall path cannot be considered in this way. The situation in glycolysis is analogous to that of a boulder rolling down a hill unaided except for a push to start it. Rolling the boulder uphill, however, is analogous to gluconeogenesis because it requires much effort. The uphill path will by necessity be different from the downhill path because the uphill path chosen should offer the least resistance: it will be erratic, at times reversing the downhill path, but, for the most part, it will seek a new course.

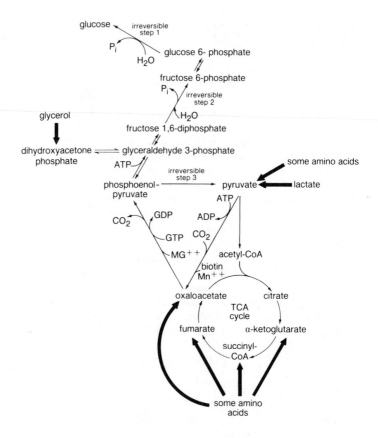

Entry of lactate, some amino acids and glycerol
into gluconeogenic pathway

Because of three places in the path "downhill" from glucose to pyruvate where cellular conditions prevent reversal of "downhill" reactions, a roundabout path must be followed that requires a net input of energy (pushing the boulder uphill), larger than that gained from glycolysis, the downhill path. These three places are (1) the step from glucose to glucose 6-phosphate where the glycolytic "downhill" enzyme is *glucokinase*; (2) the step from fructose 6-phosphate to fructose 1,6-diphosphate where the glycolytic enzyme is *phosphofructokinase*; and (3) the step from phosphoenolpyruvate to pyruvate where the glycolytic enzyme is *pyruvate kinase*.

The path uphill from pyruvate to phosphoenolpyruvate goes by way of oxaloacetate to bypass the downhill step 3. In the mitochondria, pyruvate is converted to oxaloacetate

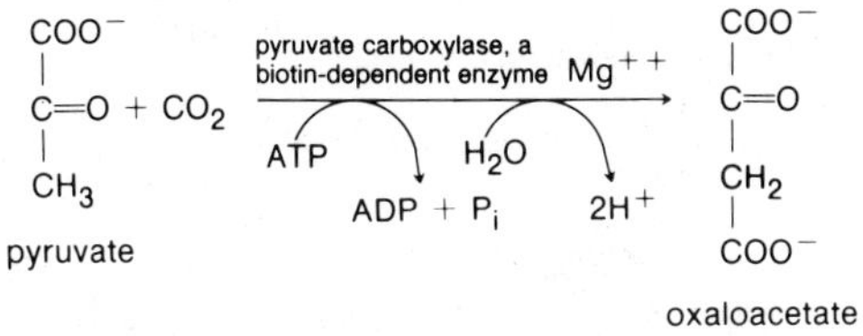

$$COO^- \quad \xrightarrow[\substack{ATP \quad\quad H_2O \\ ADP + P_i \quad 2H^+}]{\substack{\text{pyruvate carboxylase, a} \\ \text{biotin-dependent enzyme} \quad Mg^{++}}} \quad COO^-$$

The conversion of pyruvate to oxaloacetate

by the addition of a carboxyl group, a reaction catalyzed by a biotin-dependent enzyme, *pyruvate carboxylase*. In order to move oxaloacetate into the cytosol, it is reduced by an NADH-linked enzyme, forming malate which is able to cross into the cytosol. Once in the cytosol, malate is reoxidized to oxaloacetate. Oxaloacetate then is acted upon by *phosphoenolpyruvate carboxylase* to yield phosphoenolpyruvate and carbon dioxide.

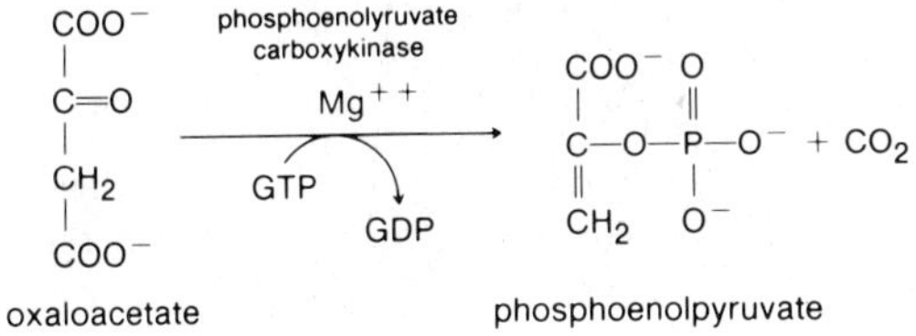

The synthesis of phosphoenolpyruvate

The path uphill from fructose 1,6-diphosphate to fructose 6-phosphate in order to bypass the downhill step 2 involves the simple removal of one phosphate. The enzyme *fructose 1,6-diphosphatase* catalyzes the removal of the phosphate on carbon 1 leaving fructose 6-phosphate to continue the climb toward glucose.

$$\text{fructose 1,6-diphosphate} + H_2O \xrightarrow{\text{fructose 1,6-diphosphatase}}$$
$$\text{fructose 6-phosphate} + P_i$$

The synthesis of fructose 6-phosphate

The final uphill step from glucose 6-phosphate to free glucose to bypass the downhill step 1 involves the removal of another phosphate. The enzyme *glucose 6-phosphatase*

$$\text{glucose 6-phosphate} + H_2O \xrightarrow[\text{Mg}^{++}]{\text{glucose 6-phosphatase}^*}$$

$$\text{glucose} + P_i$$

The synthesis of glucose

*Enzyme not present in brain or muscle cells.

catalyzes the removal of the last phosphate, yielding free glucose.

Thus, glycolysis going downhill from glucose to pyruvate yields a net of two ATP and gluconeogenesis going uphill from pyruvate to glucose requires an input of 6 ATP. See also: CORI CYCLE, for the way muscle lactate is converted into glucose; GLUCOGENIC AMINO ACIDS, for the way amino acids are converted to glucose; BIOTIN, THE COENZYME, for how biotin transfers a carbon dioxide; topics listed under each glucogenic amino acid.

SUGGESTED READINGS

Hers, H. G., and L. Hue. 1983. Gluconeogenesis and related aspects of glycolysis. *Ann. Rev. Biochem.* 52:617–653.

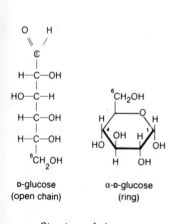

D-glucose
(open chain)

α-D-glucose
(ring)

Structure of glucose

Glutamate
(Glu)

glucose. A six-carbon sugar derived from the digestion of carbohydrate or synthesized from carbons from the degradation of other compounds, particularly GLUCOGENIC AMINO ACIDS.

Glucose is one of the principal fuels of the body, and for some tissues, such as the brain, it is the primary fuel. The concentration of glucose in the blood is under strict homeostatic control. An adult brain uses about 120 g per day whereas only about another 40 g are required for the rest of the body. About 190 g are easily obtained from the GLYCOGEN stored in the liver and muscles, which would take care of ordinary activities of the body for about a day. Therefore, foods that contribute glucose are a daily dietary requirement.

Glucose catabolism is by the anaerobic path of GLYCOLYSIS to pyruvate, which, after conversion to ACETYL-CoA, enters the aerobic path of the TCA CYCLE. See also: CARBOHYDRATE STRUCTURE; CARBOHYDRATE DIGESTION; CORI CYCLE; GLUCONEOGENESIS; GLYCOGEN; GLYCOGENESIS; GLYCOGENOLYSIS; GLYCOLYSIS.

glutamate (Glu). A five-carbon, nutritionally nonessential, glucogenic (glycogenic), α-amino acid with an acidic side chain. This amino acid is frequently referred to as glutamic acid but, since it is ionized at the PH of the cell, glutamate is a more accurate term.

Glutamate is formed during the transamination of many α-amino acids. The amino group of these AMINO ACIDS is first transferred by transamination to α-ketoglutarate (one of the intermediates of the TCA CYCLE), which then becomes glutamate. This reaction is catalyzed by the enzyme *glutamic transaminase*, which, like all transaminases, uses a VITAMIN B$_6$ coenzyme, pyridoxal phosphate.

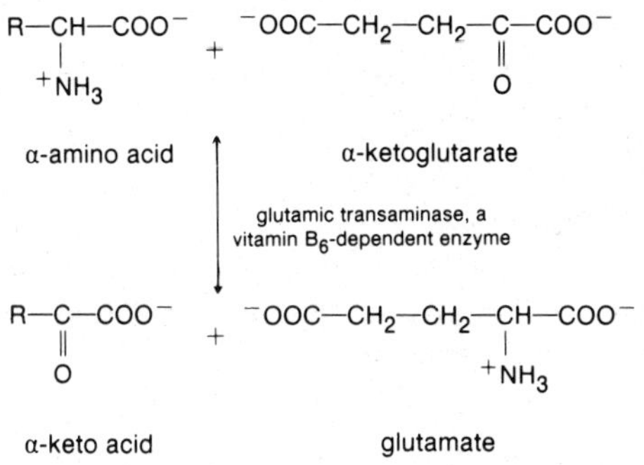

$$R\!-\!\underset{\overset{|}{^+NH_3}}{CH}\!-\!COO^- \quad + \quad {^-}OOC\!-\!CH_2\!-\!CH_2\!-\!\underset{\overset{\|}{O}}{C}\!-\!COO^-$$

α-amino acid $\qquad\qquad$ α-ketoglutarate

glutamic transaminase, a
vitamin B$_6$-dependent enzyme

$$R\!-\!\underset{\overset{\|}{O}}{C}\!-\!COO^- \quad + \quad {^-}OOC\!-\!CH_2\!-\!CH_2\!-\!\underset{\overset{|}{^+NH_3}}{CH}\!-\!COO^-$$

α-keto acid $\qquad\qquad$ glutamate

Glutamate is formed during transamination of many amino acids

Glutamate dehydrogenase catalyzes the oxidative deamination of glutamate, and α-ketoglutarate is re-formed, ready to accept an amino group from another amino acid. The ammonium ion is removed by being incorporated into a molecule of urea, which is excreted. *Glutamate dehydrogenase* is unusual in that it uses either NAD$^+$ or NADP$^+$, whereas most ENZYMES are highly specific for NAD$^+$ or for NADP$^+$.

This cycle of transaminations and oxidative deaminations involving α-ketoglutarate, glutamate, GLUTAMINE, and other amino acids is the pivotal series of reactions in amino acid metabolism. The importance of these actions is shown by the fact that the two major enzymes, *glutamate dehydrogenase* and *glutamine synthetase*, are present in all living organisms.

Glutamate is precursor of the neurotransmitter γ-aminobutyric acid (GABA) and of two non-essential amino acids, glutamine and PROLINE. Glutamine is produced when ammonia is added to glutamate in a *glutamine synthetase* catalyzed reaction powered by hydrolysis of ATP and requiring MAGNESIUM. Proline results when glutamate is converted to glutamate γ-semialdehyde, using ATP and NADH, followed by a rearrangement that uses NADPH as coenzyme.

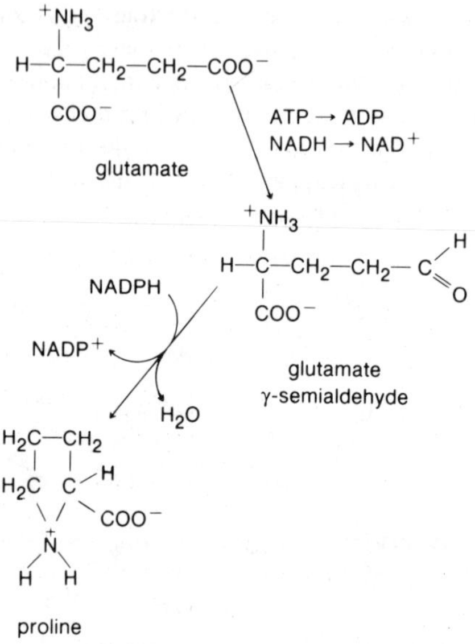

$$^+NH_3$$
$$H-C-CH_2-CH_2-COO^-$$
$$COO^-$$

glutamate

ATP $\rightarrow$ ADP
NADH $\rightarrow$ NAD$^+$

$$^+NH_3$$
$$H-C-CH_2-CH_2-C\overset{H}{\underset{O}{}}$$
$$COO^-$$

glutamate
γ-semialdehyde

NADPH

NADP$^+$

H_2O

$$H_2C-CH_2$$
$$H_2C \quad C\overset{H}{\diagdown}$$
$$\diagdown N \diagup COO^-$$
$$H \quad H$$

proline

The synthesis of proline

    Glutamate is responsible for gathering both the ammonia molecules from the amino acids incorporated into urea. The first ammonia comes directly from glutamate by oxidative deamination catalyzed by *glutamate dehydrogenase*. The second ammonia ion comes from ASPARTATE, which acquired it

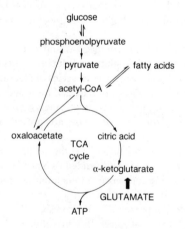

The carbons of glutamate
enter the metabolic pathways

from other amino acids via glutamate in an *aspartate trans-aminase* catalyzed reaction.

If the carbon skeleton of glutamate were to be used for energy, all 5 carbons of glutamate (like those of glutamine and proline) would enter the TCA cycle at α-ketoglutarate by the action of *glutamate dehydrogenase*. Then these carbons can exit the cycle at oxaloacetate and be converted to glucose via phosphoenolpyruvate (PEP). See also: GAMMA AMINOBUTYRATE; UREA CYCLE.

glutamic acid. See GLUTAMATE.

glutamine (Gln). A five-carbon, non-essential, glucogenic (glycogenic) α-amino acid that has an amino group on the terminal carbon of its side chain.

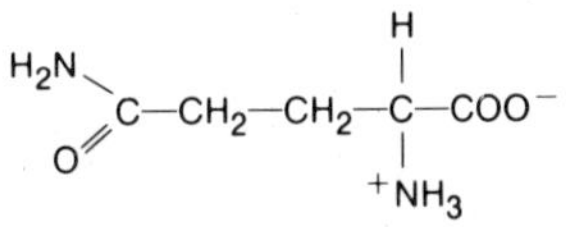

This terminal amino group is the key to its important function of collecting toxic ammonia molecules from the deamination of AMINO ACIDS and carrying them safely in the body fluids to the liver. Glutamine also functions as a donor of amino groups for the synthesis of a large number of compounds.

Glutamine is synthesized by the addition of two ammonia molecules to α-ketoglutarate. *Glutamate dehydrogenase* is the catalyst and NADPH provides the reducing power for the addition of one ammonia to α-ketoglutarate to form glutamate. Then *glutamine synthetase*, using ATP:Mg^{++} to provide the energy for the anabolism, incorporates ammonia into glutamate, resulting in glutamine. In a reversal of these reactions, all five carbons of glutamine enter the TCA CYCLE at α-ketoglutarate when glutamine is degraded for energy.

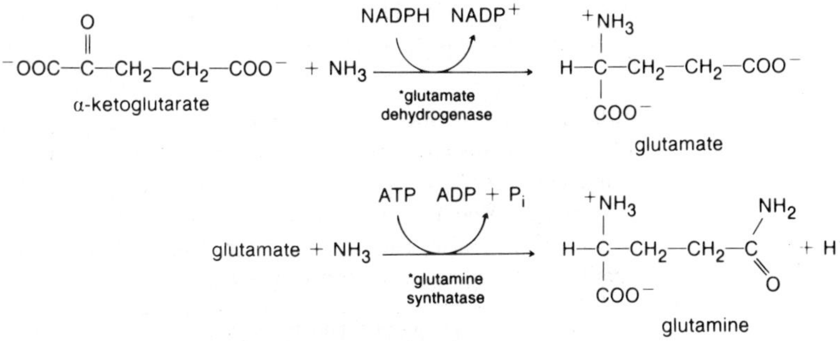

$$H_2N{-}\!\!\overset{\displaystyle O}{\underset{}{C}}{-}CH_2{-}CH_2{-}\overset{\displaystyle H}{\underset{\displaystyle +NH_3}{C}}{-}COO^-$$

Glutamine
(Gln)

Synthesis of glutamine
*(These two enzymes are present in all life forms.)

123

Glutamine plays an interesting part in blood clot formation. When the clot first forms, it is easily broken; however, with time, the side chains of glutamine and LYSINE form an unusual cross-link in the fibrin that functions to stabilize the clot.

from TCA cycle:

$$^-OOC-\overset{\overset{\textstyle O}{\|}}{C}-CH_2-CH_2-COO^-$$

α-ketoglutarate

$$H-\overset{\overset{\textstyle +NH_3}{|}}{C}-CH_2-CH_2-COO^-$$
$$\overset{|}{COO^-}$$

glutamate

$$H-\overset{\overset{\textstyle +NH_3}{|}}{C}-CH_2-CH_2-C\overset{NH_2}{\diagdown}\underset{O}{}$$
$$\overset{|}{COO^-}$$

glutamine

Glutamine carries two toxic ammonia
molecules out of brain

Elsewhere, glutamine provides a means whereby excessive ammonia can be removed from the brain. The conversion of glutamate to glutamine lowers the level of ammonia in neural tissue since glutamine holds two amino groups. In addition, glutamine, unlike glutamate, can diffuse freely out of the brain into the bloodstream or the cerebrospinal fluid carrying the two toxic ammonia molecules with it.

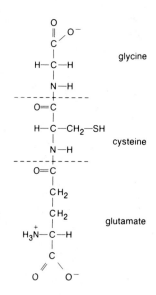

glycine

cysteine

glutamate

Reduced glutathione

glutathione. A tripeptide with a free sulfhydryl group that, in its reduced state, helps maintain the IRON in hemoglobin in the ferrous state. Red blood cells deficient in glutathione are more susceptible to hemolysis. The principal task of NADPH in the red blood cells is to reduce glutathione. See also: SICKLE CELL ANEMIA.

SUGGESTED READINGS

Meister, A., and M. E. Anderson. 1983. Glutathione. *Ann. Rev. Biochem.* 52:711–760.

glycerol.   A trihydroxy alcohol to which three FATTY ACIDS are attached to form the TRIACYLGLYCEROLS.   See also: FATTY ACIDS; TRIACYLGLYCEROLS.

glycerol phosphate shuttle.   One pathway that is responsible for the regeneration of NAD^+ from NADH so that GLYCOLYSIS may continue. The shuttle is most active in the skeletal muscle and the brain.

NADH is generated in the cytoplasm during glycolysis when glyceraldehyde 3-phosphate is oxidized. NADH must be oxidized to NAD^+ by the RESPIRATORY CHAIN so that more glyceraldehyde 3-phosphate can be processed; however, a problem exists in that the respiratory chain is in the mitochondria whose membrane is impermeable to both NADH and NAD^+. The problem is solved by the transfer of electrons to dihydroxyacetone phosphate to form glycerol 3-phosphate, which is able to cross the mitochondrial membrane. Once in the mitochondria, the dihydroxyacetone phosphate is re-formed by an FAD-linked enzyme and diffuses back into the cytosol, to complete the glycerol phosphate shuttle.

$$
\begin{array}{c}
H \\
| \\
H\!-\!C\!-\!OH \\
| \\
H\!-\!C\!-\!OH \\
| \\
H\!-\!C\!-\!OH \\
| \\
H
\end{array}
$$

Glycerol

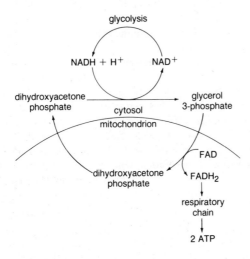

The glycerol phosphate shuttle carries two hydrogens (with their electrons) into the mitochondrion for conversion to ATP

The price of transporting two electrons across the mitochondrial membrane is one molecule of ATP since the FAD that accepts the electrons in the mitochondria yields only two ATP from the respiratory chain whereas the NADH would have yielded three ATP.

Another way that the electrons from NADH can be carried to the respiratory chain is by the MALATE-ASPARTATE SHUTTLE, which is most active in liver, kidney, and heart. This method does not cost an ATP. See also: ASPARTATE; MALATE-ASPARTATE SHUTTLE; RESPIRATORY CHAIN.

$$H-\overset{\displaystyle H}{\underset{\displaystyle {}^+NH_3}{C}}-COO^-$$

Glycine
(Gly)

glycine (Gly). A two-carbon, non-essential, glucogenic (glycogenic) α-amino acid. It is the simplest of the amino acids, having only a hydrogen atom as its side-chain.

The smallness of glycine's side chain allows it to fit comfortably in the interior of a protein chain and to make space for those amino acids with bulky side chains. Such is the case in COLLAGEN where the presence of so much glycine (every third residue in a chain of more than a thousand residues) in the slender collagen fibers allows enough room for the long side chains of PROLINE and LYSINE. These two amino acids contribute significantly to collagen's strength. Also, glycine is the hydrogen donor for the fragile hydrogen bonding that maintains the conformation of the helix. Other proteins in which glycine provides a similar function include cytochrome c, chymotrypsin, myoglobin, and hemoglobin.

Glycine is derived from the amino acid SERINE in a reaction requiring tetrahydrofolate (FH_4), a derivative of the vitamin FOLACIN and a carrier of one-carbon units. The beta carbon of serine is removed and inserted in FH_4 where it forms a bridge between nitrogens 5 and 10. FH_4 thus becomes N^5, N^{10}-methylenetetrahydrofolate and glycine is formed. This reaction is reversible so that if serine is required, it can be made from glycine and N^5,N^{10}-methylenetetrahydrofolate. In the synthesis of many other biomolecules, acceptors stand ready to use the carbon group carried in N^5, N^{10}-methylenetetrahydrofolate.

$$HO-CH_2-\underset{\displaystyle {}^+NH_3}{CH}-COO^- \xrightleftharpoons[\text{tetrahydrofolate}]{\substack{\text{serine hydroxymethyl transferase,} \\ \text{a vitamin } B_6\text{-dependent enzyme}}} \underset{\displaystyle {}^+NH_3}{CH_2}-COO^- + H_2O$$

serine N^5, N^{10}-methylenetetrahydrofolate   glycine

The synthesis of glycine

When energy is required and glycine's carbons must enter the TCA CYCLE, glycine is first converted to serine, a three-carbon amino acid, which then is deaminated and dehydrated to pyruvate. This latter reaction is catalyzed by VITAMIN B_6-dependent *serine dehydratase*. Glycine's major path of degradation, however, does not lead to the TCA cycle. In this reversible path, glycine is acted upon by *glycine synthase* to produce CO_2 and NH_4^+. In the process, FH_4 is converted to N^5,N^{10}-methylenetetrahydrofolate and NAD^+ accepts the hydrogens to become $NADH + H^+$. Vitamin B_6 in the form of pyridoxal phosphate is required for activity of the enzyme.

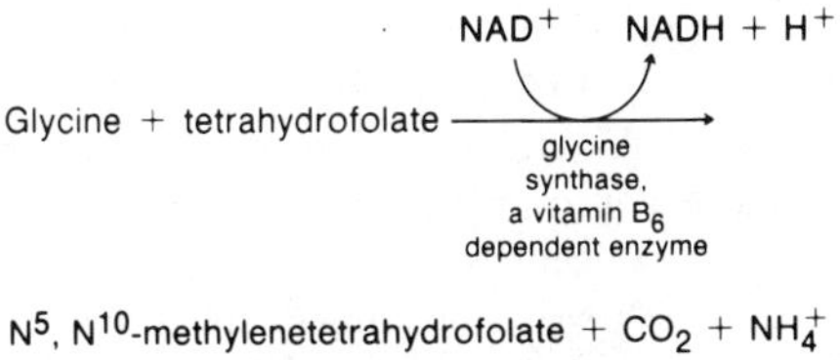

$$NAD^+ \qquad NADH + H^+$$

Glycine + tetrahydrofolate ⟶
glycine
synthase,
a vitamin B_6
dependent enzyme

N^5, N^{10}-methylenetetrahydrofolate + CO_2 + NH_4^+

The degradation of glycine

glycocholate. A bile salt made from the amino acid GLYCINE and cholic acid. It is required for fat digestion. See also: BILE SALTS.

glycogen. The storage form of GLUCOSE synthesized in human liver and muscles. Because it is constructed in the same way as plant starch, it is sometimes called "animal starch." Table meats are not a dietary glycogen source, however, because the trauma of slaughter will have degraded it.

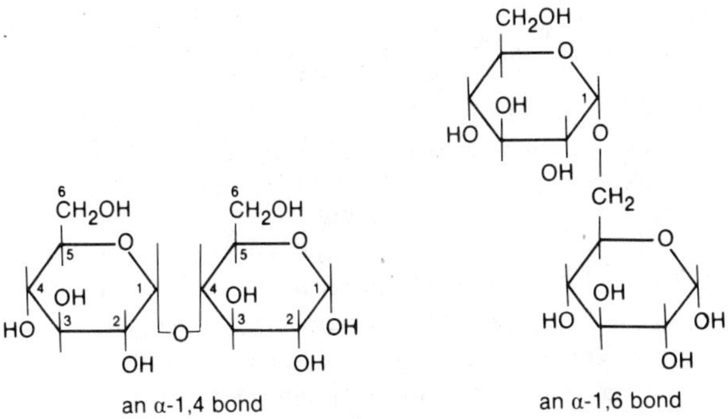

an α-1,4 bond   an α-1,6 bond

The two chemical bonds of glycogen as seen
in the union of glucose molecules

Glycogen's branched chain-structure is composed of chains of glucose molecules with branch points (α-1,6 linkages) about every 8 to 10 residues. Glycogen has more branch points than plant starch, therefore there are many end units on the periphery of the molecule. This proves especially valuable when a person needs energy suddenly. The enzyme that will cleave the last 1,4 glycosidic bond on every chain can approach these bonds easily. With that cleavage, the next glycosidic 1,4 bond is exposed to the enzyme's action. Thus a large amount of glucose can be set free almost instantly.

It is fortunate for humans that during the course of natural selection the process of storing energy from food and providing for rapid retrieval was preserved in our ancestors. Because of this storage and retrieval, humans are freed from the burden of continuous eating; glycogen sustains the blood glucose concentration between feedings, allowing people to pursue more stimulating interests. In addition, the stored glucose can be summoned for quick energy to run from or stand and fight an enemy.

Other advantages, which are not as obvious as sustaining blood glucose concentrations or providing energy for an emergency, are hidden in molecular actions. For instance, the glucose molecules that are freed from the 1,4 bonds by *phosphorylase* are phosphorylated using inorganic phosphorus which is abundant. Because these glucose molecules are already phosphorylated, they can enter the glycolytic pathway directly, saving both time and the use of high energy phosphates. On the other hand, free glucose molecules released during hydrolysis of the 1,6 bonds by the debranching enzyme must be phosphorylated by ATP in order to enter the glycolytic pathway. The ratio of free glucose to glucose 1-phosphate is about 1:10.

Another interesting way that glycogen is adapted to the needs of the body is how certain tissues with a special need for glucose are protected from loss of their glucose via GLYCOLYSIS. Skeletal muscles, for example, require that energy be available at a moment's notice for emergencies, therefore they have their own supply of glycogen. To protect this supply, they lack *glucose 6-phosphatase* that would free glucose from glucose 6-phosphate, which would allow the glucose to escape from the muscles into the blood.

In liver cells, unlike muscle cells, it is imperative that glucose escape because the liver must provide glucose for other cells. Therefore, the presence of *glucose 6-phosphatase* frees glucose that then migrates from the liver to the bloodstream where it can be acquired by other cells. See also: CARBOHYDRATE STRUCTURE; GLYCOGENESIS; GLYCOGENOLYSIS.

glycogenesis. The synthesis of GLYCOGEN. GLUCOSE produced from the digestion and metabolism of carbohydrate
and protein foods that are eaten in excess of need may be
stored in glycogen molecules in the liver and muscles. Unlike fat storage depots, which have an unlimited capacity,
these organs have limited storage capacity for glycogen.
Several minutes of strenuous exercise would deplete the
muscles' supply and twenty-four hours of fasting would deplete the liver's supply. Glycogen in the liver provides glucose for all the tissues of the body whereas glycogen in
muscles is used locally; however the supply of glycogen in
muscles is about five times as great as that in the liver due
to the large total mass of body muscle.

As in any other anabolic reaction, high energy compounds pay for glycogenesis. The synthesis of glycogen
uses ATP and uridine triphosphate (UTP), a nucleotide
that is widely used for sugar metabolism. The ATP is used
to activate the glucose to glucose 6-phosphate, the first step
of many processes, not just of glycogenesis. After the phosphate is moved from carbon 6 to carbon 1 by a mutase,
UTP donates energy through the hydrolysis of inorganic
pyrophosphate (PP_i). The rest of the molecule uridine
monophosphate (UMP) attaches to the phosphate of the
glucose 1-phosphate, forming UDP-glucose, an activated
form of glucose. (This part of the series of reactions that

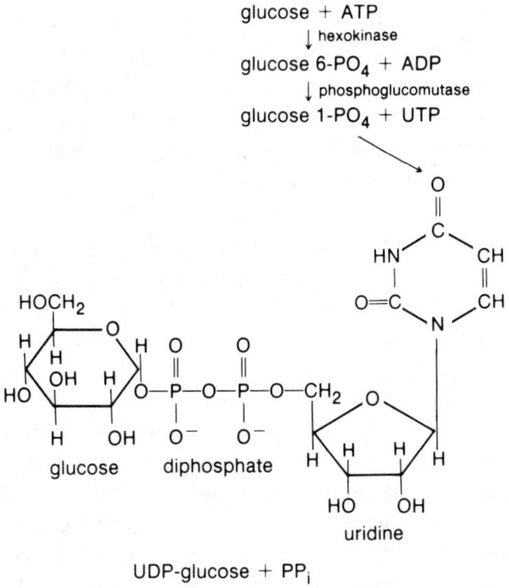

glucose + ATP
↓ hexokinase
glucose 6-PO_4 + ADP
↓ phosphoglucomutase
glucose 1-PO_4 + UTP

UDP-glucose + PP_i

Preparation for the glycogen synthase reaction

will synthesize glycogen is common to many anabolic processes. The nucleoside diphosphate sugars, such as UDP-glucose, act as glycosyl donors in pathways that generate polysaccharides.) The UDP-glucose then is transferred to the hydroxyl group on carbon 4 of a terminal glucose on the growing glycogen chain. *Glycogen synthase* forms these α-1,4 glycosidic bonds which may number in the hundreds of thousands in the glycogen molecule.

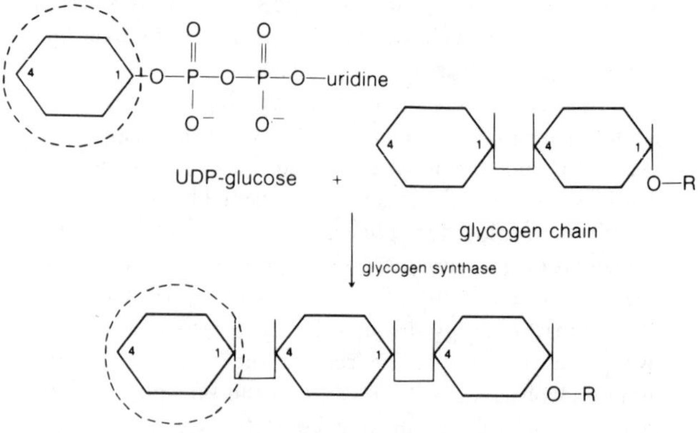

The glycogen synthase reaction
R = rest of glycogen chain

The chain made of α-1,4 bonds will not extend indefinitely, however. When a number of glucose residues have been linked, another enzyme will form the α-1,6 branch point that is crucial to glycogen. This branching enzyme,

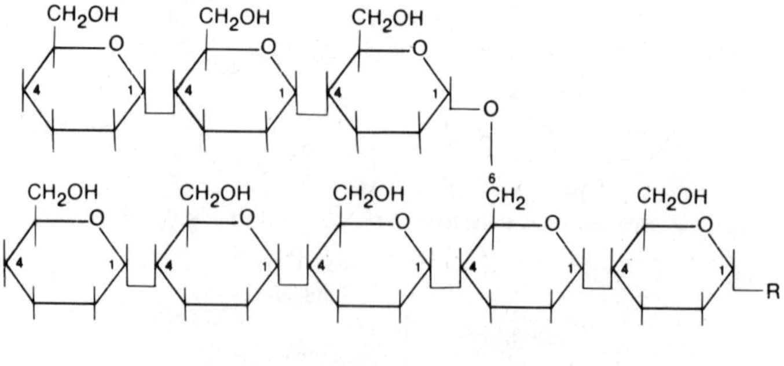

Alpha-1,6 bonds make the many branches of glycogen
R = rest of glycogen chain

glucosyl (4→6) transferase, will transfer a string of glucoses to a hydroxyl group on carbon 6 of a glucose residue on an already existing chain deeper in the molecule.

This chain then will grow in 1,4 links until the branching enzyme forms another 1,6 link, which will then grow in 1,4 links until the branching enzymes transfers a segment of the chain to form another 1,6 link. This cycle continues until the glycogen molecule becomes densely packed with branches about every 8 to 10 residues.

The many branches increase the number of end units exposed to the degradative enzyme that will break the last α-1,4 bond on each chain and deliver a large amount of glucose on demand. The many branches also increase the solubility of glycogen.

Some glycogen storage diseases are caused by genetic errors in one of the enzymes involved in the synthesis or degradation of glycogen. See also: GLYCOGEN, for the difference between α-1,4 and α-1,6 bonds; GLYCOGENOLYSIS, for mechanism of glucose release from glycogen; GLYCOGEN STORAGE DISEASES; UDP-GLUCOSE; URIDINE MONOPHOSPHATE.

SUGGESTED READINGS

Ahlborg, G. 1985. Mechanism for glycogenolysis in nonexercising human muscle during and after exercise. *Am. J. Physiol.* 248:E540–E545.

glycogenic amino acids. See GLUCOGENIC AMINO ACIDS.

glycogenolysis. The chemical process by which GLUCOSE is freed from GLYCOGEN. Glucose is a vital source of energy, especially for neural tissues, and the body has evolved an exquisite method for its storage as glycogen (GLYCOGENESIS) as well as a smooth-running process for reclaiming it from glycogen (glycogenolysis). The signal that glucose is needed (and glycogenolysis must start) is given by hormones, such as epinephrine which stimulates glycogen breakdown in muscle and glucagon which responds to low blood glucose levels by stimulating glycogenolysis in the liver.

Glycogen is perfectly constructed for its intended function as a glucose reservoir used to sustain the BLOOD GLUCOSE LEVEL between meals and to provide quick energy during an emergency. Because its branched chains of glucose residues produce many end units on the periphery of a giant molecule, *glycogen phosphorylase* can release many of these terminal glucose residues instantly.

When glucose is needed, *glycogen phosphorylase* cleaves the terminal α-1,4 glycosidic bonds and releases glucose 1-phosphate. Glucose 1-phosphate is ready to enter the

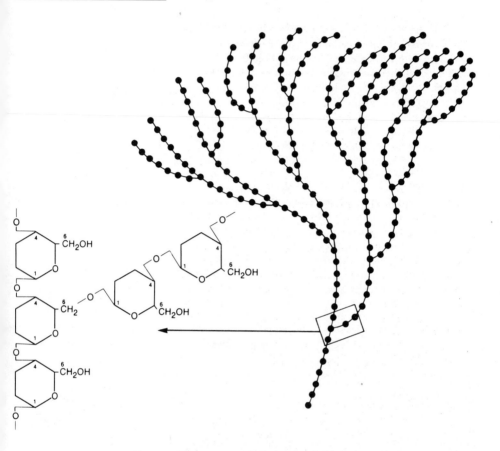

Glycogen has many terminal glucose residues
Reproduced with permission, from Martin DW Jr et al: Harper's Review of Biochemistry, 20th ed. © 1985 by Lange Medical Publications, Los Altos, California.

glycolytic pathway without any expenditure of a high energy compound. Cleaving the first glucose exposes the next α-1,4 bond and thus a large amount of glucose can be released simultaneously.

The above action will continue until the branch point is four residues away, at which time a transferase moves a block of three residues from one outer branch to another, exposing the branch point (α-1,6 bond) to the debranching enzyme that will hydrolyze it. This action releases free unphosphorylated glucose which, unlike glucose 1-phosphate or glucose 6-phosphate, is able to migrate across cell membranes and enter the bloodstream. Glucose 6-phosphate, which enters glycolysis, can be formed from glucose 1-phosphate by the action of *phosphoglucomutase*.

There is an enzyme, *glucose 6-phosphatase,* in liver and kidney (not in muscle) that removes the phosphate so that glucose is set free to migrate into the blood stream. These enzymes will continue dismantling the glycogen molecule until the glycogen is exhausted or until the signal is received that no more glucose is needed.

Glycogenolysis and glycogenesis take place in the cytosol where all the ingredients for these two processes occur together. This situation demands rigid controls, otherwise a futile cycle will occur that would wastefully use ATP to regenerate UTP. From the accompanying table it can be seen that all the reactants needed for the synthesis and breakdown of glycogen, except ATP, are produced by another reaction. If these equations were added together, all reactants and products would cancel and the sum would be a futile cycle; however, this does not occur. The controls are so well coordinated that when the demand for glucose is high and the enzymes of glycogenolysis are active, the enzymes for the synthesis of glycogen are inactive.

$$ATP \leftrightarrows ADP + P_i$$

Futile cycle

Glycogenesis and Glycogenolysis Occur in the Cytosol Where All Reactants and Products Occur Together[*]

Reactants	Products
Glycogenesis:	
glucose 1-phosphate + UTP	UDP-glucose + PP_i
UDP-glucose + $glycogen_{(n)}$	UDP + $glycogen_{(n + 1)}$
Glycogenolysis:	
$glycogen_{(n + 1)}$ + P_i	glucose 1-phosphate + $glycogen_{(n)}$
UDP + ATP	UTP + ADP

[*]Without strict controls these would cancel each other, except for ATP.

CYCLIC AMP ensures that the enzymes of glycogen metabolism will respond to demands. Glycogen synthesis will be turned on if no demands for glucose are being made and if abundant UTP is available to activate the incoming glucose. When glucose is demanded, glycogen synthesis is turned off and the phosphorylases are turned on. When enough glucose has been funneled into the glycolytic path to build up the supply of ATP, the cyclic AMP concentration will fall and this will turn off the degradative process.

Muscle glycogen responds to CALCIUM ions. Stimulation of the nerves calling for muscular action releases calcium ions that start the contraction. At the same time these ions activate the phosphorylase and inhibit the synthase. When stimulation of the nerves ceases, calcium ions are removed and the other processes reverse.

133

Muscle glycogen is the source of energy for muscles after the first thirty seconds of an activity, such as a sprint, during which the muscles use up their tiny supply of ATP. For the next two or three minutes, glycogen provides the only source of energy until the CORI CYCLE begins to operate in the liver to regenerate glucose from the lactate that accumulates during exercise. See also: CORI CYCLE; GLYCOGENESIS.

glycogen storage diseases. See VON GIERKE'S DISEASE; POMPE'S DISEASE; CORI'S DISEASE; ANDERSEN'S DISEASE; MCARDLE'S DISEASE; HERS' DISEASE; TARUI'S DISEASE.

SUGGESTED READINGS

Howell, R. R., and J. C. Williams. 1983. The glycogen storage diseases. In *The metabolic basis of inherited disease*, 5th ed., ed. J. B. Stanbury et al., 146–166. New York: McGraw-Hill.

glycolipid. A compound consisting of both FATTY ACIDS and carbohydrates, yet also containing NITROGEN. Glycolipids are found in the myelin sheath that covers and protects the nerves.

glycolysis (Embden-Meyerhof pathway). A group of chemical reactions responsible for converting GLUCOSE to lactate and ATP without the consumption of oxygen, an anaerobic path. This glycolytic pathway takes place in the cytosol where glucose is converted to pyruvate unless oxygen is in short supply, in which case lactate is produced. With sufficient oxygen, pyruvate will be prepared for entry into the mitochondria where it will be converted into ACETYL-COA that will be oxidized through the TCA CYCLE.

Glycolysis is an ancient energy-producing process, present before there was oxygen blanketing the earth. After the earth was covered by plants that produced oxygen through photosynthesis, forms of life emerged that utilized oxygen to produce energy; these aerobic processes produced much greater amounts of energy. Today, both aerobic and anaerobic processes can be found in the same cell, usually kept apart by a barrier such as the mitochondrial membrane which separates glycolysis and the TCA cycle in animal cells.

The reactions of glycolysis can be thought of as occurring in three stages. In the first, the gathering stage, all the monosaccharides are phosphorylated and enter the pathway at various points. At the close of this stage the monosaccharides will be indistinguishable. In the next stage, the 6-carbon compound will be phosphorylated on another carbon so that it can be split into 2 interchangeable, 3-carbon,

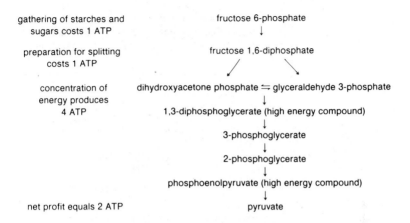

gathering of starches and sugars costs 1 ATP

preparation for splitting costs 1 ATP

concentration of energy produces 4 ATP

net profit equals 2 ATP

fructose 6-phosphate
↓
fructose 1,6-diphosphate

dihydroxyacetone phosphate ⇌ glyceraldehyde 3-phosphate
↓
1,3-diphosphoglycerate (high energy compound)
↓
3-phosphoglycerate
↓
2-phosphoglycerate
↓
phosphoenolpyruvate (high energy compound)
↓
pyruvate

Glycolysis outlined as a series of energy-costing
or energy-producing stages

phosphorylated compounds. In the third stage, the energy carried in the various bonds is concentrated during several steps, finally producing two high-energy compounds from which ATP will be produced. The following discussion gives the details of each of these stages.

In the gathering stage, glucose is phosphorylated so that it can enter the pathway as glucose 6-phosphate while glucose from glycogen breakdown enters as glucose 1-phosphate. Mannose and some fructose enter as fructose 6-phosphate, the final compound of this stage.

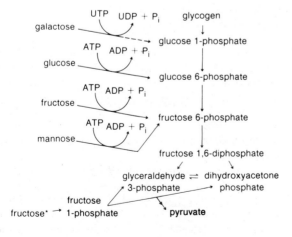

The first stage of glycolysis is the gathering of sugars
* may be a major pathway of catabolism in some tissues

In the preparation stage, fructose 6-phosphate is phosphorylated at carbon #1 by the enzyme *phosphofructokinase* in an irreversible reaction that requires ATP and MAGNESIUM (Mg^{++}).

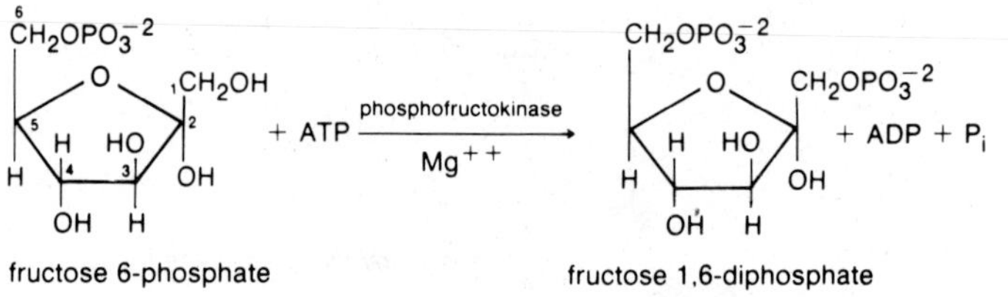

Phosphorylation of fructose 6-phosphate

The enzyme *aldolase* then cleaves the fructose 1, 6-diphosphate into two 3-carbon compounds: dihydroxyacetone phosphate (the entry point for glycerol from the degradation of TRIACYLGLYCEROLS) and glyceraldehyde 3-phosphate. The two cleavage compounds are easily interconvertible by *triose phosphate isomerase* but only one, the glyceraldehyde 3-phosphate, continues in the path to the next stage.

In the final stage of glycolysis, successive oxidations and reductions concentrate the energy of the bonds and produce

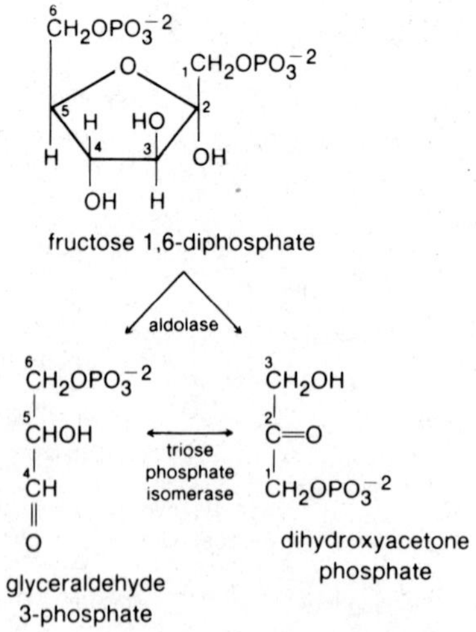

The fate of fructose 1,6-diphosphate in glycolysis

ATP. (Recall that "oxidation" means "loss of electrons" not always including the process of uniting with oxygen.) To this point, glycolysis has been costly; two high-energy phosphates have been used and no energy has been produced. Two molecules of glyceraldehyde 3-phosphate are now oxidized to 1,3-diphosphoglycerate which has a higher group transfer potential than ATP, thus ensuring the production of ATP.

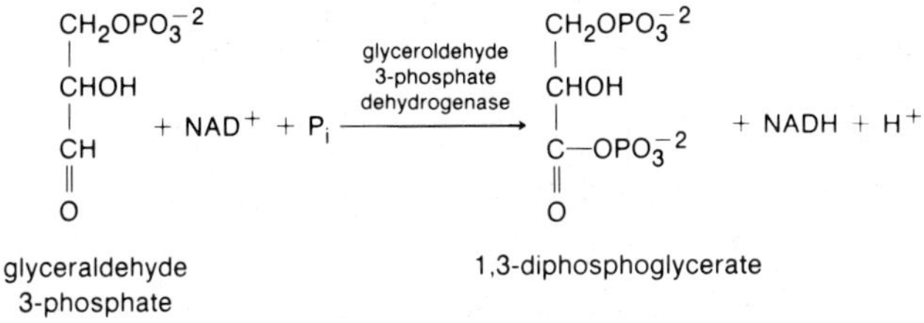

$$CH_2OPO_3^{-2} \quad\quad\quad\quad\quad\quad CH_2OPO_3^{-2}$$

$$\begin{array}{l} CH_2OPO_3^{-2} \\ | \\ CHOH \\ | \quad\quad + NAD^+ + P_i \\ CH \\ \| \\ O \end{array} \xrightarrow{\begin{array}{c}\text{glyceroldehyde}\\\text{3-phosphate}\\\text{dehydrogenase}\end{array}} \begin{array}{l} CH_2OPO_3^{-2} \\ | \\ CHOH \\ | \quad\quad + NADH + H^+ \\ C-OPO_3^{-2} \\ \| \\ O \end{array}$$

glyceraldehyde 3-phosphate \quad\quad 1,3-diphosphoglycerate

Oxidation of glyceraldehyde 3-phosphate

With the 1,3-diphosphoglycerate loaded with the energy of two phosphate bonds, the productive phase of glycolysis is ready to begin. *Phosphoglycerate kinase* catalyzes the transfer of high-energy phosphate to ADP.

The two ATP produced (one from each of the two molecules of 1,3-diphosphoglycerate) pay the debt of the two ATP used earlier. When the phosphate group of the product, 3-phosphoglycerate, is shifted to carbon-2 in a reaction

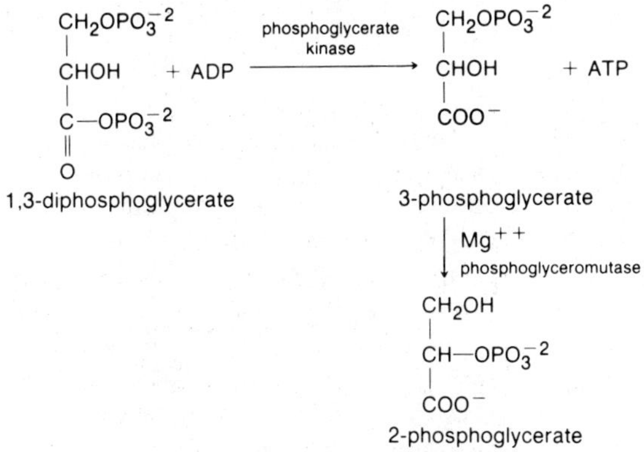

$$\begin{array}{l} CH_2OPO_3^{-2} \\ | \\ CHOH \quad\quad + ADP \\ | \\ C-OPO_3^{-2} \\ \| \\ O \end{array} \xrightarrow{\begin{array}{c}\text{phosphoglycerate}\\\text{kinase}\end{array}} \begin{array}{l} CH_2OPO_3^{-2} \\ | \\ CHOH \quad\quad + ATP \\ | \\ COO^- \end{array}$$

1,3-diphosphoglycerate \quad\quad\quad\quad 3-phosphoglycerate

$$\downarrow \begin{array}{l} Mg^{++} \\ \text{phosphoglyceromutase} \end{array}$$

$$\begin{array}{l} CH_2OH \\ | \\ CH-OPO_3^{-2} \\ | \\ COO^- \end{array}$$

2-phosphoglycerate

Production of ATP in glycolysis

137

catalyzed by *phosphoglyceromutase* that requires magnesium (Mg^{++}), the product is 2-phosphoglycerate.

In the next reaction phosphoenolpyruvate, another high-energy compound, is produced by the action of *enolase* on 2-phosphoglycerate. *Enolase,* that requires either magnesium (Mg^{++}) or MANGANESE (Mn^{++}), evidently brings about a large internal change because phosphoenolpyruvate has considerably more energy of hydrolysis than 2-phosphoglycerate from which it came.

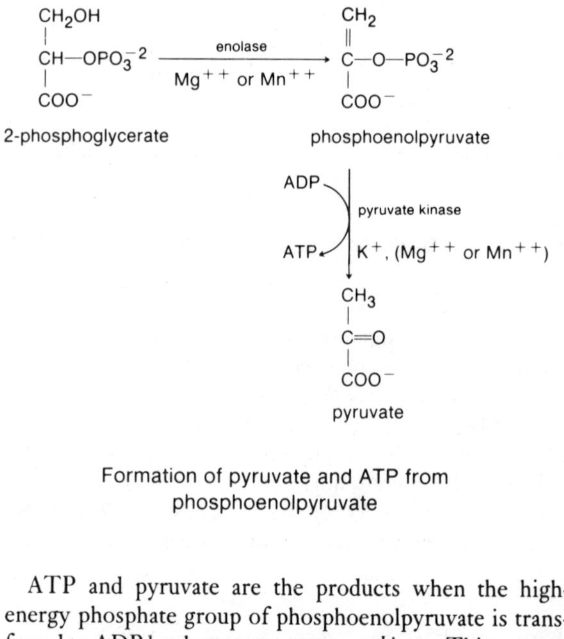

Formation of pyruvate and ATP from
phosphoenolpyruvate

ATP and pyruvate are the products when the high-energy phosphate group of phosphoenolpyruvate is transferred to ADP by the enzyme *pyruvate kinase.* This enzyme requires POTASSIUM (K^+) and either manganese (Mn^{++}) or magnesium (Mg^{++}). Another divalent molecule, CALCIUM (Ca^{++}), competes for this enzyme's active site and, if calcium is successful, the enzyme will be inactivated.

With the production of pyruvate, glycolysis is complete unless there is a shortage of oxygen as there may be in skeletal muscles during the early minutes of vigorous exercise. In that instance, pyruvate is converted to lactate by *lactate dehydrogenase,* an enzyme that uses NADH as carrier of the needed hydrogens, producing NAD^+. The conversion of NADH to NAD^+ is useful for it resupplies the glycolytic path with NAD^+.

The lactate formed leaves the muscles and participates in the Cori cycle, that is, it is carried by the blood to the liver

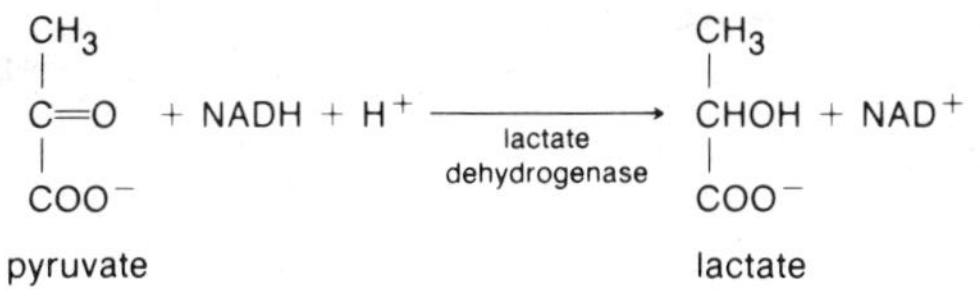

$$\begin{array}{c} CH_3 \\ | \\ C{=}O \\ | \\ COO^- \end{array} + NADH + H^+ \xrightarrow[\text{dehydrogenase}]{\text{lactate}} \begin{array}{c} CH_3 \\ | \\ CHOH \\ | \\ COO^- \end{array} + NAD^+$$

pyruvate   lactate

The anaerobic conversion of pyruvate to lactate
and regeneration of NAD$^+$

where it is converted to glucose that returns via the blood
to the muscles for fuel. One of the reasons for the warm-up
period before vigorous exercise is to assure that the Cori
cycle is functioning so that there will be no accumulation of
lactate, the substance that causes the discomfort of muscle
fatigue.

Glycolysis produces a net of 2 ATP in the conversion of
glucose to pyruvate or lactate. Two ATP are used in the
early stages and four are generated in the final oxidation and
reduction reactions. See also: CORI CYCLE; GLUCOSE;
GLYCOGEN.

SUGGESTED READINGS

Hers, H. G., and L. Hue. 1983. Gluconeogenesis and related aspects of glycolysis. *Ann. Rev. Biochem.*
52:617–653.

glycoprotein. A protein in which oligosaccharide chains
are covalently attached to the polypeptide backbone. Glycoproteins include structural molecules, lubricants, and
transport molecules for vitamins, LIPIDS, hormones, and
ENZYMES.

GMP. See GUANOSINE MONOPHOSPHATE.

GTP. See GUANOSINE TRIPHOSPHATE.

guanine. A purine base. See also: DNA; PURINE, PYRIMIDINE
BASES.

guanosine. A nucleoside containing guanine (a purine) and
ribose. See also: NUCLEOSIDES, NUCLEOTIDES.

guanosine diphosphate (GDP). A nucleotide containing
guanine (a purine), ribose, and two phosphates. See also:
NUCLEOSIDES, NUCLEOTIDES.

guanosine monophosphate (GMP, guanylate). A nucleotide containing guanine (a purine), ribose, and one
phosphate. See also: NUCLEOSIDES, NUCLEOTIDES.

guanosine triphosphate (GTP). A nucleotide containing
guanine (a purine), ribose, and three phosphates. See also:
NUCLEOSIDES, NUCLEOTIDES; TCA CYCLE.

139

half-life (t$_{1/2}$). The time required for half of a substance to disappear from a system. This disappearance could be loss of a radioisotope as it decays to become another radioisotope or to become a stable element. The disappearance could be that of molecules which formerly were present in tissues but have been degraded into other metabolites. See also: ISOTOPIC DILUTION TECHNIQUE.

HDL. See HIGH DENSITY LIPOPROTEIN; LIPOPROTEINS.

heme. The portion of hemoglobin, myoglobin, and cytochromes that is responsible for their ability to carry and release oxygen and electrons. Heme results from a joining of IRON with a porphyrin ring to produce the familiar bright

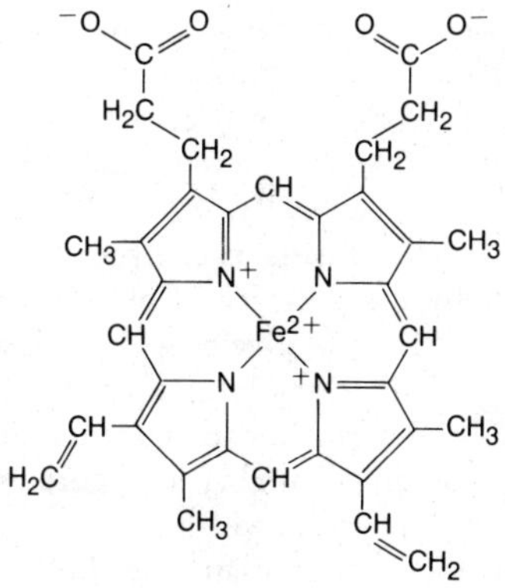

Heme

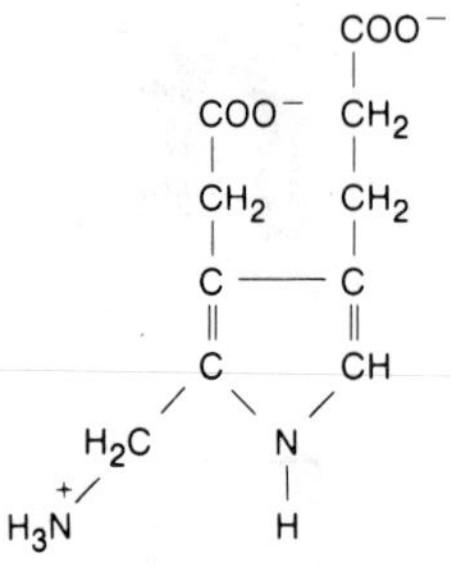

Porphobilinogen

red complex. The liver is the crucial organ in heme metabolism, although bone marrow and spleen play important secondary roles.

Heme is made from two molecules that are readily available in the body: GLYCINE, a nonessential amino acid, provides all the nitrogens, and succinyl-CoA, a TCA CYCLE intermediate, provides most of the carbons in the porphyrin rings. Glycine and succinyl-CoA condense in the mitochondria under the influence of a VITAMIN B_6-dependent enzyme to form δ-aminolevulinate. Two molecules of δ-aminolevulinate join in such a way that the first of the rings is formed, resulting in the compound porphobilinogen.

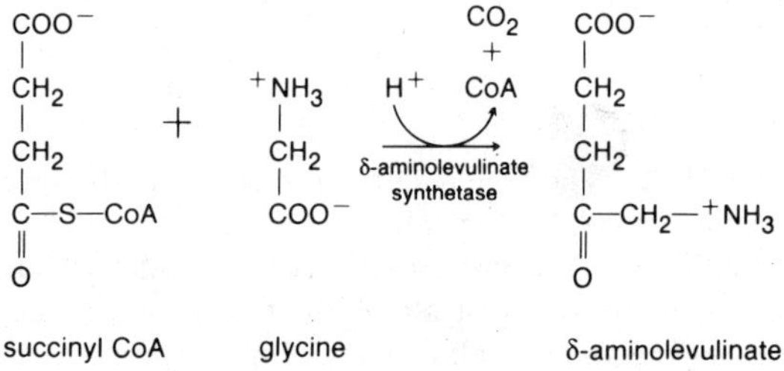

succinyl CoA   glycine   δ-aminolevulinate

The synthesis of δ-aminolevulinate

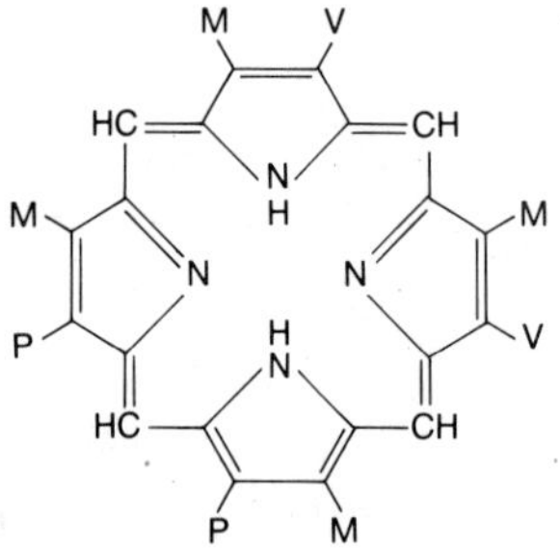

Protoporphyrin IX

M – methyl
V – vinyl
P – propionate

Four molecules of porphobilinogen condense in a linear sequence to form tetrapyrrole, which is still bound to the enzyme. When these cyclize, the familiar pattern of a heme emerges, and, after some rearrangements on the side chains, protoporphyrin IX, the immediate precursor of heme, results.

The final, heme-yielding step involves the insertion of a ferrous ion in the center of the structure where it joins four NITROGEN atoms. Both the final and first steps take place in the mitochondria, but the intermediate steps occur in the cytosol.

The manufacture of heme is controlled by its own production whereby the presence of heme inhibits the first step, the condensation of glycine and succinyl-CoA. Certain drugs, especially the barbiturates and sulfanomides, as well as the steroid hormones stimulate the first step.

Genetic disorders involving the porphyrins include erythropoietic porphyria in which there is an accumulation of some of the intermediate metabolites, including uroporphinogen I. These spill into the urine causing it to be bright red and to fluoresce under ultra-violet light, a reaction that is the basis for diagnosis. Photosensitivity is also observed in afflicted persons. Most of the symptoms are caused by the destruction of erythrocytes. In acute intermittent porphyria, where the liver, rather than the erythrocytes, is involved, acute abdominal pain is accompanied by neurologic disorders.

When heme is degraded, its iron is conserved and the protein to which heme is attached is split into AMINO ACIDS, which may be incorporated in new proteins. The porphyrin ring is broken apart and excreted, some of the degradation products lending their colors to the excretion products. In the presence of oxygen and NADPH, a cytochrome will oxidize one of the carbons that forms a bridge in the rings, remaking the linear tetrapyrrole (biliverdin) that was one of the early intermediates during its formation. Biliverdin is a bile pigment that gives the green color often seen in a bruise.

Biliverdin is reduced quickly to bilirubin by a reductase that requires NADPH. This action takes place in the reticuloendothelial cells. Because bilirubin is lipid soluble, it diffuses through the cell membrane into the bloodstream where it combines with albumin with which it is carried through the bloodstream.

When bilirubin reaches the liver, two UDP-glucose molecules become attached resulting in the conjugated form of the bile pigment, bilirubin diglucuronide. Both this form and free bilirubin will find their way into bile. Bile will be released into the duodenum where it will emulsify dietary fats, and the bilirubin will be converted to urobilin which is excreted in the feces. These pigments impart their typical color to fecal matter.

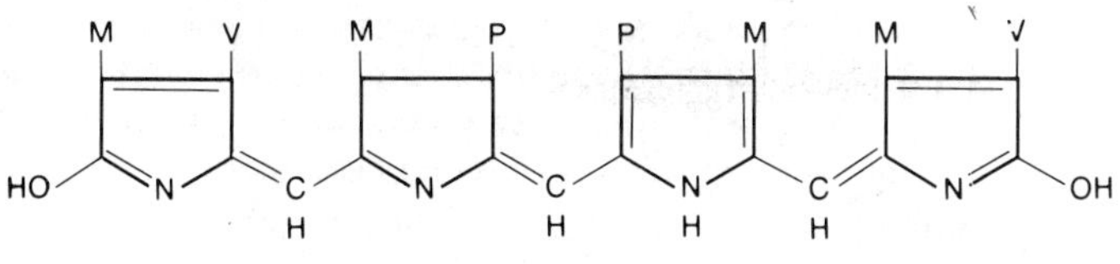

Biliverdin

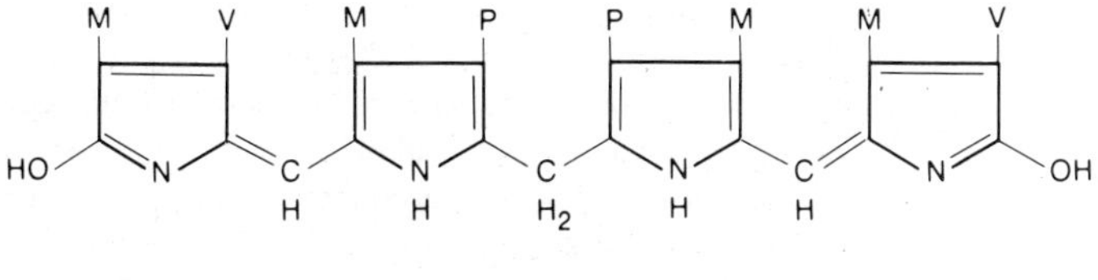

Bilirubin

hemochromatosis. A rare disease of IRON metabolism in which iron accumulates in body tissues. The liver becomes enlarged, the skin takes on a bronze hue, DIABETES MELLITUS may develop, and cardiac failure is common. Usually primary hemochromatosis starts after age forty, more often in men than in women. The condition may also develop as a consequence of other diseases that require frequent blood transfusions.

SUGGESTED READINGS

Bothwell, T. H., and R. W. Charlton, and A. G. Motulsky. 1983. Idiopathic hemochromatosis. In *The metabolic basis of inherited disease,* 5th ed., ed. J. B. Stanbury et al., 1269–1300. New York: McGraw-Hill.

Powell, L. W., M. L. Bassett, and J. W. Halliday. 1980. Hemochromatosis: 1980. Update. *Gastroenterology* 78:374–381.

Simon, M., et al. 1980. Idiopathic hemochromatosis: A study of biochemical expression in 247 heterozygous members of 63 families: Evidence for a single major HLA-linked gene. *Gastroenterology* 78:703–708.

hemoglobin. A heme protein that acts as a carrier of oxygen from the lungs to the cells, and of hydrogen ions and carbon dioxide from the cells to the lungs for excretion. Hemoglobin contains four polypeptide chains, two alphas and two betas, and four heme groups, one on each chain. Its ability to carry and release compounds depends on the presence of ferrous IRON in each heme group.

Analysis of amino acid sequences found in the hemoglobin of various species has shown wide variability at most positions. There are nine positions, however, in which the same amino acid is found: histidine occupies two of these positions. In all species studied, nonpolar AMINO ACIDS are concentrated in the interior near the location of the heme portion, protecting it from water, but there is no distinct sequence. See also: HEME; SICKLE CELL ANEMIA.

hemolysis. Rupture of red blood cells, resulting in anemia.

hemorrhagic disease of the newborn. See VITAMIN K.

$$pH = pK' + \log \frac{[A^-]}{[HA]}$$

Henderson-Hasselbalch equation

Henderson-Hasselbalch equation. An equation relating the pH, the pK', and the ratio of the concentrations of a weak base (proton acceptor, "A⁻") to that of a weak acid (proton donor, "HA"). This equation is useful in evaluating the buffering systems of the blood. A buffering system, consisting of a weak acid and its conjugate base, tends to resist changes in pH when acidic or basic ions are added. The brackets in the equation denote concentrations. See also: PH; PK'; BUFFER.

Hers' disease (glycogen storage disease: type VI). A disease caused by the absence of hepatic *phosphorylase*, resulting in excessive deposition of GLYCOGEN in the liver.

SUGGESTED READINGS

Howell, R. R., and J. C. Williams. 1983. The glycogen storage diseases. In *The metabolic basis of inherited disease*, 5th ed., ed. J. B. Stanbury et al., 141–166. New York: McGraw-Hill.

hexose. A 6-carbon sugar. See also: CARBOHYDRATE STRUCTURE.

hexose monophosphate shunt. See PENTOSE PHOSPHATE PATHWAY.

high density lipoprotein (HDL). One of the LIPOPROTEINS in which LIPIDS are carried in the watery fluids of the body. HDL is synthesized in the liver and possibly in the intestine and contains primarily protein, as well as phospholipids and CHOLESTEROL. HDL mainly is responsible for the transport of cholesterol from the peripheral tissues to the liver for oxidation to BILE SALTS. The blood level of HDL has an inverse relationship with the risk for developing atherosclerosis. See also: LIPOPROTEINS.

high energy compound. A substance whose hydrolysis results in the release of a large amount of energy. A high energy compound is one which has a negative free energy change ($\Delta G^{\circ\prime}$) of more than -5 kcal/mol under standard conditions. The best-known high energy compound is ATP, which has a $\Delta G^{\circ\prime}$ in the hydrolysis of its terminal phosphate group of -8.8 kcal/mol. A compound that has a greater negative standard free energy of hydrolysis than ATP is PEP (phosphoenolpyruvate) whose $\Delta G^{\circ\prime}$ is -14.8 kcal/mol. PEP is a key intermediate in GLUCONEOGENESIS, the path from pyruvate to GLUCOSE. See also: ENERGETICS.

histidine (His). A glucogenic (glycogenic), six-carbon α-amino acid that, along with LYSINE and ARGININE, has a positively charged side group. Also, unlike the other two, histidine's side chain can be neutral, the shift in charge depending on the PH of the environment. Histidine forms part of the active center of many ENZYMES, is an important amino acid in hemoglobin structure, and is valuable as a buffer.

Although histidine is usually classified as an ESSENTIAL AMINO ACID for infants, there is growing evidence that it may also be essential for adults because humans cannot synthesize the imidazole ring.

During degradation histidine is first deaminated, then its imidazole ring opens so that it becomes N-formimingluta-

Histidine
(His)

145

mate (Figlu). The formimino group (encircled in the diagram) is picked up by tetrahydrofolate, the coenzyme form of the vitamin FOLACIN. The remaining part of the molecule is GLUTAMATE, which enters the TCA CYCLE at α-ketoglutarate.

In patients with folacin deficiency, the degradation of histidine to glutamate is blocked, causing N-formiminoglutamate to be excreted in the urine. The presence of Figlu in

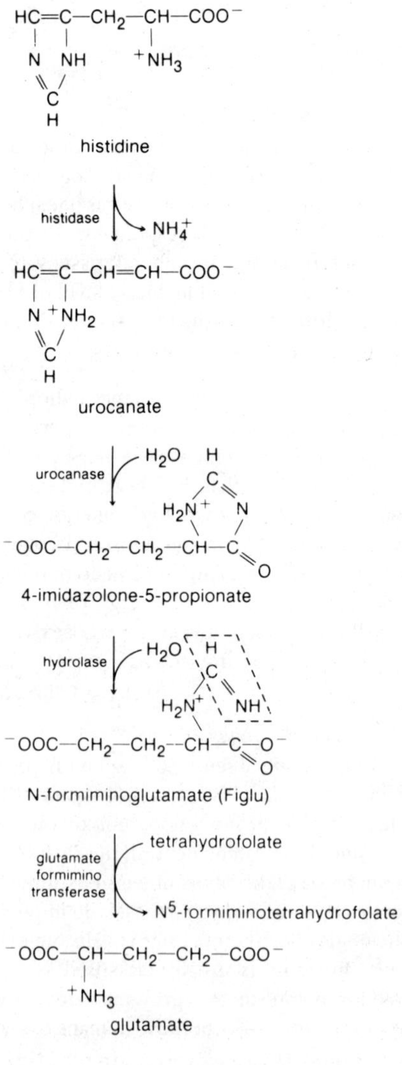

$$HC=C-CH_2-CH-COO^-$$

histidine

histidase ↘ NH_4^+

$$HC=C-CH=CH-COO^-$$

urocanate

urocanase / H_2O

4-imidazolone-5-propionate

hydrolase / H_2O

N-formiminoglutamate (Figlu)

glutamate formimino transferase / tetrahydrofolate ↘ N^5-formiminotetrahydrofolate

$$^-OOC-CH-CH_2-CH_2-COO^-$$
$$^+NH_3$$

glutamate

The conversion of histidine to glutamate

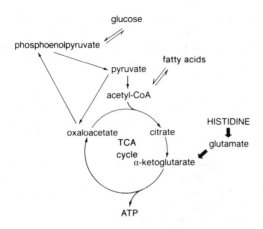

The carbons of histidine enter metabolic pathways

$$HC\!=\!C\!-\!CH_2\!-\!CH_2\!-\!^+NH_3$$

histamine

Histamine is a derivative
of histidine

the urine after a large dose of histidine is a test for folacin deficiency.

Histamine, a well-known vasodilator and stimulant of gastric secretion, is derived from histidine by decarboxylation. See also: HEMOGLOBIN for histidine's role in hemoglobin structure.

histidinemia. An accumulation of HISTIDINE in the blood and other tissues, resulting from the absence of *histidase.*

holoenzyme. The complete, active ENZYME. The protein part, called the apoenzyme, plus the catalytic part, called the cofactor or coenzyme, make up the holoenzyme, which has biologic activity.

homeostasis. A state of physiological equilibrium produced by a balance of functions and of chemical composition within an organism. In other words, when a stress is placed on a tissue, the tissue attempts to restore itself to its "normal" condition. This concept of homeostasis was first presented in 1932 by Walter B. Cannon, a professor in the medical college of Harvard University, in a book entitled, "The Wisdom of the Body." There is a variety of chemical processes available to tissues to keep them in a state of homeostasis for each parameter that is under homeostasic control. One parameter of the blood that is under homeostatic control is the glucose concentration. See also: BLOOD GLUCOSE LEVEL.

homocystinuria. An inherited disease characterized by a high level of homocysteine excreted in the urine. The disease is caused by an absence of the VITAMIN B_6-dependent enzyme, *cystathionine synthetase*, that converts homocysteine to cystathionine during METHIONINE metabolism. Affected persons are mentally retarded and fail to grow normally. In some cases the disorder will respond to vitamin B_6 supplements.

SUGGESTED READINGS

Mudd, S. H., and H. L. Levy. 1983. Disorders of transsulfuration. In *The metabolic basis of inherited disease*, 5th ed., ed. J. B. Stanbury et al., 522–560. New York: McGraw-Hill.

Smolin, L. A., N. S. Benevenga, and S. Berlow. 1981. The use of betaine for the treatment of homocystinuria. *J. Pediatr.* 99:467–472.

See suggested readings for INBORN ERRORS OF METABOLISM.

homogentisic acid. An intermediate in the pathway that converts PHENYLALANINE and TYROSINE to fumarate and acetoacetic acid. Persons with the genetic defect alkaptonuria lack *homogentisic acid oxidase* so that homogentisic acid is excreted in the urine. When the urine is made alkaline and exposed to oxygen, it turns black. See also: ALKAPTONURIA.

hormone. A chemical substance synthesized in one organ or gland that acts as a messenger to stimulate or inhibit the reactions in another organ or tissue. Hormones may be steroids, proteins, or protein derivatives.

hydrogenation. The process of adding hydrogen atoms to a substance to alter its physical or chemical characteristics. Hydrogen is most often added to a TRIACYLGLYCEROL (fat) that contains unsaturated FATTY ACIDS. Complete hydrogenation of the unsaturated fatty acids yields saturated fatty acids. This alteration would make the fat more solid at room temperature by raising its melting point.

hydrolase. A class of ENZYMES which catalyze the addition of the elements of water to a substance, thus breaking it into two substances. A hydrolase hydrolyzes a specific bond. For example, *thrombin*, one of the blood clotting enzymes, will only hydrolyze the bond between the carboxyl side of ARGININE and the amino side of GLYCINE in the fibrinogen chain. *Thrombin* will not act on a bond between arginine and glycine when their positions in the chain are reversed. Under the influence of *thrombin*, a hydroxyl ion from an ionized water molecule will be added to arginine and a hydrogen ion will be added to glycine, cleaving the fibrinogen chain at that point. See also: HYDROLYSIS.

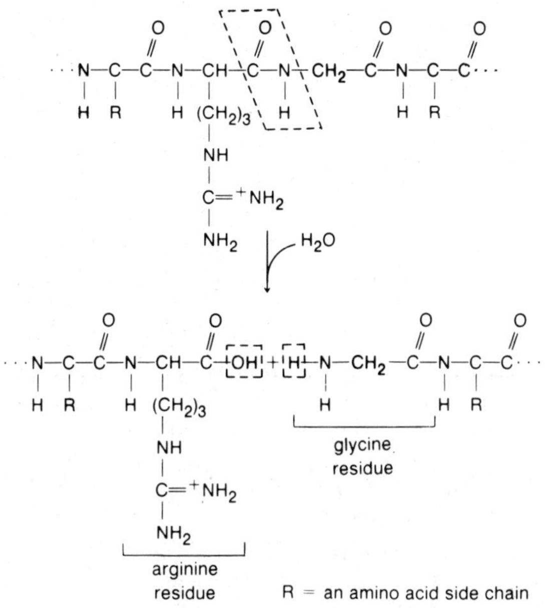

During the clotting process, thrombin hydrolyzes the peptide bond between arginine and glycine in the fibrinogen chain

hydrolysis. The process by which a molecule is broken apart with the addition of water. Hydrolysis occurs under the influence of ENZYMES, known as hydrolases, which are involved in a wide variety of catabolic processes. During hydrolysis, the hydroxyl ion of an ionized water molecule is added to the "residue" on one side of a bond while a hydrogen ion is added to the "residue" on the other side. Thus the substrate molecule, for example, a disaccharide, is broken into two molecules, in this case two monosaccharides. See also: HYDROLASE.

hydrophilic. A descriptive term indicating that a molecule is polar (has regions of opposing charges) and associates with water molecules.

hydrophobic. A descriptive term indicating that a molecule is nonpolar and is repelled by water molecules.

hydroxylysine (Hyl). A special amino acid formed from LYSINE after incorporation in the COLLAGEN fibers by the action of *lysyl hydroxylase*. Molecular oxygen is necessary for hydroxylation to occur. One oxygen atom is attached at carbon-5 and the other is added to α-ketoglutarate. Hydroxylysine is rarely found in any other protein.

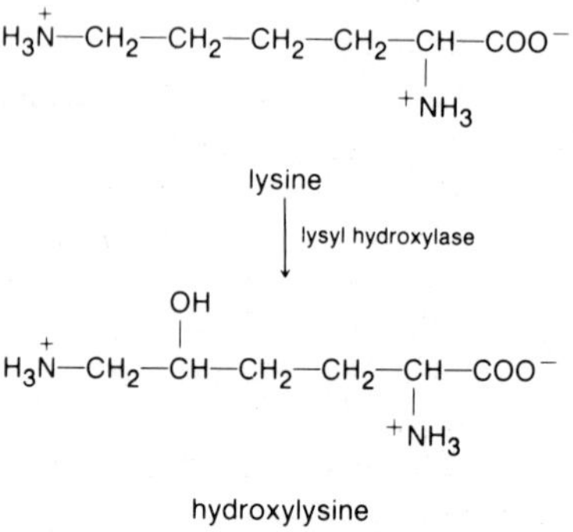

$$H_3\overset{+}{N}-CH_2-CH_2-CH_2-CH_2-CH-COO^-$$
$$\overset{+}{N}H_3$$

lysine

lysyl hydroxylase

$$OH$$
$$H_3\overset{+}{N}-CH_2-CH-CH_2-CH_2-CH-COO^-$$
$$\overset{+}{N}H_3$$

hydroxylysine

Formation of hydroxylysine

hydroxyproline (Hyp). A special amino acid formed from PROLINE by hydroxylation after it has been incorporated in a COLLAGEN chain. This reaction is catalyzed by *prolyl hydroxylase*, which has a ferrous ion at its active site and requires VITAMIN C to keep the IRON in the ferrous state. Molecular oxygen is also necessary if hydroxylation is to occur. One oxygen atom is attached at carbon-4 of proline; the other atom is added to α-ketoglutarate converting it to succinate. Hydroxyproline, rarely found in any other protein, favors the packing together of collagen fibers.

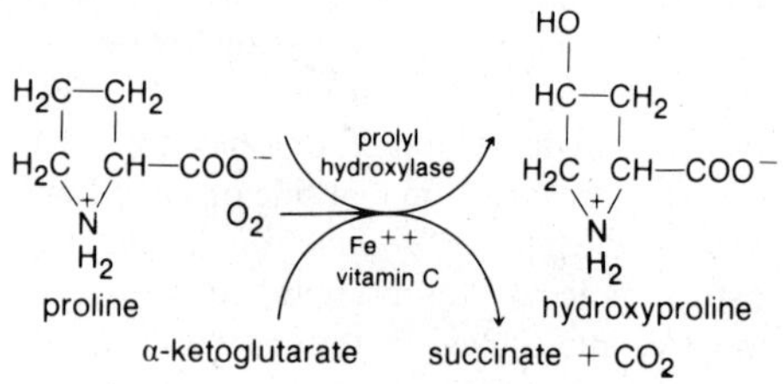

Formation of hydroxyproline

hyperammonemia type I (carbamoyl-phosphate synthetase deficiency). A rare genetic disorder characterized by accumulation of ammonia (NH_3) in the blood causing marked hyperammonemia.

hyperammonemia type II (ornithine-carbamoyl transferase deficiency). The most common of UREA CYCLE disorders. The defect is an x-linked, dominant trait characterized by a low level of citrulline and a high level of ammonia in the blood.

hyperkalemia.   A serum POTASSIUM level above 6 mEq/L. A level of 7 mEq/L is considered an emergency situation.

hyperuricemia.   An increase in the serum level of uric acid. Several disorders involving purine degradation may result in hyperuricemia. This increase in levels of uric acid predates or accompanies the painful symptoms of arthritis or uric acid stones. The condition may begin during adolescence for males but usually does not appear in females until the onset of menopause. If the uricemia is caused by a genetic defect in an enzyme, uricemia may be present at birth.   See also: PURINE, PYRIMIDINE BASES.

hypokalemia.   A serum POTASSIUM level below 3.5 mEq/L.

i

iatrogenic. A condition that is caused by a medical or hospital regimen. Originally, the word meant physician-induced but usage has broadened its definition. For example, iatrogenic malnutrition may result from not eating during such medical regimens as diagnostic testing, chemotherapy, or following surgery.

idiopathic. A disease without recognizable cause, as if of spontaneous origin.

immunoprotein (antibody, immunoglobulin). A protein, usually found in the gamma globulin fraction of blood plasma, that develops in response to an antigen (such as a bacteria or toxin) and reacts with the antigen to cause its destruction.

SUGGESTED READINGS

Beisel, W. R. 1982. Single nutrients and immunity. *Am. J. Clin. Nutr.* 35:417–468.

Feigin, R. D. 1977. Interaction of nutrition and infection. *Am. J. Clin. Nutr.* 30:1553–1563.

Gross, R. L., and P. M. Newberne, 1980. Role of nutrition in immunologic function. *Physiol. Rev.* 60:188–302.

McMurray, D. N., et al. 1981. Development of impaired cell-mediated immunity in milk and moderate malnutrition. *Am. J. Clin. Nutr.* 34:68–77.

Mullin, T. J., and J. R. Kirkpatrick. 1981. The effect of nutritional support on immune competency in patients suffering from trauma, sepsis, or malignant disease. *Surgery* 90:610–615.

inborn errors of metabolism. A genetic disorder in which the directions for making an enzyme are missing or altered in the DNA. When an enzyme that converts compound A to compound B is missing or defective, the amount

153

of compound A will increase and that of compound B will decrease. Either or both of these results may be critical: compound A may reach toxic levels or the absence of compound B may interfere with a crucial, life-supporting reaction. Such a situation occurs in phenylketonuria (PKU). See also: PHENYLALANINE.

SUGGESTED READINGS

Batshaw, M. L., et al. 1982. Treatment of inborn errors of urea synthesis. *N. Engl. J. Med.* 306:1387–1392.

Batshaw, M. L., G. H. Thomas, and S. W. Brusilow. 1981. New approaches to the diagnosis and treatment of inborn errors of urea synthesis. *Pediatrics* 68:290–297.

Clow, C. L., T. M. Reade, and C. R. Scriver. 1981. Outcome of early and long term management of classical maple syrup urine disease. *Pediatrics* 68:856–862.

Collins, F. S., et al. 1980. Neonatal argininosuccinic aciduria—survival after early diagnosis and dietary management. *J. Pediatr.* 96:429–431.

Elsas, L. J., and D. J. Danner, 1982. The role of thiamin in maple syrup urine disease. *Ann. N.Y. Acad. Sci.* 378:404–421.

Frimpter, G. W. 1973. Aminoacidurias due to inherited disorders of metabolism. Part 2. *N. Engl. J. Med.* 289:895–901.

Goodman, S. I. 1981. Antenatal diagnosis of defects of ureagenesis. *Pediatrics* 68:446–447, 459–462.

Mohoney, M. J., and L. E. Rosenberg, 1980. Inherited defects of B$_{12}$ metabolism. *Am. J. Med.* 48:584–593.

Stanbury, J. B., et al., eds. 1983. *The metabolic basis of inherited disease,* 5th ed. New York: McGraw-Hill.

Wellner, D., and A. Meister. 1981. A survey of inborn errors of amino acid metabolism and transport in man. *Ann. Rev. Biochem.* 50:911–968.

Wolf, B., et al. 1981. Propionic acidemia: A clinical update. *J. Pediatr.* 99:835–846.

inositol. An alcohol (carbohydrate) that is a part of a phosphoglyceride in cell MEMBRANE structures.

insulin. A hormone, secreted by the beta cells of the islets of Langerhans in the pancreas, that enhances the uptake of GLUCOSE by the peripheral tissues and thus maintains the BLOOD GLUCOSE LEVEL within normal limits. Insulin also increases the synthesis of GLYCOGEN from glucose, decreases GLUCONEOGENESIS, and promotes lipogenesis in the fat cells.

Without sufficient insulin, the blood glucose concentration following a high-carbohydrate meal may increase tremendously, perhaps above 220 mg/100ml. If the kidneys were unable to reabsorb the glucose, it would "spill" into

Inositol

the urine, causing glucosuria. In DIABETES MELLITUS, the failure to produce sufficient insulin may result in chronic hyperglycemia and in glucosuria. Counter-regulatory hormones of insulin include the glucocorticoids such as cortisol, a steroid hormone of the adrenal cortex, and glucagon, a pancreatic hormone that increases gluconeogenesis and lipolysis.

The action of insulin is thought to be potentiated, in part, by chromium, which functions as part of an organic compound called "glucose tolerance factor." Chromium supplements have been shown to improve impaired glucose tolerance.   See also: BLOOD GLUCOSE LEVEL; DIABETES MELLITUS; GLUCAGON.

SUGGESTED READINGS

Stanbury, J. B., et al., eds. 1983. *The metabolic basis of inherited disease*, 5th ed. New York: McGraw-Hill.

intrinsic factor.   A protein secreted by the gastric cells and required for the absorption of vitamin B_{12}.   See also: VITAMIN B_{12}.

iodide (I^-).   An ion of the element iodine. Iodine exists naturally as iodate and as iodide salts with SODIUM, POTASSIUM, or COPPER. Sources of iodine include sea foods, vegetables grown in iodine-rich soil, and foods seasoned with iodized salt. In the intestinal tract, iodine is reduced to iodide and absorbed in the small intestine. In the body, inorganic iodide is distributed in extracellular fluid, plasma, and red blood cells, as well as concentrated in higher amounts in the salivary glands and the gastric mucosa. In the thyroid gland, as well as in the blood, iodine occurs in an organic form.

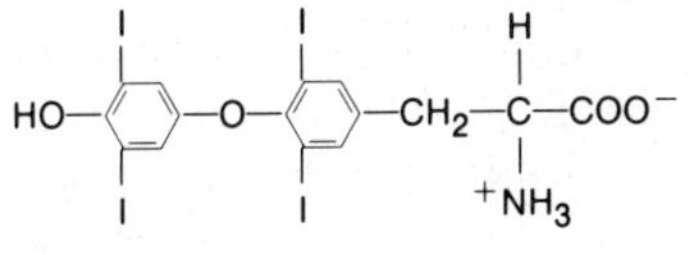

Thyroxine (T_4)

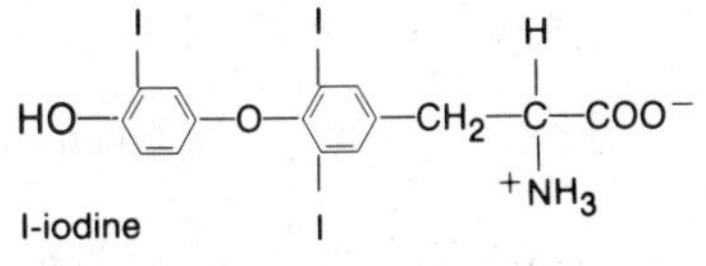

I-iodine

Triiodothyronine (T_3)

Iodine is extracted from the blood by the thyroid gland for the synthesis of two hormones, thyroxine (T_4), also called 3,5,3',5'-tetraiodothyronine, and 3,5,3'-triiodothyronine (T_3). By stimulating processes that increase oxygen consumption and heat production the thyroid hormones have a profound effect on the level of activity of every tissue of the body. It is not entirely clear how thyroid hormones function although their effects on the basal metabolic rate (BMR) have been known for many years. BMR is the rate, determined at least twelve hours after a meal, at which a resting person consumes oxygen when awake. BMR is expressed either in terms of kilocalories of heat produced per kilogram of body weight per time or of liters of oxygen consumed/ kg /time. It is a function of body surface plus the activity of the thyroid gland.

Hyperthyroidism leads to an increase in the BMR and to the stimulation of all activities in cells. (Brain tissue and some reproductive tissues are not stimulated by increased thyroid hormone secretion.) Nervousness, inability to sleep, and weight loss are some of the presenting symptoms. In hyperthyroidism and/or a deficiency of iodine, the thyroid gland enlarges in an effort to trap more iodine from the capillaries coursing through it. The enlargement is goiter which is sometimes visible on the neck. Radical treatment of goiter is removal of some of the thyroid tissue by surgery or radiation.

Hypothyroidism, also called myxedema, leads to a decrease in oxygen consumption. Sluggish behavior, fatigue and other physical complaints accompany the slowing down of activity. The treatment for hypothyroidism is administration of thyroid hormone.

The synthesis of these hormones in the thyroid gland involves iodination of TYROSINE residues found in the molecule thyroglobulin, a glycoprotein. Iodine reacts with tryosine to form 3-monoiodotyrosine (MIT) or 3,5-diiodotryosine (DIT). Two molecules of DIT may then react to form 3,5,3',5'-tetraiodothyronine (T_4) or DIT and MIT may react to form 3,5,3'-triiodothyronine (T_3). These reactions are catalyzed by peroxidases. T_4 is the major hormone produced, although T_3 is more metabolically active.

In the blood, T_4 and T_3 are found free or bound to thyroxine-binding globulin, pre-albumin and albumin. The liver may catalyze T_4 to T_3, reverse T_3 (rT_3), an inactive compound, and tetraiodothyroacetic acid, an excretory product.

Both T_4 and T_3 are secreted into the bloodstream in response to a message from the TSH (thyroid-stimulating hormone, also called thyrotropin) which is secreted by the pituitary gland. The body's response to the secretion of the thyroid hormones is: stimulated growth, increased protein synthesis, increased production of the oxidative enzymes and overall increased oxygen consumption.

SUGGESTED READINGS

Oppenheimer, J. H. 1979. Thyroid hormone action at the cellular level. *Science* 203:971–979.
Oppenheimer, J. H. 1985. Thyroid hormone action at the nuclear level. *Ann. Intern. Med.* 102:374–384.

iron (ferrous, Fe^{++}, ferric, Fe^{+++}). A metallic ion whose central role in the body is in the transport of oxygen and electrons. Ferrous, reduced iron, is designated as Fe(II) or Fe^{++}; ferric, oxidized iron is designated as Fe(III) or Fe^{+++}. Iron forms a part of HEME, hemoglobin, myoglobin, cytochromes, iron-sulfur protein, and many ENZYMES, such as *prolyl hydroxylase* required in the formation of COLLAGEN.

In cytochromes, which are electron carriers, iron changes valence as the cytochromes pick up and deliver electrons in the RESPIRATORY CHAIN. However, in hemoglobin and myoglobin, which are oxygen carriers, iron does not change valence. Only reduced iron becomes incorporated in these two molecules and it remains reduced during pick up and delivery of oxygen.

The only electron carrier in the respiratory chain that is not a cytochrome is an iron-sulfur protein. MoFe protein, another iron-sulfur protein, is joined by two molecules of MOLYBDENUM (Mo). This protein is necessary for inert nitrogen to undergo fixation into ammonia by nitrogen-fixing bacteria. These reactions occur in the soil and are important for the synthesis of amino acids in plants.

The body absorbs only a small percentage of the iron that is brought to it in food but it saves and recycles most of this amount. Absorption of iron is enhanced by the presence of VITAMIN C-containing foods consumed in the same meal. It is inhibited by CALCIUM salts as well as by phytates which are found in whole grain cereals and in some vegetables. The best food sources of iron are of animal origin. Although legumes, prunes, raisins, and molasses also contain iron, it is less absorbable than that present in animal foods.

Despite the body's preservation of iron, iron-deficiency anemia is common. This anemia is characterized by small, red blood cells, known as "microcytic, hypochromic cells," that are pink rather than red. Anemia is prevalent among children and adolecents as well as in menstruating or pregnant women.

Excess iron may occur because of the body's conservation. The danger here is that iron will be deposited in the soft tissues of the body, a condition likely to occur in patients with thalassemia, idiopathic hemochromatosis, or in those who have had frequent blood transfusions. See also: COLLAGEN; CYTOCHROMES; HEME; HEMOCHROMATOSIS; HYDROXY-PROLINE, PHENYLALANINE, TRYPTOPHAN, TRYOSINE, for iron's involvement as a cofactor.

SUGGESTED READINGS

Aisen, P., and I. Listowsky. 1980. Iron transport and storage proteins. *Ann. Rev. Biochem.* 49:357–393.

Bottomley, S. S. 1983. Iron and Vitamin B_6 metabolism in the sideroblastic anemias. In *Nutrition and hematology*, ed. J. Lindenbaum, 203–224. New York: Churchill Livingstone.

Cook, J. D., T. A. Morck, and S. R. Lynch. 1981. The inhibitory effect of soy products on non-heme iron absorption in man. *Am. J. Clin. Nutr.* 34:2622–2629.

Disler, P. B., et al. 1975. The effect of tea on iron absorption. *Gut* 16:193–200.

Finch, C. A., and H. Huebers. 1982. Perspectives in iron metabolism. *N. Engl. J. Med.* 306: 1520–1528.

Hallberg, L. 1981. Bioavailability of dietary iron in man. *Ann. Rev. Nutr.* 1:123–147.

Leigh, M. J., and D. D. Miller. 1983. Effect of pH and chelating agents on iron binding by dietary fiber: Implications for iron availability. *Am. J. Clin. Nutr.* 38:202–213.

Lynch, S. R., and T. A Morck. 1983. Iron deficiency anemia. In *Nutrition and hematology*, ed. J. Lindenbaum, 143–166. New York: Churchill Livingstone.

Morck, T. A., S. R. Lynch, and J. D. Cook. 1983. Inhibition of food iron absorption by coffee. *Am. J. Clin. Nutr.* 37:416–420.

Simpson, K. M., E. R. Morris, and J. D. Cook. 1981. The inhibitory effect of bran on iron absorption in man. *Am. J. Clin. Nutr.* 34:1469–1478.

Skikne, B..S., S. R. Lynch, and J. D. Cook. 1981. Role of gastric acid in food iron absorption. *Gastroenterology* 81:1068–1071.

Solomons, N. W., et al. 1983. Studies on the bioavailability of zinc in humans: Mechanism of the intestinal interaction of non-heme iron and zinc. *J. Nutr.* 113:337–349.

isoelectric point.   The pH of the solution at which a protein will possess an equal number of positively and negatively charged groups, i.e., the protein possesses no net charge.

isoleucine (Ile). A six-carbon, essential, α-amino acid with a branched hydrocarbon side chain. Isoleucine is both glucogenic and ketogenic because during degradation, four of its carbons enter the TCA CYCLE at succinyl-CoA (leading to synthesis of GLUCOSE) and two enter at ACETYL-CoA (leading to synthesis of FATTY ACIDS or KETONE BODIES).

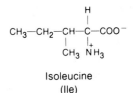

Isoleucine
(Ile)

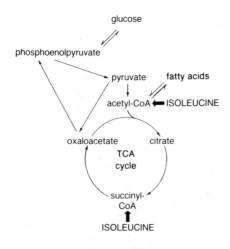

The carbons of isoleucine
enter metabolic pathways

During degradation isoleucine is first transaminated to its α-keto acid and then oxidatively decarboxylated to propionyl-CoA and acetyl-CoA. Propionyl-CoA is converted to D-methyl malonyl-CoA by *propionyl-CoA carboxylase*, a BIOTIN dependent enzyme. L-methyl malonyl-CoA, derived from D-methyl malonyl CoA, is then converted to succinyl-CoA. This reaction is catalyzed by *methylmalonyl mutase*, one of the rare enzymes which uses VITAMIN B_{12} as a coenzyme. Acetyl-CoA either will enter the TCA cycle for oxidation or will proceed to the synthesis of LIPIDS or ketone bodies, depending on the conditions within the cells.

An inborn error of metabolism affecting the oxidative decarboxylation step in the degradation of isoleucine, as well as of LEUCINE and VALINE, results in maple syrup urine disease. See also: BRANCHED CHAIN AMINO ACIDS; MAPLE SYRUP URINE DISEASE.

SUGGESTED READINGS

See suggested readings for BRANCHED-CHAIN AMINO ACIDS; INBORN ERRORS OF METABOLISM.

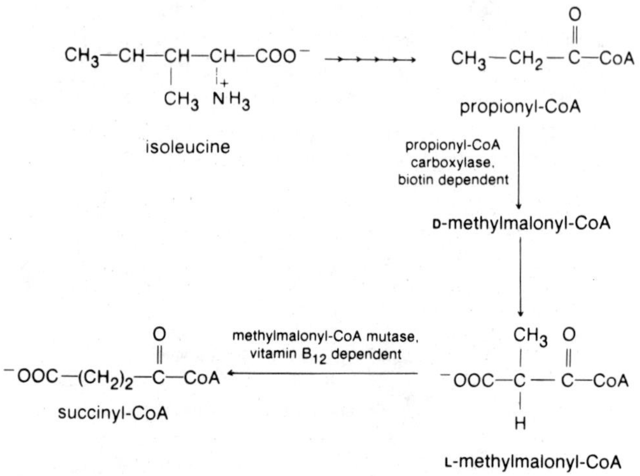

$$CH_3-CH-CH-CH-COO^- \longrightarrow\ \longrightarrow\quad CH_3-CH_2-\overset{\overset{\displaystyle O}{\|}}{C}-CoA$$

$$\qquad\qquad \underset{CH_3}{|}\ \underset{\overset{+}{N}H_3}{|}$$

isoleucine

propionyl-CoA

propionyl-CoA
carboxylase,
biotin dependent

D-methylmalonyl-CoA

$$^-OOC-(CH_2)_2-\overset{\overset{\displaystyle O}{\|}}{C}-CoA \longleftarrow \quad \underset{\text{vitamin } B_{12} \text{ dependent}}{\text{methylmalonyl-CoA mutase,}} \quad ^-OOC-\overset{\overset{\displaystyle CH_3}{|}}{\underset{\underset{\displaystyle H}{|}}{C}}-\overset{\overset{\displaystyle O}{\|}}{C}-CoA$$

succinyl-CoA

L-methylmalonyl-CoA

The conversion of isoleucine to succinyl-CoA.

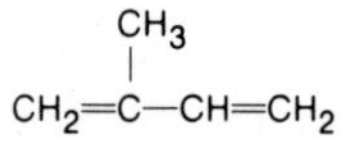

isoprene. A five-carbon unit important in the synthesis of many biomolecules known for their fragrance, such as bay leaves or menthol, and other molecules some of which lend color to tomatoes and carrots. Isoprene is the basic unit in the synthesis of CHOLESTEROL, the side chain of vitamin K_2, and of coenzyme Q_{10} in the mitochondrial RESPIRATORY CHAIN.

$$\underset{\text{Isoprene}}{CH_2{=}\overset{\overset{\displaystyle CH_3}{|}}{C}-CH{=}CH_2}$$

isotopic dilution technique. A method by which the path of a compound can be traced through an organism to its final form and destination. In this method a radioactive isotope is incorporated in a compound that is then introduced into a living organism. From samples of various tissues taken at intervals, chemical analysis reveals what compounds in what amounts are present. The development of this technique contributed to our present understanding of the enzymatic synthesis of many biomolecules.

j

jaundice. A yellow color in the skin that is evidence of an accumulation of bilirubin, a bile pigment produced in the spleen during the breakdown of the HEME portion of hemoglobin, myoglobin, and cytochromes. Usually the liver is able to metabolize the bilirubin as it accumulates and to send it into the upper intestinal tract with bile. In the lower intestine, bilirubin is converted to urobilin prior to excretion in the feces. Jaundice can result from an overproduction of bilirubin or from an inability of the liver to accept, metabolize, and/or secrete this pigment properly so that it backs up in the bloodstream.

Bilirubin's toxicity relates to its effect on developing brain cells. Since newborn infants do not have fully developed systems for eliminating bilirubin, their brain cells are especially vulnerable to attack.

k

K'_{eq}. See EQUILIBRIUM CONSTANT.

ketogenic amino acids. Those AMINO ACIDS whose carbon atoms are converted to ACETYL-CoA and/or acetoacetyl-CoA when they are degraded for energy. Acetyl-CoA and acetoacetyl-CoA are precursors of the KETONE BODIES acetoacetate, β-hydroxybutyrate, and acetone.

LEUCINE is the only completely ketogenic amino acid. Two of its carbons are converted to acetyl-CoA while the other four form acetoacetyl-CoA. PHENYLALANINE and TYROSINE are both gluco- and ketogenic since fumarate, an intermediate of the TCA CYCLE, and acetoacetate, which leads to

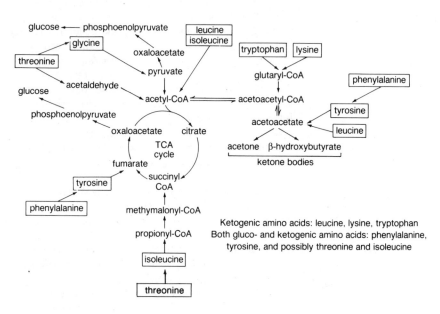

Ketogenic amino acids: leucine, lysine, tryptophan
Both gluco- and ketogenic amino acids: phenylalanine, tyrosine, and possibly threonine and isoleucine

Entry into TCA cycle of carbons of ketogenic amino acids

$$O$$
$$\|$$
$$CH_3-C-CH_2-COO^-$$

acetoacetate

$$OH$$
$$|$$
$$CH_3-C-CH_2-COO^-$$
$$|$$
$$H$$

β-hydroxybutyrate

$$O$$
$$\|$$
$$CH_3-C-CH_3$$

acetone

Ketone bodies

acetoacetyl-CoA, are the products of their degradation. ISO-LEUCINE and THREONINE also may be classified as both gluco- and ketogenic; however, they are more often classified as glucogenic. The remaining ketogenic amino acids are LYSINE and TRYPTOPHAN.

ketone bodies. Acetoacetate, β-hydroxybutyrate, and acetone.

Through the formation of ketone bodies in the liver, other parts of the body are supplied with an energy source. Because the liver cannot oxidize ketone bodies for energy, it exports them to the bloodstream for distribution to other body cells. Skeletal and heart muscles, the brain, and other tissues can oxidize ketone bodies to ACETYL-CoA, which is further oxidized through the TCA CYCLE and RESPIRATORY CHAIN to ATP.

When the liver produces more ketone bodies than the peripheral tissues can oxidize, the level of ketone bodies in the blood can reach toxic levels, resulting in ketosis. The rise in the level of ketone bodies will lower the pH and produce the condition of metabolic ACIDOSIS. Ketosis and metabolic acidosis occur in nutritionally oriented crises such as STARVATION, fasting, low-carbohydrate diet, or uncontrolled DIABETES MELLITUS.

Ketone bodies are produced in the MITOCHONDRIA of liver cells from acetyl-CoA which primarily results from excessive FATTY ACID OXIDATION (in the presence of a low supply of glucose). Among the metabolic and endocrine factors that influence the production of ketone bodies are: the relative concentrations of insulin and glucagon, opposing hormones that respond to the BLOOD GLUCOSE LEVEL and influence the fate of GLUCOSE molecules; the concentration of malonyl-CoA, the product of the committed step in FATTY ACID SYNTHESIS; the concentration of carnitine and *carnitine acyl transferase I*, both of which are required for the transport of FATTY ACIDS from the cytosol to the mitochondria for oxidation; and the supply of oxaloacetate (OAA).

One of the first factors influencing ketogenesis is the ratio of glucagon to insulin in the blood. When this ratio rises (as may occur with fasting, starvation, or low-carbohydrate diets), GLUCONEOGENESIS is stimulated and GLYCOLYSIS is inhibited. In addition, lipolysis, the breakdown of fat deposits mainly in adipose tissues, is stimulated, causing a rise in the level of fatty acids in the blood; the fatty acids are then taken up by the liver.

Two paths are open to fatty acids in the liver: they may be used to synthesize TRIACYLGLYCEROLS in the cytosol, or they may be oxidized to acetyl-CoA in the mitochondria.

Which path is followed is thought to be controlled, in part at least, by the concentration of malonyl-CoA in the cytosol. High levels of malonyl-CoA, generated from a high level of carbohydrate and insulin, inhibit fatty acid oxidation by suppressing the enzyme *carnitine acyl transferase I* that would carry the fatty acids into the mitochondrial matrix for oxidation. Low levels of malonyl-CoA, on the other hand, stimulate the enzyme and encourage fatty acid oxidation causing the level of acetyl-CoA in the mitochondria to rise.

Several theories have been proposed to explain why acetyl-CoA accumulates in the mitochondria. One suggests that a low level of glucose from dietary carbohydrate is responsible since glucose is needed to supply the oxaloacetate (OAA) that will join with the acetate portion of acetyl-CoA to form citrate. Normally, citrate proceeds through the TCA cycle to complete oxidation of the acetate, reforming OAA. Or, if energy (ATP) is not needed, citrate enters the cytosol where it will release the acetate to undergo fatty acid synthesis. Without OAA, however, citrate will not be formed. Thus, in the situation of a high level of acetyl-CoA in the mitochondria with both exit paths—oxidation and fatty acid synthesis—blocked by insufficient glucose, the liver forms ketone bodies.

The first step in ketone body formation is the condensation of two molecules of acetyl-CoA to form acetoacetyl-CoA, a reaction catalyzed by *thiolase*. The CoA attached to

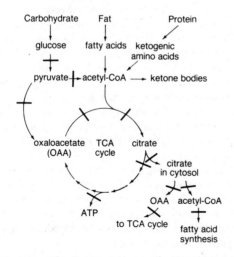

Effect of low glucose supply on
paths available to acetyl-CoA

$$CH_3-\overset{\overset{\displaystyle O}{\|}}{C}-CoA \ + \ CH_3-\overset{\overset{\displaystyle O}{\|}}{C}-CoA \ \xrightarrow{\quad CoA \quad} \ CH_3-\overset{\overset{\displaystyle O}{\|}}{C}-CH_2-\overset{\overset{\displaystyle O}{\|}}{C}-CoA$$

acetyl-CoA   acetyl-CoA   acetoacetyl-CoA

acetyl-CoA
+
H_2O

CoA

$$\overset{\overset{\displaystyle O}{\|}}{^-OOC-CH_2-C-CH_3} \quad \xleftarrow[\text{glutaryl-CoA lyase}]{\text{hydroxymethyl-}} \quad ^-OOC-CH_2-\overset{\overset{\displaystyle OH}{|}}{\underset{\underset{\displaystyle CH_3}{|}}{C}}-CH_2-\overset{\overset{\displaystyle O}{\|}}{C}-CoA$$

acetoacetate*   acetyl-CoA

β-hydroxy-β-methylglutaryl-CoA
(HMG-CoA)

NADH + H⁺

dehydrogenase

NAD⁺

H⁺

CO_2

$$CH_3-\overset{\overset{\displaystyle O}{\|}}{C}-CH_3$$

acetone*

$$^-OOC-CH_2-\overset{\overset{\displaystyle OH}{|}}{CH}-CH_3$$

β-hydroxybutyrate*

The formation of ketone bodies*

the acetoacetyl-CoA is removed by a process called deacylation that results in the formation of β-hydroxy-β-methylglutaryl-CoA (HMG-CoA). When this intermediate is acted upon by *hydroxymethylglutaryl-CoA lyase*, free acetoacetate, a ketone body, is produced.

Another ketone body, β-hydroxybutyrate, results from the action of an NADH-dependent dehydrogenase on the acetoacetate that was formed from acetoacetyl-CoA. The third ketone body, acetone, is produced by the spontaneous decarboxylation of acetoacetate. Because acetone is volatile it is excreted primarily via the lungs imparting a unique, sweet odor to the breath of diabetics or other persons who have a high level of acetoacetate. The other two ketone bodies diffuse into the bloodstream and are picked up by the peripheral tissues.

When ketone bodies arrive in the peripheral tissues, β-hydroxybutyrate is oxidized by an NAD⁺-dependent dehydrogenase to form acetoacetate. Both the acetoacetate that diffused from the liver and that which was produced in the peripheral tissues then react with succinyl-CoA under the influence of a transferase to form acetoacetyl-CoA. Subsequently, the acetoacetyl-CoA is cleaved by *thiolase* to form two acetyl-CoA molecules, which enter the TCA cycle to

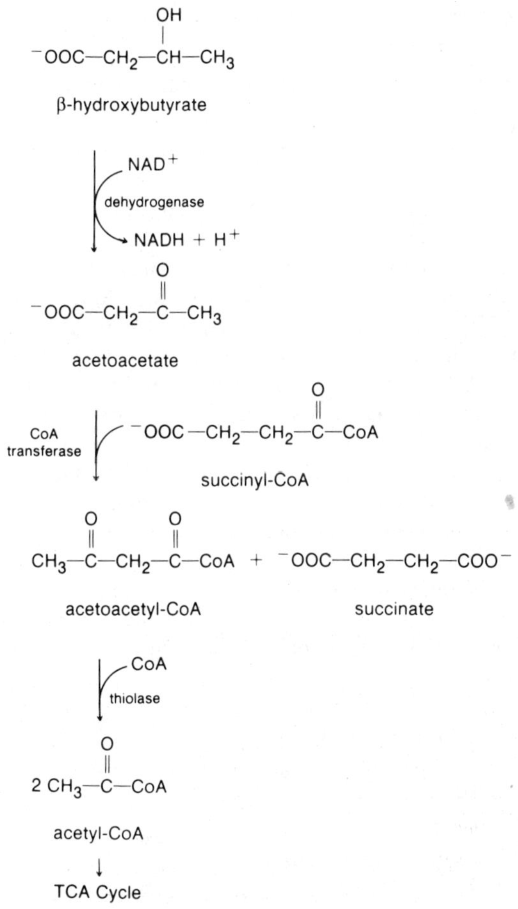

$$OOC-CH_2-\overset{\overset{\displaystyle OH}{|}}{C}H-CH_3$$

β-hydroxybutyrate

NAD$^+$

dehydrogenase

NADH + H$^+$

$$OOC-CH_2-\overset{\overset{\displaystyle O}{\|}}{C}-CH_3$$

acetoacetate

CoA transferase

$$OOC-CH_2-CH_2-\overset{\overset{\displaystyle O}{\|}}{C}-CoA$$

succinyl-CoA

$$CH_3-\overset{\overset{\displaystyle O}{\|}}{C}-CH_2-\overset{\overset{\displaystyle O}{\|}}{C}-CoA \ + \ ^-OOC-CH_2-CH_2-COO^-$$

acetoacetyl-CoA   succinate

CoA

thiolase

$$2 \ CH_3-\overset{\overset{\displaystyle O}{\|}}{C}-CoA$$

acetyl-CoA

↓

TCA Cycle

The degradation of ketone bodies for energy

be oxidized to CO_2, H_2O, and ATP. See also: ACIDOSIS; DIABETES MELLITUS; KETOSIS; STARVATION.

SUGGESTED READINGS

Foster, D. W. 1984. From glycogen to ketones—and back. *Diabetes* 33:1188–1199.

McGarry, J. D., and D. W. Foster. 1980. Regulation of hepatic fatty acid oxidation and ketone body production. *Ann. Rev. Biochem.* 49:395–420.

Robinson, A. M., and D. H. Williamson. 1980. Physiological roles of ketone bodies as substrates and signals in mammalian tissues. *Physiol. Rev.* 60:143–187.

ketonemia. A high level of ketone bodies in the blood. See also: KETOSIS.

ketonuria. A high level of ketone bodies in the urine. See also: KETOSIS.

ketosis (ketoacidosis). Metabolic ACIDOSIS caused by a rise in the plasma level of the acids, acetoacetate and β-hydroxybutyrate. This rise is caused by a shift in fuel usage from GLUCOSE to FATTY ACIDS as the body adapts to a crisis such as STARVATION or uncontrolled DIABETES MELLITUS.

Acetoacetate and β-hydroxybutyrate, along with acetone, known collectively as KETONE BODIES, are formed mostly in the liver from ACETYL-COA. The liver secretes the ketone bodies into the bloodstream where they are extracted by peripheral tissues and oxidized for energy. Ketosis, an abnormal condition, results when the peripheral tissues cannot use the circulating ketone bodies as fast as they are made. The accumulation causes the level of ketone bodies in the blood to rise and the PH of the blood to drop.

If the high level of ketone bodies in the blood (ketonemia) continues to rise, some will spill into the urine (ketonuria). Excretion of the ketone bodies is accompanied by increased loss of water and of the electolytes SODIUM and POTASSIUM. These losses, as well as the drop in pH, are life threatening. See also: ACIDOSIS for more about the dangers of a shift in pH; DIABETES MELLITUS for a further discussion of the shifts in fuel from glucose to ketone bodies and fatty acids in diabetes mellitus; and KETONE BODIES for more about the formation of the ketone bodies.

Krebs cycle. See TCA CYCLE.

L. A small capital L preceding the name of a compound indicates that the compound is a stereoisomer and has an absolute configuration like that of L-glyceraldehyde. See also: AMINO ACIDS.

lactate (lactic acid). See CORI CYCLE; GLYCOLYSIS.

lactose. A disaccharide composed of GLUCOSE and galactose. Lactose is found primarily in dairy products. See also: CARBOHYDRATE STRUCTURE.

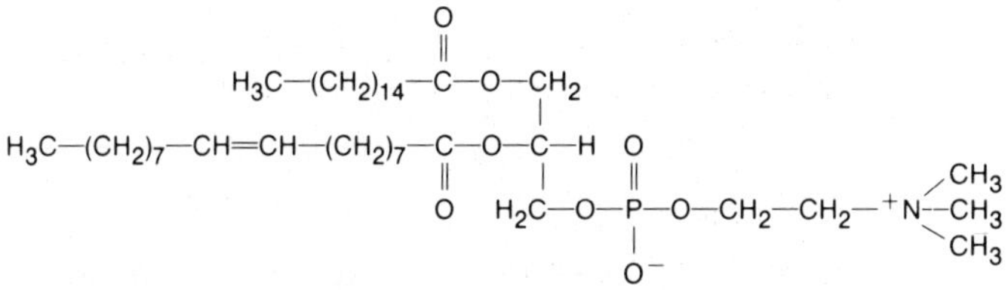

Phosphatidylcholine (lecithin)

LDL. See LOW DENSITY LIPOPROTEINS.

lecithin. The trivial name of a phosphoglyceride whose correct name is phosphatidylcholine. In phosphotidylcholine, the hydroxyl groups at carbons 1 and 2 of glycerol are esterified to the carboxyl groups of a 16-carbon and an 18-carbon fatty acid, respectively. The carbon 3 hydroxyl group of the glycerol is esterified to phosphorylcholine.

Lecithin is a polar lipid and a major component of animal cell MEMBRANES. It also acts as an emulsifier. See also: LIPIDS; LIPID DIGESTION; MEMBRANES.

Lesch-Nyhan syndrome. An inherited metabolic disease, affecting only males, that is characterized by mental retardation, self-mutilation, and renal failure. Biochemically, there is excess uric acid production due to the absence of *hypoxanthine-guanine phosphoribosyl transferase,* which is essential for purine metabolism. See also: PURINE, PYRIMIDINE BASES.

SUGGESTED READINGS

Kelley, W. N., and J. B. Wyngaarden. 1983. Clinical syndromes associated with hypoxanthine-guanine phosphoribosyl transferase deficiency. In *The metabolic basis of inherited disease,* 5th ed., ed. J. B. Stanbury et al, 1115–1143. New York: McGraw-Hill.

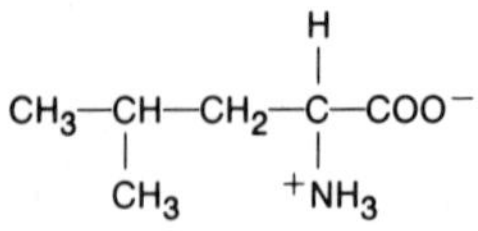

leucine (Leu). An essential, completely ketogenic, six-carbon α-amino acid. Leucine is abundant in globulins and albumins.

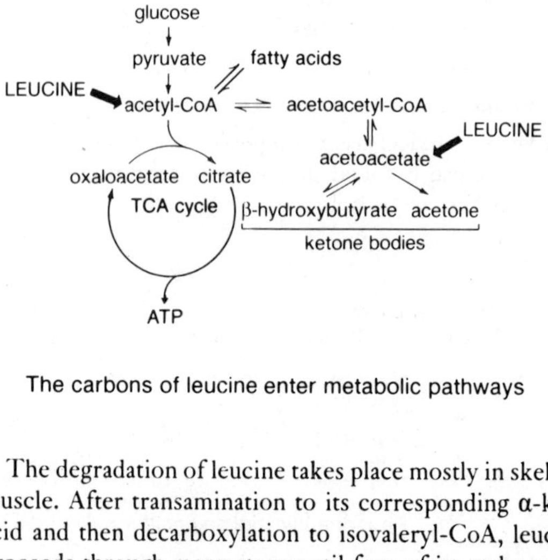

$$CH_3-CH-CH_2-\overset{\overset{\displaystyle H}{|}}{C}-COO^-$$
$$\underset{\displaystyle CH_3}{|} \qquad \underset{\displaystyle {}^+NH_3}{|}$$

Leucine (Leu)

The carbons of leucine enter metabolic pathways

The degradation of leucine takes place mostly in skeletal muscle. After transamination to its corresponding α-keto acid and then decarboxylation to isovaleryl-CoA, leucine proceeds through many steps until four of its carbons are converted to acetoacetate and the other two are converted to ACETYL-COA. In the next-to-last step of this complex degradative process, the intermediate compound formed is β-hydroxy-β-methylglutaryl-CoA (HMG-CoA) which, as a precursor of mevalonate, makes leucine a precursor of CHOLESTEROL. HMG-CoA is cleaved to acetoacetate and acetyl-CoA, which may lead to the formation of KETONE BODIES, thus explaining leucine's strong ketogenic effect.

Many vitamins participate in these degradation steps. In the oxidative decarboxylation steps, THIAMIN (TPP), RIBOFLAVIN (FAD), and NIACIN (NAD$^+$) are required. VITAMIN B$_6$

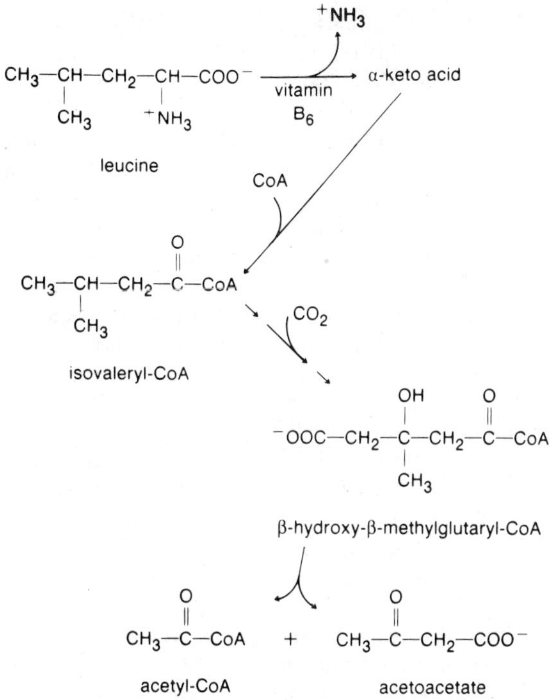

$$\underset{\underset{CH_3}{|}}{CH_3-CH-CH_2-}\underset{\underset{^+NH_3}{|}}{CH-COO^-} \xrightarrow[\text{vitamin B}_6]{^+NH_3} \alpha\text{-keto acid}$$

leucine

CoA

$$\underset{\underset{CH_3}{|}}{CH_3-CH-CH_2-}\overset{\overset{O}{||}}{C}-CoA$$

isovaleryl-CoA

CO_2

$$^-OOC-CH_2-\underset{\underset{CH_3}{|}}{\overset{\overset{OH}{|}}{C}}-CH_2-\overset{\overset{O}{||}}{C}-CoA$$

β-hydroxy-β-methylglutaryl-CoA

$$CH_3-\overset{\overset{O}{||}}{C}-CoA \quad + \quad CH_3-\overset{\overset{O}{||}}{C}-CH_2-COO^-$$

acetyl-CoA   acetoacetate

Degradation of leucine

is required in the transamination step; riboflavin (FAD) is required in the dehydrogenation step. BIOTIN is involved in carboxylation and COENZYME A (made from PANTOTHENIC ACID) is the acyl carrier.

SUGGESTED READINGS

Hutson, S. M., et al. 1980. Regulation of leucine and alpha keto isocaproic acid metabolism in skeletal muscle. *J. Biol. Chem.* 255:2418–2426.

See suggested readings for BRANCHED-CHAIN AMINO ACIDS; IN-BORN ERRORS OF METABOLISM.

linoleic acid. See ESSENTIAL FATTY ACIDS.

linolenic acid. See ESSENTIAL FATTY ACIDS.

lipid digestion. The process by which dietary LIPIDS, especially TRIACYLGLYCEROLS, are broken down so they can be absorbed in the intestine. The principal action in lipid, or fat, digestion that differs from protein and carbohydrate digestion is that of making the hydrophobic fats compatible with the watery fluids of the body. Before chemical action of enzymes (lipases) on the bonds of triacylglycerols can occur, the physical action of emulsification must take place.

No significant digestive action on fats occurs in the mouth except, of course, the warming of the fat and the physical breakup of large bites of fatty food. A lingual lipase that acts on fat in milk has been reported. Also, there is a lipase in the stomach that breaks some bonds on short-chain FATTY ACIDS. However, these actions are thought to be insignificant.

Thus, the fats linger in the stomach while other nutrients, principally protein, are digested. Small boluses of food containing some carbohydrate and protein fragments plus fat are released from the stomach into the top part of the small intestine, the duodenum. As the fats arrive in the duodenum, the cells of the small intestine detect their presence and secrete a hormone, cholecystokinin, which triggers the release of bile from the gallbladder. (Bile is synthesized in the liver from CHOLESTEROL that is first converted to bile acids, then bound to GLYCINE or taurine, and stored in the gallbladder.)

BILE SALTS are the detergents that break up the large aggregations of fats into small droplets in a process called emulsification. The fat droplets, in turn, are surrounded by fluid that contains lipases. The hydrophobic, nonpolar region of the bile salt is attracted to the fat and the hydrophilic polar region is attracted to the fluid, thus stabilizing the suspension of the fat droplets in the fluid. When the droplets are in close contact with the fluid, the lipases can "reach" the chemical bonds and hydrolyze the lipids.

Most of the fat in food is in the form of triacylglycerols. *Pancreatic lipase* hydrolyzes the bonds between the fatty acids of carbon 1 and 3 of glycerol, leaving a 2-monoglyceride. The end products of fat digestion, primarily fatty acids, glycerol, and monoglycerides, form micelles that are then absorbed into the intestinal cells. The bile salts are absorbed lower in the small intestinal tract and are returned to the liver via the lymph system, a path known as enterohepatic circulation.

Within the intestinal cell, the longer-chain fatty acids and the monoglycerides are re-formed into triacylglycerols, a process requiring ATP, CoA, and MAGNESIUM (Mg^{++}). The triacylglycerols are then incorporated into chylomicrons, which contain cholesterol and have a hydrophilic coat of phospholipids and protein. The chylomicrons then enter the lymphatic system and are carried to the thoracic duct, which empties into the subclavian vein.

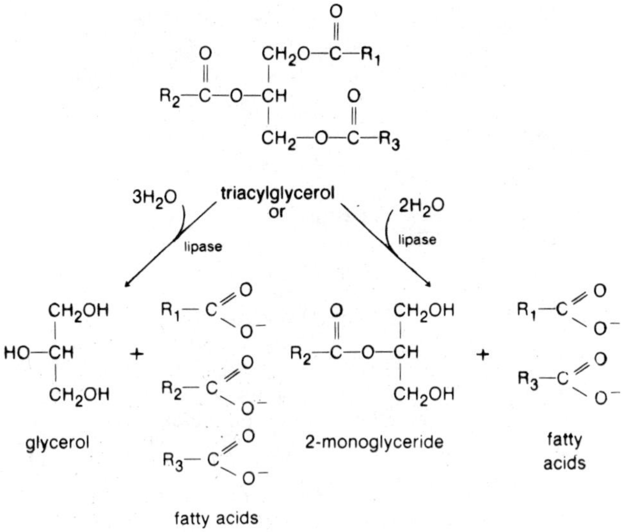

Digestion of triacylglycerol to glycerol and 3 fatty acids
or to 2-monoglyceride and 2 fatty acids
R_1, R_2, R_3 = hydrocarbon tails of fatty acids

The short-chain and medium-chain fatty acids, that is, those that contain fewer than twelve carbons, are transported from the intestinal cell to the bloodstream, where they may be bound to albumin. Free glycerol may also pass directly into the portal blood.

Lecithin, the phosphoglyceride present in food, is hydrolyzed by *phosphorylase A₂* in the number 2 position, yielding free fatty acid and a lysolecithin, both of which are absorbed. In food, cholesterol is joined in an ester linkage to fatty acids and also occurs as free cholesterol. In the intestinal tract, esterified cholesterol is hydrolyzed by *cholesterol esterase;* the free cholesterol, along with the fatty acid, is absorbed. Both the cholesterol and the phospholipids are incorporated into the chylomicron for transport through the body.

lipids. A class of biomolecules that have as their common properties their insolubility in water and their solubility in organic solvents such as benzene, chloroform, or ether. Lipids act as important constituents in membrane structures, as concentrated metabolic fuels, as coatings for surfaces, as insulating or padding for internal organs, and some, such as the fat-soluble vitamins and steroid hormones, have highly specialized roles to perform.

In the diet, some lipids provide calories (9 kcal/g) and enhance the taste and smell of food (recall the distinctive odor of breakfast bacon frying). Fat-rich foods in the diet introduce a number of essential nutrients that the human body cannot synthesize: vitamins A, D, E, and K, as well as the ESSENTIAL FATTY ACIDS, linoleic and linolenic. Dietary fat as well as other fuel nutrients eaten in excess of need are stored in the body as fat (mostly triacylglycerol).

Lipids are classified as simple, compound, and derived. Some of these also are classified as neutral lipids, meaning that they are uncharged molecules. Simple lipids include the familiar fats, oils, and waxes.

Fats are compounds that have a glycerol (a three-carbon alcohol) backbone with FATTY ACIDS, which replace the hydroxyl groups, joined in an ester linkage to one or more of the three carbons. These have the chemical designation of mono-, di-, or triacylglycerols.

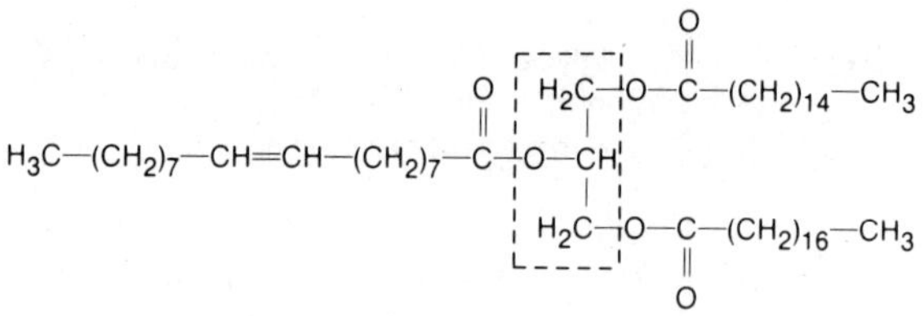

$$H_3C-(CH_2)_7-CH=CH-(CH_2)_7-C-O-CH$$

Triacyglycerol (triglyceride)

Oils have the same general chemical structure as fats but are more fluid at the same temperature. This ability of the molecules to flow over each other (as in corn oil used for cooking) rather than to be packed together (as in lard) is due to "kinks" in the fatty acid chains that are attached to the glycerol backbone. The kinks are caused by rigidity in the chain where a double bond between carbons appears. Such fatty acids are said to be unsaturated. Most unsaturated fatty acids come from plant foods rather than from animal foods; an exception is coconut oil, which is saturated. Another oil should be singled out for mention: mineral oil. Mineral oil cannot be absorbed and because of this attribute and its lubricating properties is advertised as a laxative. However, health professionals do not usually recommend that mineral oil be used in this way, and it is no longer allowed in commercially prepared foods such as salad dressings, since it dissolves the fat-soluble vitamins and carries them out of the body.

Waxes are composed of fatty acids joined in ester linkage to a long-chain alcohol. The alcohol in this instance may have as many as 36 carbons, or it may be cyclic, such as CHOLESTEROL. Waxes are secreted by skin glands to keep the skin pliable and lubricated.

Compound lipids have groups besides fatty acids joined to the alcohol. They are named according to the kind of group that is attached to the fatty acid and alcohol. Prominent compound lipids are the phospholipids, glycolipids, and LIPOPROTEINS.

Phospholipids, because they possess a hydrophilic polar head (the phosphoric acid end) and a long, hydrophobic, hydrocarbon tail, are the major components of MEMBRANES in all biological systems. Because phospholipids are both hydrophilic and hydrophobic they are said to be amphipathic.

The major phospholipids found in membranes are the phosphoglycerides. The phosphoglycerides have a glycerol backbone with fatty acids attached at carbons 1 and 2 and phosphoric acid attached at carbon 3. All phosphoglycerides contain two non-polar tails from their long-chain fatty acids. In addition, phosphoglycerides have an alcohol attached to the phosphoric acid. The parent compound of phosphoglycerides is phosphatidic acid which is an intermediate in the biosynthesis of phosphoglycerides.

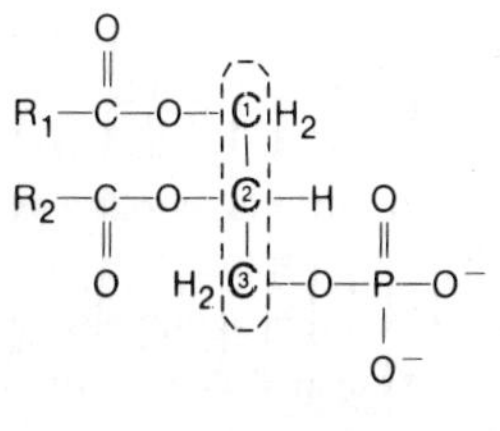

Phosphatidate
(phosphatidic acid, a phospholipid)

R_1 and R_2 = fatty acids
glycerol backbone is circled

The other phosphoglycerides have the same glycerol backbone and, in addition, attach other alcohols in an ester linkage to the phosphoric acid group. These are named according to the alcohol attached; for example, phosphatidylethanolamine, phosphatidylcholine, phosphatidylserine, or phosphatidylinositol. Of these, phosphatidylethanolamine (also known as ethanolamine phosphoglyceride or cephalin) and phosphatidylcholine (also known as choline phosphoglyceride or lecithin) are the most prominent in animal membranes.

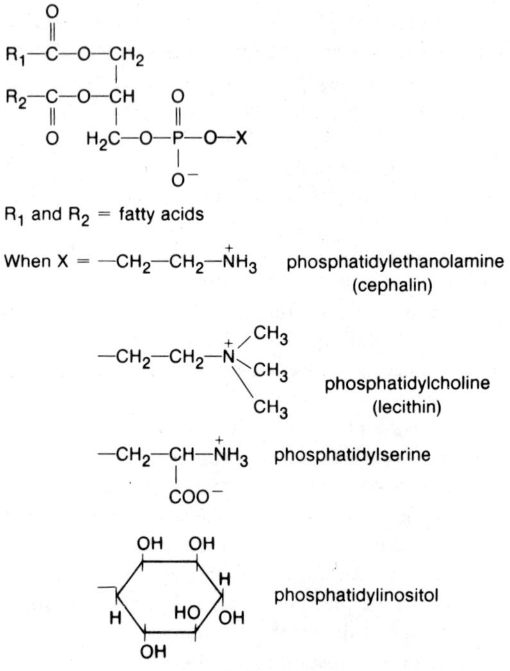

$$R_1-\overset{\overset{\textstyle O}{\|}}{C}-O-CH_2$$

$$R_2-\underset{\underset{\textstyle O}{\|}}{C}-O-\underset{\underset{\textstyle H_2C-O-\overset{\overset{\textstyle O}{\|}}{P}-O-X}{|}}{CH}$$

$$\overset{|}{O^-}$$

R_1 and R_2 = fatty acids

When X = $-CH_2-CH_2-\overset{+}{N}H_3$ phosphatidylethanolamine
(cephalin)

$-CH_2-CH_2-\overset{+}{N}\Big\langle\begin{matrix}CH_3\\CH_3\\CH_3\end{matrix}$ phosphatidylcholine
(lecithin)

$-CH_2-\underset{\underset{\textstyle COO^-}{|}}{CH}-\overset{+}{N}H_3$ phosphatidylserine

phosphatidylinositol

Some phosphoglycerides

In sphingomyelin, the glycerol backbone is replaced by sphingosine. A fatty acid is attached at the amino group of sphingosine and choline phosphoglyceride is attached to the terminal hydroxyl group.

The glycolipids, like sphingomyelin, have a sphingosine backbone but have a sugar linked to the terminal hydroxyl

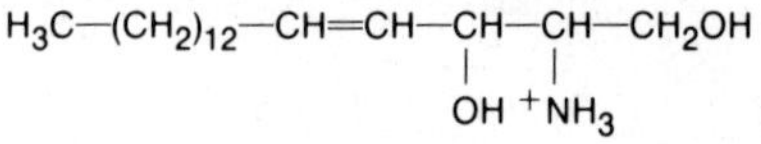

$$H_3C-(CH_2)_{12}-CH=CH-\underset{\underset{\textstyle OH}{|}}{CH}-\underset{\underset{\textstyle {}^+NH_3}{|}}{CH}-CH_2OH$$

Sphingosine

$$H_3C-(CH_2)_{12}-CH=CH-\underset{\underset{\textstyle OH}{|}}{CH}-\underset{\underset{\textstyle NH}{|}}{CH}-CH_2-O-\overset{\overset{\textstyle O}{\|}}{\underset{\underset{\textstyle O^-}{|}}{P}}-O-(CH_2)_2-\overset{+}{N}\Big\langle\begin{matrix}CH_3\\CH_3\\CH_3\end{matrix}$$

$$\underset{\underset{\textstyle R}{|}}{C=O}$$ fatty acid unit   phosphorylcholine unit

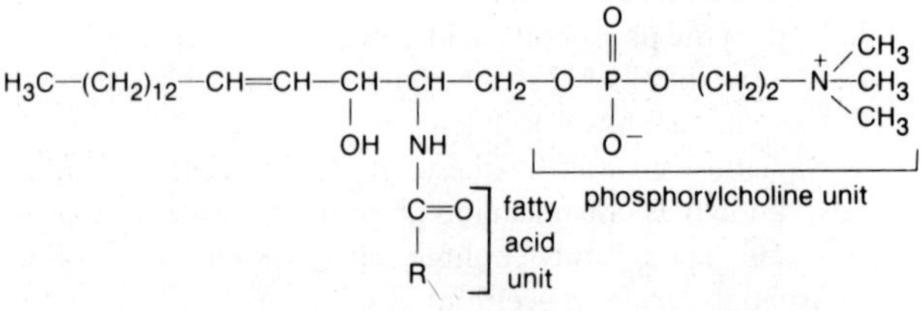

Sphingomyelin

of sphingosine. The cerebrosides, a prominent group of glycolipids abundant in neural tissues, especially the myelin sheaths, have either glucose or galactose as the sugar. Gangliosides are a complex group of glycolipids with large, negatively charged heads. These are found on the outer surface of membranes, particularly those of nerve cells.

Lipoproteins are composed of triglycerides, cholesterol, phospholipids, and protein in various concentrations. The best known of the lipoproteins are in mammalian blood plasma and function to carry hydrophobic lipids throughout the body in the lymphatic fluid and the blood.

Derived lipids are those which are derived by hydrolysis of the lipids above. Derived lipids include fatty acids, steroids, fatty aldehydes and KETONE BODIES.

The steroids, including BILE SALTS, cholesterol, adrenocorticoid hormones, sex hormones, and VITAMIN D, have a cyclopentane ring (D) attached to three phenanthrene rings (A, B, C). See also: BILE SALTS; CHOLESTEROL; CIS-, TRANS-BONDS; FAT-SOLUBLE VITAMINS; FATTY ACID OXIDATION; FATTY ACID SYNTHESIS; FATTY ACIDS; KETONE BODIES; LIPOPROTEINS; MEMBRANES; TRIACYLGLYCEROLS; VITAMIN D.

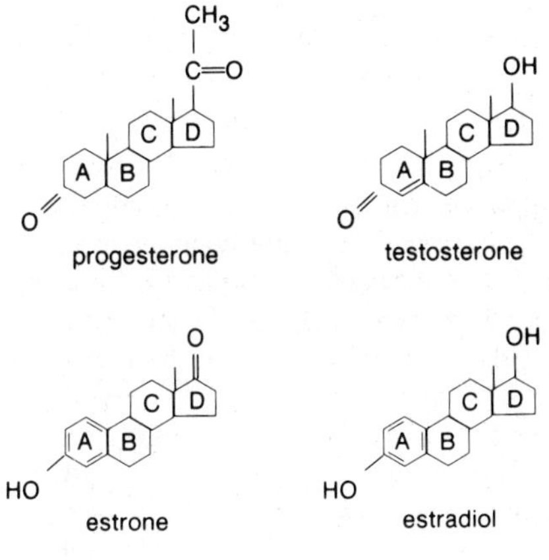

progesterone

testosterone

estrone

estradiol

Steroids

lipogenesis. The synthesis of LIPIDS. See also: BIOTIN, THE COENZYME; CHOLESTEROL; FATTY ACID SYNTHESIS; TRIACYLGLYCEROLS.

SUGGESTED READINGS

Schroepfer, G. J., Jr. 1981. Sterol biosynthesis. *Ann. Rev. Biochem.* 50:585–621.

Wakil, S. J., J. K. Stoops, and V. C. Joshi. 1983. Fatty acid synthesis and its regulation. *Ann. Rev. Biochem.* 52:537–579.

lipoic acid (thioctic acid).   A critical compound in the oxidative decarboxylation of pyruvate and α-ketoglutarate. As part of the pyruvate dehydrogenase complex, which assists in the conversion of pyruvate to ACETYL-COA, the long carbon chain of lipoic acid reaches out like an arm to pick up an acetyl group and transfer it to the next enzyme in the complex. The long arm attaches to a LYSINE of an enzyme in an ester linkage forming lipoamide. The coenzyme forms of THIAMIN, NIACIN, and RIBOFLAVIN (TPP, NAD$^+$, FAD) are cofactors; PANTOTHENIC ACID is important to this reaction since it is a part of CoA.   See also: THIAMIN PYROPHOSPHATE for a more thorough discussion of the role of lipoic acid.

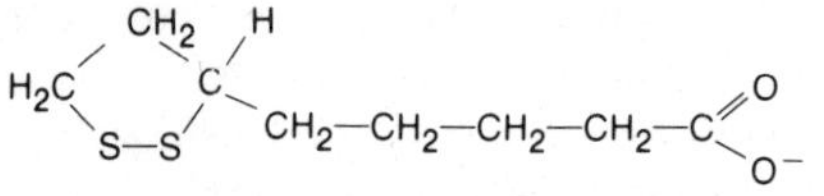

Lipoic acid (thioctic acid)

lipolysis.   The hydrolysis of LIPIDS by ENZYMES termed "lipases." Lipases act on dietary fats as well as on the fat in storage depots.

lipoproteins.   Conjugated proteins consisting of simple proteins combined with lipid components, the latter including CHOLESTEROL, phospholipids, or TRIACYLGLYCEROLS. Lipoproteins are classified according to their density: those with a higher percentage of lipid have a lower density; those with a higher percentage of protein have a higher density. The classification includes chylomicrons, very low density lipoprotein (VLDL), low density lipoprotein (LDL), high density lipoprotein (HDL), or very high density lipoprotein (VHDL) (this class may be included in high density lipoproteins).

Lipoprotein	Density (g/cm^3)
Chylomicrons	< 0.960
VLDL	0.960 - 1.006
LDL	1.006 - 1.059
HDL	1.059 - 1.210
VHDL	> 1.210

Lipoproteins consist of a central region of highly hydrophobic LIPIDS that is surrounded by hydrophilic polar lipids.

Proteins on the outside of the polar lipids "cover" the structure. The polar lipids are arranged such that the charged portion of the molecule lies in the protein and the hydrocarbon tail lies in the lipid. Because of this arrangement, dietary lipids, such as the highly hydrophobic triacylglycerols, may be transported through the watery fluids of the blood plasma after absorption from the intestine.

Some of the proteins, termed "apoproteins," in the lipoproteins have been identified as short peptides, others as very long polypeptides, and some are rich in particular AMINO ACIDS. The two major apoproteins of HDL have been named A-I and A-II. The main apoprotein of LDL is apo-B, which is also found in VLDL and chylomicrons, although the apo-B of chylomicrons has a different amino acid sequence and is smaller than apo-B of LDL or VLDL. The C-apoproteins are thought to be transferred between VLDL, HDL, and chylomicrons. D-apoprotein is found in certain subfractions of HDL, and the arginine-rich E-apoprotein is found in chylomicrons, VLDL, and HDL. Some of these apoproteins have the ability to activate various lipases or have other metabolic functions.

Chylomicrons are produced in the intestinal mucosa and primarily transport dietary lipids, mostly triacylglycerols, some cholesterol, and fat-soluble vitamins to the target tissues: adipose tissue, heart, muscle, and liver cells. After lipids have been extracted from the chylomicron by the various tissues, the chylomicron remnant is taken up by the liver after binding to a membrane receptor specific for apoprotein E.

Very low density lipoproteins are synthesized primarily in the liver and contain cholesterol and triacylglycerols. The triacylglycerols may be derived from carbohydrates, free fatty acids, and/or the chylomicron remnant. Various tissues, such as adipose tissue, may utilize the components of VLDL.

Low density lipoproteins are thought to be derived primarily from the catabolism of VLDL and to contain mostly cholesterol. LDLs are removed from the blood after binding to specific receptors on cell MEMBRANES. Both the LDL and its receptor are taken up by the cells. Within the cell, the cholesterol and other LDL components may be used. The receptor is normally returned to the cell surface.

High density lipoproteins are synthesized primarily in the liver and contain predominantly protein, as well as phospholipids and cholesterol. HDLs are thought to function in the transport of cholesterol from peripheral tissues to the liver.

High HDL concentrations have been shown to be inversely related to the incidence of atherosclerosis. This relationship may be due to HDL "scavenger" activity as they transport cholesterol out of "storage" and to the liver where it may be used, for example, to synthesize bile. High LDL concentrations, on the other hand, have been shown to be directly related to an increased incidence of atherosclerosis. This relationship may be due to LDL roles in transporting cholesterol into storage and in regulating cholesterol metabolism.

SUGGESTED READINGS

Brown, M. S., and J. L. Goldstein. 1983. Lipoprotein metabolism in the macrophage: Implications for cholesterol deposition in atherosclerosis. *Ann. Rev. Biochem.* 52:223–261.

Feldman, E. B. 1983. Diet and plasma lipids and lipoproteins. In *Nutrition and heart disease,* ed. E. B. Feldman, 45–58. New York: Churchill Livingstone.

Scanu, A., and F. R. Landsberger, 1980. Lipoprotein structure. *Ann. N.Y. Acad. Sci.* 348:1–434.

low density lipoprotein (LDL). One of the LIPOPROTEINS that carries lipids in the watery fluids of the body. LDLs are synthesized in the liver from the catabolism of VLDLs (very low density lipoprotein) and contain mostly CHOLESTEROL that they deliver to the tissues of the body to be used or stored. A high level of LDL is thought to indicate a higher risk of atherosclerosis. See also: LIPOPROTEINS.

lysine (Lys). An essential, mainly ketogenic six-carbon α-amino acid that, like ARGININE and HISTIDINE, has a positively charged side chain.

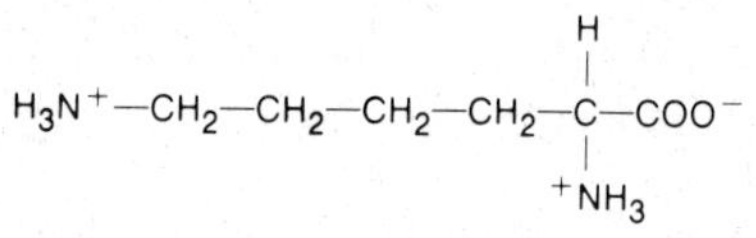

$$H_3N^+—CH_2—CH_2—CH_2—CH_2—\overset{\displaystyle H}{\underset{\displaystyle {}^+NH_3}{C}}—COO^-$$

Lysine (Lys)

Lysine is an important constituent of COLLAGEN and elastin in which it is hydroxylated to hydroxylysine, a compound that stabilizes cross-links after the amino acid sequence is established. These cross-links occur by the action of *lysine oxidase,* a COPPER-containing enzyme. Like THREONINE, lysine does not participate in transaminations.

Upon its complex degradation, four of lysine's skeletal carbons end up in acetoacetyl-CoA and the other two are lost as CO_2 after decarboxylations. Because acetoacetyl-CoA is the precursor of KETONE BODIES, lysine is ketogenic. If acetoacetyl-CoA is cleaved to ACETYL-COA, however, then some carbons may be incorporated randomly into GLUCOSE through GLUCONEOGENESIS and, to that extent, lysine will be glucogenic. The steps of degradation require the co-enzyme forms of the vitamins NIACIN and RIBOFLAVIN.

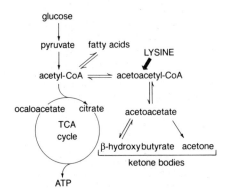

**The carbons of lysine enter
the metabolic pathways**

Lysine is the limiting amino acid in many cereals. This is of interest to vegans, who rely heavily on cereals for their daily supply of protein, and to those who are concerned with malnutrition in low-income populations in which the principal staple food is a cereal. The world's poor have been offered hope by the development of new high-lysine strains of both wheat and maize.

Loss of some of the available lysine can occur from mild heat treatment of protein when a reducing sugar such as lactose is present. During milk processing, for example, the sugar lactose reacts with the side chains of lysine rendering some lysine unavailable to digestive ENZYMES. This loss is negligible when compared to the health advantages of the long shelf life of irradiated evaporated and dry skim milk.

181

m

macrocytic anemia (megaloblastic anemia). See VITA-
MIN B$_{12}$; FOLACIN.

magnesium (Mg^{++}). A divalent ion that is a cofactor for
the ENZYMES that hydrolyze ATP and ADP and transfer
their phosphate groups to acceptor molecules. ATP is always present as a magnesium: ATP complex.

Magnesium plays important roles in PROTEIN BIOSYNTHE-
SIS. It is necessary for the activation of AMINO ACIDS by
aminoacyl-tRNA synthetase and the attachment of mRNA
to the ribosome. Magnesium is present in high concentration in intracellular fluid and in bone. Because magnesium
occurs as the central ion in chlorophyll, the key pigment in
green leaves that uses the energy of the sun to synthesize
GLUCOSE, it plays a fundamental role in the food chain.

Dietary intake is difficult to assess because the amount of
magnesium in foods varies greatly. Absorption is carrier-
mediated and is influenced by transit time through the gut,
dietary intake of magnesium, and the amounts of CALCIUM
and PHOSPHORUS in the diet. These divalent minerals compete for absorption sites in the proximal intestinal mucosa.
As magnesium intake increases, absorption decreases. Excess magnesium, not deposited in bone or retained in new
tissue, is excreted in the urine. Percent excreted decreases
as the intake decreases.

In healthy individuals, both the intestine and the kidneys
function to maintain magnesium homeostasis. Deficiencies
have been seen during prolonged fasting, in malnourished
alcoholics, in the newborn, in persons with renal tubule defects, and in hospital patients on prolonged magnesium-
free parenteral feeding. Signs and symptoms of magnesium
deficiency include apathy, anorexia, nausea, and neurologic

Mg^{++}: ATP complex

problems. Also present along with hypomagnesemia are hypocalcemia and hypokalemia.

SUGGESTED READINGS

Aikawa, J. K. 1976. Biochemistry and physiology of magnesium. In *Trace elements in human health and disease,* ed. A. S. Prasad, 47–48. New York: Academic Press.

Hodgkinson, A. D., H. Marshall, and B. E. C. Nordin. 1979. Vitamin D and magnesium absorption in man. *Clin. Sci.* 57:121–123.

Schwartz, R., H. Spencer, and J. J. Welsh. 1984. Magnesium absorption in human subjects from leafy vegetables, intrinsically labeled with stable ^{26}Mg. *Am. J. Clin. Nutr.* 39:571–576.

Wilz, D. R., et al. 1979. Plasma 1,25 (OH)$_2$ Vitamin D concentrations and net intestinal calcium, phosphate and magnesium absorption in humans. *Am. J. Clin. Nutr.* 32:2052–2060.

malate.   One of the carbohydrate intermediates of the TCA CYCLE.   See also: MALATE-ASPARTATE SHUTTLE; TCA CYCLE.

malate-aspartate shuttle.   A system, found mainly in the liver, kidney, and heart, whereby the reducing equivalents (electrons) gleaned from GLYCOLYSIS in the cytosol and carried by NADH can be transported into the MITOCHONDRION where they can be passed to the RESPIRATORY CHAIN. NADH cannot cross the membrane barrier but its electrons, carried in malate, can be transported across.

To form malate, the reducing equivalents (electrons) in the cytosol are transferred from NADH to oxaloacetate (OAA). This transfer yields NAD$^+$ and malate by the action of *malate dehydrogenase.* After being transported into the mitochondrion, malate gives up its electrons to mitochondrial NAD$^+$ by the action of *malate dehydrogenase* to re-form oxaloacetate and NADH. The NADH thus formed can give its electrons directly to the respiratory chain in the inner membrane. Three ATPs are generated as the pair of electrons is passed to oxygen.

The OAA, however, cannot pass from the mitochondrion back to the cytosol. But, by transamination, OAA can be converted to ASPARTATE and the aspartate can be transported from the mitochondrion to the cytosol. Within the cytosol, the aspartate may be reconverted to OAA and the OAA may, once again, accept electrons from NADH.

maltose.   A disaccharide composed of two molecules of glucose joined in an α1-4 linkage.   See also: CARBOHYDRATE STRUCTURE.

manganese (Mn^{++}). An essential mineral. While research findings are primarily confined to animal studies, it appears that in humans manganese is involved in the activation of transferases, lyases, isomerases, and hydrolases. Two important manganese-containing metalloenzymes found intracellularly are *pyruvate carboxylase* and *superoxide dismutase. Pyruvate carboxylase* catalyzes the conversion of pyruvate to oxaloacetate; *superoxide dismutase,* which also requires COPPER, converts superoxide radicals to hydrogen peroxide.

In addition, manganese is required for the incorporation of galactose into glycoproteins and it may be involved in steroid synthesis. In the UREA CYCLE, manganese is tightly bound to all four subunits of *arginase,* the enzyme that cleaves urea from ARGININE.

Manganese is found in wheat germ, seeds, nuts, and leafy vegetables; meat, fish, and poultry are relatively poor sources. This mineral is poorly absorbed from the intestinal tract especially when dietary intakes of CALCIUM, PHOSPHORUS, or IRON are high. Excretion of manganese is primarily via the bile.

A deficiency of manganese in humans has been shown to result in hypocholesterolemia, weight loss, transient dermatitis, nausea, and vomiting, as well as changes in hair growth and color. Toxicity, when reported, generally results from inhalation of manganese-containing dusts or fumes, not from dietary ingestion.

SUGGESTED READINGS

De Rosa, G., et al. 1980. Regulation of superoxide dismutase activity by dietary manganese. *J. Nutr.* 110:795–804.

Hurley, L. S. 1981. Teratogenic aspects of manganese, zinc and copper nutrition. *Physiol. Rev.* 61:249–295.

Leach, R. M., and M. S. Lilburn. 1978. Manganese metabolism and its function. *World Rev. Nutr. Diet.* 32:123–134.

maple syrup urine disease (branched-chain ketoacidosis). An inborn error of metabolism in which the infant with the typical, classical form of the disease fails to thrive within days after birth, feeds poorly, and vomits. Some other signs include convulsions, stupor, and irregular respiration. The levels of the three branched-chain amino acids, LEUCINE, ISOLEUCINE, and VALINE, and their α-keto acids are elevated in the blood and urine. The disease gets its name from the odor, color and viscosity of the urine of the patients.

SUGGESTED READINGS

See suggested readings for INBORN ERRORS OF METABOLISM.

McArdle's disease (glycogen storage disease: type V).
This disease results from the lack of the enzyme, *phosphorylase*, in muscle. Consequently, GLYCOGEN accumulates within muscle resulting in pain and fatigue after exertion. The hepatic phosphorylase, however, functions normally.

SUGGESTED READINGS

Howell, R. R., and J. C. Williams, 1983. The glycogen storage diseases. In *The metabolic basis of inherited disease*, 5th ed., ed. J. B. Stanbury et al., 141–166. New York: McGraw-Hill.

melanin. The pigment of the skin and hair. It is derived from TYROSINE through the action of the enzyme *tyrosinase* to produce DOPA (3,4-dihydroxyphenylalanine). DOPA, through a series of reactions, is used to produce melanin.

membranes. Cellular structures that form a protective barrier around cells and around organelles within cells in order to maintain their individuality and integrity.

Membranes are composed mainly of lipid bilayers and proteins. The lipid bilayers are permeable to water but do not allow the passage of ions, such as Na^+, Cl^-, or H^+, or the passage of polar, but uncharged, substances, such as sugar. The proteins embedded in the lipid layer carry out specific duties of the cell, such as the ferrying through of certain water-soluble substances.

Membrane structures have the quality of selective permeability by which the composition of the interior of the cell can be monitored and kept constant in spite of fluctuations in the environment just outside the cell. These structures can receive hormonal signals through specific receptor sites on their exterior and some can even send hormonal signals. Some membranes contain a series of ENZYMES attached to the membrane in the same order in which the chemical process occurs so that the process goes forward with economy of time and accuracy.

Membranes surrounding cell organelles serve to keep various cellular processes in separate compartments while allowing some compounds to cross the barrier. When a compound is produced in one compartment but is needed in another, it must be converted to one that can traverse the membrane. Oxaloacetate (OAA), for example, is produced in the mitochondria and used both in the mitochondria and in the cytosol. However, for OAA to be used in the cytosol, it must be aminated to ASPARTATE. Aspartate, carrying the carbons from OAA, is able to cross the membrane to the cytosol where it may become part of a pyrimidine ring or

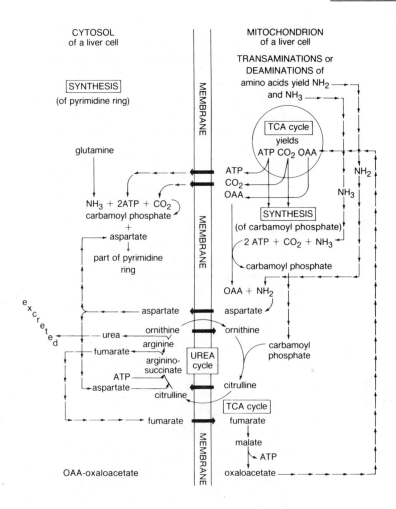

CYTOSOL
of a liver cell

SYNTHESIS
(of pyrimidine ring)

glutamine

NH_3 + 2ATP + CO_2
carbamoyl phosphate
+
aspartate
↓
part of pyrimidine
ring

excreted

aspartate

urea
ornithine
arginine
fumarate
arginino-
succinate
ATP
aspartate
citrulline

fumarate

OAA-oxaloacetate

MEMBRANE

MEMBRANE

UREA
cycle

MEMBRANE

MITOCHONDRION
of a liver cell

TRANSAMINATIONS or
DEAMINATIONS of
amino acids yield NH_2
and NH_3

TCA cycle
yields
ATP CO_2 OAA

ATP
CO_2
OAA

SYNTHESIS
(of carbamoyl phosphate)
2 ATP + CO_2 + NH_3

carbamoyl phosphate

OAA + NH_2

aspartate

ornithine

carbamoyl
phosphate

citrulline

TCA cycle
fumarate

malate
ATP
oxaloacetate

NH_2

NH_3

A compound produced in one compartment but needed in another
may have to be converted to a compound that is able to
traverse the membrane. Trace OAA, CO_2, and NH_2 as they
pass across the membrane barrier.

enter the UREA CYCLE. In the urea cycle, aspartate's amino
group will be incorporated into ARGININE and then into urea
for excretion; its carbons will exit the cycle in fumarate.
Fumarate will return to the mitochondrion, enter the TCA
cycle and re-form oxaloacetate.

Some of the most exciting biochemical findings of the
last two decades have taken place during the search for the
particulars of membrane structure. It has been determined,
for example, that the lipid molecules making up a membrane are not bound to each other by covalent bonds. The

membrane that surrounds the basic unit of life and has life-or-death control over what substances enter or leave the cell, is made of molecules standing in an orderly array without being firmly bonded to one another. Because of their own physical characteristics, they assembly themselves in the order required by the tissue. They are compacted and held together by van der Waals forces (between the hydrocarbon tails) and simple hydrogen bonding (between the ionized heads and the water).

The key to the self-assembly of the membrane components lies primarily in the twin characteristics of lipid molecules: hydrophobia and hydrophilia. Such molecules are said to be "amphipathic." In lipid-water mixtures, the hydrophobic "tails" of LIPIDS tend to orient themselves as far away as possible from the watery fluid of the interior and exterior of the cell. On the other hand, the ionized "heads" of lipids are attracted to the water molecules. These two characteristics of lipids operate to form a bilayer sheet in the presence of water.

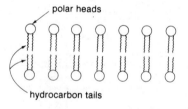

polar heads

hydrocarbon tails

Diagram of phospholipids
assembled into a bilayer.

Phospholipids and glycolipids are lipids that form these membrane bilayers. Phospholipids are esters of glycerol, a three-hydroxyl alcohol. In the simplest phospholipid, two of the carbons of glycerol are esterified to FATTY ACIDS (saturated or unsaturated) and the third is bonded to a phosphate to form phosphatidate. In the more complex molecules of this class, other alcohols become esterified to the phosphate radical. One of the most common of these in membranes is phosphatidylcholine, better known as lecithin.

Sphingomyelin is a phospholipid crucial to the membranes that protect neural cells. It differs from other phospholipids in that it uses sphingosine in place of glycerol as a backbone. Sphingosine has a long hydrocarbon tail, and at the other end an amide group occurs on one of the carbons.

$$H_3C-(CH_2)_{14}-\overset{\overset{\displaystyle O}{\|}}{C}-O-CH_2$$

$$H_3C-(CH_2)_7-\underset{\underset{\displaystyle H}{H}}{C}=\underset{\displaystyle H}{C}-(CH_2)_7-\overset{\overset{\displaystyle O}{\|}}{C}-O-\overset{\displaystyle |}{C}-H$$

$$H_2C-O-\overset{\overset{\displaystyle O}{\|}}{\underset{\underset{\displaystyle O^-}{|}}{P}}-O-CH_2-CH_2-\overset{+}{N}\overset{\nearrow CH_3}{\underset{\searrow CH_3}{-CH_3}}$$

Lecithin (phosphatidylcholine)

$$H_3C-(CH_2)_{12}-\underset{\displaystyle H}{\overset{\displaystyle H}{C}}=C-\underset{\underset{\displaystyle OH}{|}}{\overset{\overset{\displaystyle H}{|}}{C}}-\underset{\underset{\displaystyle NH}{|}}{\overset{\overset{\displaystyle H}{|}}{C}}-CH_2-O-\overset{\overset{\displaystyle O}{\|}}{\underset{\underset{\displaystyle O^-}{|}}{P}}-O-CH_2-CH_2-\overset{+}{N}\overset{\nearrow CH_3}{\underset{\searrow CH_3}{-CH_3}}$$

$$O=\overset{\displaystyle |}{C}$$
$$\overset{\displaystyle |}{R}$$

Sphingomyelin

R-long, hydrophobic tail of a fatty acid

In sphingomyelin, the amide group of sphingosine is attached to a fatty acid and one of the hydroxyl groups is attached to a phosphorylated choline. These attachments produce two nonpolarized hydrocarbon tails and a polar head, necessary attributes for a molecule to form a membrane bilayer.

Glycolipids also will use sphingosine as the backbone and form bilayers. Sugars are attached to the primary hydroxyl group in glycolipids, whereas in sphingomyelin, a phosphatidylcholine is attached at that point.

CHOLESTEROL, another substance important in membrane structure, does not participate in the formation of the bilayers. Cholesterol functions to maintain the fluidity of the membrane by packing in between the long hydrocarbon tails.

Proteins attached to or embedded in the membrane perform the work of the cell. Some proteins attach themselves to the exterior of the membrane and function as a receptor to recognize and bind hormones. Other proteins must necessarily span both surfaces of the lipid bilayer because their function is to pick up molecules on the exterior and transfer them to the interior of the cell or vice versa. Many of these proteins are the energy-requiring pumps that maintain concentrations of vital electrolytes.

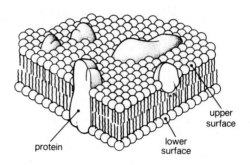

protein

lower
surface

upper
surface

Proteins embedded in lipid bilayer

SUGGESTED READINGS

Dautry-Varsat, A., and H. F. Lodish. 1984. How receptors bring proteins and particles into cells. *Sci. Am.* 250:52–58.

Kreil, G. Transfer of proteins across membranes. 1981. *Ann. Rev. Biochem.* 50:317–348.

Kummerow, F. A. 1983. Modification of cell membrane composition by dietary lipids and its implications for atherosclerosis. *Ann. N.Y. Acad. Sci.* 414:29–43.

Lefkowitz, R. J., M. G. Caron, and G. L. Stiles. 1984. Mechanisms of membrane-receptor regulation. *N. Engl. J. Med.* 310:1570–1579.

Op den Kamp, J. A. F. 1979. Lipid asymmetry in membranes. *Ann. Rev. Biochem.* 48:47–71.

Singer, S. J., and G. L. Nicolson. 1972. The fluid mosaic model of the structure of cell membranes. *Science* 175:720–731.

menaquinone (K_2). See VITAMIN K.

mEq. See MILLIEQUIVALENT.

mEq/L. See MILLIEQUIVALENTS PER LITER.

messenger RNA (mRNA, messenger ribonucleic acid). A single strand of genetic material synthesized in the nucleus so that its base sequence is complementary to one of the strands of DNA. Unlike DNA, it is able to leave the nucleus and enter the cytosol. Each molecule of mRNA carries the directions for synthesizing a protein and serves as a template for its construction. See also: DNA; GENETIC CODE; RNA.

metabolism. The sum of all the biochemical changes that take place in a living organism. Those changes in compounds that release energy to the organism or to the environment and that produce simpler compounds are termed "catabolic reactions," and the process is called "catabolism." Those alterations that require energy and result in the synthesis of more complex molecules are "anabolic reactions," and the process is called "anabolism."

In living organisms, catabolism takes place in small steps each of which is controlled by a specific enzyme. The parcels of energy released are mostly conserved in the phosphate-bond energy of adenosine triphosphate (ATP).

Some catabolic pathways include the breakdown of GLYCOGEN to GLUCOSE (GLYCOGENOLYSIS), of protein to AMINO ACIDS, and of TRIACYLGLYCEROLS to FATTY ACIDS and glycerol. However, most of the ATP (energy) derived from catabolism is obtained by the further degradation of glucose, amino acids, glycerol, and fatty acids through specific pathways, including GLYCOLYSIS, TCA CYCLE, RESPIRATORY CHAIN, beta oxidation, and the PENTOSE PHOSPHATE PATHWAY. During catabolism, electrons are channeled to electron-carrying coenzymes such as NAD^+ and FAD; then the electrons carried in $NADH + H^+$ and $FADH_2$ are transferred to the respiratory chain, which utilizes the energy to produce ATP.

Anabolism is performed in stepwise reactions, catalyzed by specific ENZYMES. ATP that is produced during the catabolic reactions provides the energy needed for the anabolic reactions, including PROTEIN BIOSYNTHESIS, GLYCOGENESIS, GLUCONEOGENESIS, as well as FATTY ACID SYNTHESIS. The steps taken along the path of anabolism (going "uphill") may not be identical to the ones of catabolism (going "downhill"), but some of the steps may be shared. Often, the two paths, catabolism and anabolism, take place in different parts of the cell.   See also: ATP, ADP, AMP; GLUCONEOGENESIS, for a more detailed discussion of anabolic and catabolic pathways; ENERGETICS; NAD^+, $NADP^+$; RESPIRATORY CHAIN; TCA CYCLE.

metabolite.   Any intermediate compound produced during the catabolism of a biological substance. For example, pyruvate is a metabolite of the catabolism of GLUCOSE.

methionine (Met).   An essential, glucogenic (glycogenic), five-carbon α-amino acid. Like CYSTEINE, it has a SULFUR atom in its side chain. Because of the presence of a sulfur atom and a methyl group at the end of its side chain, methionine functions as a methyl donor in the synthesis of many compounds. Methionine and cysteine are the main contributors of sulfur to the many sulfur-containing structures (cartilage, tendons, bone matrix, hair) and compounds (insulin, heparin) of the body.

$$CH_3-S-CH_2-CH_2-\overset{\overset{\displaystyle H}{|}}{\underset{\underset{\displaystyle {}^+NH_3}{|}}{C}}-COO^-$$

Methionine (Met)

The derivative of methionine which acts as the methyl donor in most biosyntheses is S-adenosylmethionine (SAM). SAM is synthesized by attaching an adenosyl group from ATP to the sulfur atom of methionine, an addition effected by *methionine adenosyl transferase.* This high energy methyl donor is an intermediate in a series of reactions that converts methionine, with the addition of SERINE, into the other sulfur-containing amino acid, cysteine. Ammonia and α-ketobutyrate are also produced in this series; the butyrate undergoes oxidative decarboxylation to become propionyl-CoA. *Alpha keto acid dehydrogenase,* using NAD^+ as coenzyme, facilitates this reaction.

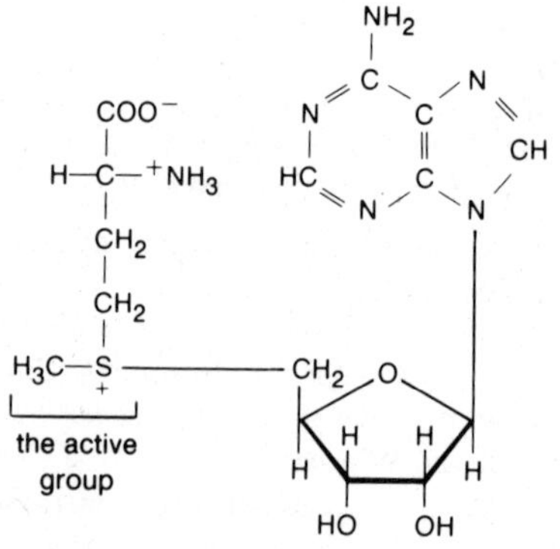

S-adenosylmethionine

The path from propionyl-CoA to succinyl-CoA is the degradative path also followed by VALINE, THEONINE, and ISOLEUCINE. A BIOTIN-dependent enzyme, *propionyl-CoA carboxylase,* incorporates a carboxyl group into the propionyl-CoA, converting it into D-methylmalonyl-CoA. A racemase converts the D-form of methyl-malonyl-CoA into the L-form. Then a vitamin B_{12}-dependent enzyme, *methylmalonyl-CoA mutase,* performs some internal rearrangements to produce succinyl-CoA.

Methionine is the precursor of taurine, which combines with cholyl-CoA to form one of the BILE SALTS, taurocholate. This is a FOLACIN-requiring reaction. Bile salts are important for the emulsification of fats in the digestive tract.

As can be seen from the foregoing discussion, the degradation of methionine is not a simple deamination followed by entry of the carbon skeleton into the TCA CYCLE. Along the way, many important intermediates are produced that

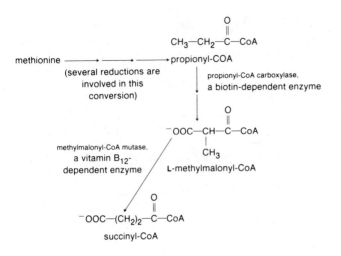

The conversion of methionine to succinyl-CoA

lead to the synthesis of many biomolecules, only a few of which have been mentioned here.

SUGGESTED READINGS

Benevenga, N. J. 1984. Evidence for alternative pathways of methionine catabolism. *Adv. Nutr. Res.* 6:1–18.

Cooper, A. J. L. 1983. Biochemistry of sulfur-containing amino acids. *Ann. Rev. Biochem.* 52:187–222.

Wolf, B., et. al. 1981. Propionic acidemia: A clinical update. *J. Pediatr.* 99:835–846.

See suggested readings for INBORN ERRORS OF METABOLISM.

methylmalonic acidemia. An acidosis appearing in the first year of life due to an inherited disorder of methylmalonyl-CoA metabolism. Some patients respond when massive doses of vitamin B_{12} are administered. See also: VITAMIN B_{12}.

SUGGESTED READINGS

See suggested readings for INBORN ERRORS OF METABOLISM.

mg/ml. See MILLIGRAMS PER MILLILITER.

micelle. A very fine, colloidal dispersion of polar LIPIDS, usually as a parallel array within a liquid phase, which fails to form a true solution of the molecules. This aggregation makes it possible for FATTY ACIDS and other lipids that contain polar groups to travel through the aqueous fluids of the body.

Michaelis-Menten equation. The kinetic expression for the dependence of enzyme velocity (V) upon substrate concentration (S) where V_{max} is the maximal rate with saturating substrate concentration and K_m is the Michaelis-Menton constant, which is the substrate concentration that yields ½ of V_{max}.

$$V_o = V_{max} \frac{[S]}{[S] + K_M}$$

micrograms per millimeter (μg/ml). Also known as parts per million.

milliequivalent (mEq). The milligrams of a substance, for example, sodium (Na), divided by the substance's atomic weight (Na = 23) multiplied by the valence of the substance (Na valence = +1).

milliequivalents per liter (mEq/L). The concentration of electrolytes in a certain volume of solution. It is calculated by multiplying milligrams per liter by the valence of the electrolyte and dividing by its molecular weight:

$$\frac{(mg/L) \times valence}{molecular\ weight}$$

milligrams per milliliter (mg/ml). A unit with which to express density, the weight of a substance per unit volume.

mitochondrion. An organelle found in an aerobic eukaryotic cell. The mitochondria are often spoken of as the "power houses" of the cell because the catabolic pathway known as the TCA CYCLE, the largest producer of ATP, takes place there.

Depending on the energy needs of the cell, as many as several hundred mitochondria can occur in a single cell. Mitochondria contain the electron carriers of the RESPIRATORY CHAIN and the ENZYMES for the TCA cycle, the oxidation and carboxylation of pyruvate, FATTY ACID OXIDATION, the UREA CYCLE, and for many metabolic pathways involving AMINO ACIDS.

The mitochondrion has two membranes, a smooth outer membrane and an inner membrane with many finger-like infoldings called "cristae." Contained within the boundary of the inner membrane is a gel-like substance called the "matrix," in which are suspended the enzymes for the TCA cycle and fatty acid oxidation. The carriers for the electrons of the respiratory chain are fixed sequentially in the inner membrane.

All along the inner membrane are mushroom-like projections called "inner membrane spheres" that contain the enzymes for phosphorylating ADP to ATP. The inner membrane is not freely permeable, yet many molecules must move across this barrier. Transport systems are available in the membrane for this purpose. One such system moves ATP out of the mitochondria to the cytoplasm where it is needed, and, in the other direction, moves ADP into the mitochondria to be phosphorylated. Another system employs carnitine to transport fatty acids from the cytosol where they are synthesized to the mitochondrial matrix where they are oxidized.

mole (gram molecular weight). A quantity of a substance measured in grams equal to the substance's molecular weight. For example, a mole of GLUCOSE ($C_6H_{12}O_6$) is 180 grams ($6 \times 12 + 12 \times 1 + 6 \times 16$). A mole of water ($H_2O$) is 18 grams ($2 \times 1 + 1 \times 16$).

molybdenum (Mo). A trace element present in animal and plant tissues. Molybdenum is a cofactor for ENZYMES such as *xanthine oxidase, aldehyde oxidase,* and *sulfite oxidase.* High dietary molybdenum intake by humans results in increased *xanthine oxidase* activity, which converts hypoxanthine to xanthine and subsequently to uric acid. High intakes also appear to increase COPPER excretion in humans.

In laboratory animals, a dietary deficiency decreases *xanthine oxidase* activity; in plants, Mo is essential for NITROGEN fixation. One step of the complex fixation process, which precedes the synthesis of AMINO ACIDS, is carried out by the nitrogenase complex in which molybdenum is a component along with IRON and SULFUR—this protein is named the MoFe protein. See also: FAD, FMN; IRON.

SUGGESTED READINGS

Abumrad, N. N. 1984. Molybdenum—is it an essential trace metal. *Bull. N.Y. Acad. Med.* 60:163–171.

Deosthale, Y. G., and C. Gopalan. 1974. The effect of molybdenum levels in sorghum on uric acid and copper excretion in man. *Br. J. Nutr.* 31:351–355.

monoacylglycerol. A glycerol that has one fatty acid substituted for a hydroxyl. See also: LIPIDS.

monounsaturated fatty acid. A fatty acid with one double bond between carbon atoms. See also: LIPIDS.

mutation. Chemical modification of a gene such that one or more of the bases in the DNA is deleted or altered or a new base is inserted, thus changing the base sequence. With the modification, the protein coded by the gene either is produced with an altered amino acid sequence or is not produced at all. See also: SICKLE-CELL ANEMIA, which describes a mutation that confers protection from another disease (malaria) as well as causing the primary disease (hemolytic anemia).

mutual supplementation. A dietary strategy, especially for vegetarians, in which two different protein foods, each lacking an essential amino acid that the other possesses, are eaten at the same meal. These two foods thus contribute the equivalent of a complete protein in that meal.

myoglobin. A HEME protein that is abundant in muscles. Unlike hemoglobin that has four atoms of IRON, myoglobin has only one. Myoglobin is more abundant in those muscles that contract slowly but must sustain the contraction, such as the flight muscles of birds. In contrast, myoglobin is less abundant in muscles that are responsible for sudden bursts of activity for short periods of time.

Na⁺—K⁺ pump (sodium-potassium pump). An active transport system in cell membranes that requires both SO-DIUM and POTASSIUM as well as energy (ATP). See also: SO-DIUM PUMP.

NAD⁺ (nicotinamide adenine dinucleotide). A coenzyme form of the vitamin NIACIN. See also: NAD⁺, NADP⁺.

NAD⁺, NADP⁺ (nicotinamide adenine dinucleotide, nico-tinamide adenine dinucleotide phosphate). Two co-enzyme forms of the vitamin, NIACIN. NAD^+ is a major elec-tron acceptor in the conversion of energy of the fuel nutrients into ATP, while $NADP^+$ in its reduced form (NADPH) is the major electron donor in most reductive biosyntheses.

NAD^+ and $NADP^+$ serve as coenzymes for the dehy-drogenases, ENZYMES that remove two hydrogen atoms (pro-ton plus electron) from their substrates. One of these pro-tons is released into the surrounding medium (H^+) and the other proton and the two electrons are transferred to the coenzyme, which becomes NADH in the case of reduced NAD^+, or NADPH in the case of reduced $NADP^+$.

Molecules of NAD^+ are composed of nicotinamide, D-ribose (a five-carbon sugar), phosphoric acid, and ade-nine (a purine base). $NADP^+$ has the same structure with an extra phosphate group attached to the ribose of the aden-osine moiety.

Nicotinamide is the physiologically active form of the B-vitamin, niacin, which is found in yeast, lean meats, liver, and poultry. In addition to being brought into the body pre-formed in foods, niacin can be derived in the body from the amino acid, TRYPTOPHAN.

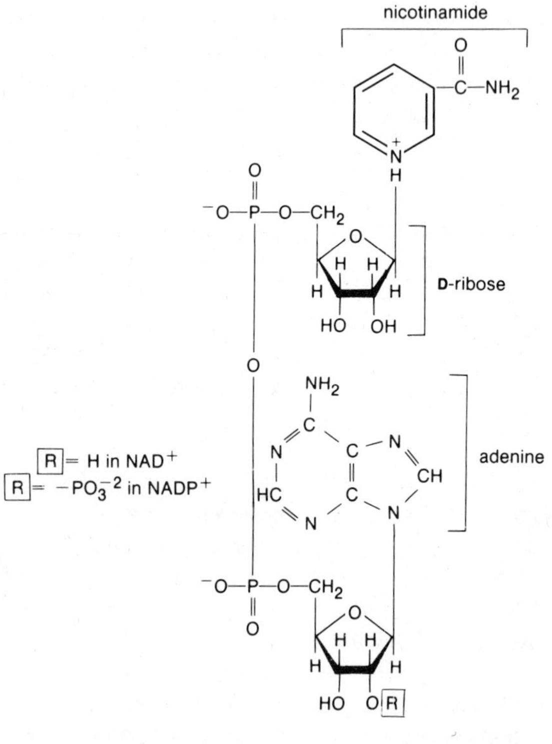

NAD⁺ and NADP⁺

The two coenzyme forms are used differently by the cell. NAD⁺ is most involved in catabolic reactions resulting in ATP production. Its special task is to "pull" hydrogens and electrons from substrates. When hydrogen and electrons are removed, more of the valence of the carbon atoms can be used to combine with oxygen, therefore the substrate becomes more oxidized. Oxidation of nutrients is the source of the energy needed to run the cell.

NADP⁺, on the other hand, is involved in anabolic reactions. The cell stores its reduced form, NADPH. This storehouse of reducing power is then used to "pluck" oxygen from carbons so that the reduced carbon can combine with other carbons and hydrogens to form the large biological molecules needed by the cell.

NAD⁺ is essential to the stepwise transfer of hydrogens and electrons in GLYCOLYSIS and the TCA CYCLE. After NAD⁺ has picked up a hydrogen ion and two electrons, it becomes NADH + H$^+$. The NADH transfers its hydrogens and electrons to the cytochromes in the cell's RESPIRATORY CHAIN. By the actions of the respiratory chain, the energy will be used to phosphorylate ADP to ATP. NADPH is generated in the PENTOSE PHOSPHATE PATHWAY and donates its hydrogens and electrons to intermediates in many biosynthetic pathways.

NADP$^+$ (nicotinamide adenine dinucleotide phosphate). A coenzyme form of the vitamin NIACIN. See also: NAD$^+$, NADP$^+$.

niacin (nicotinic acid). A B-vitamin first isolated as an oxidation product of nicotine. Niacin is a beta-pyridine carboxylic acid that is easily converted in the body to its physiologically active form, nicotinamide.

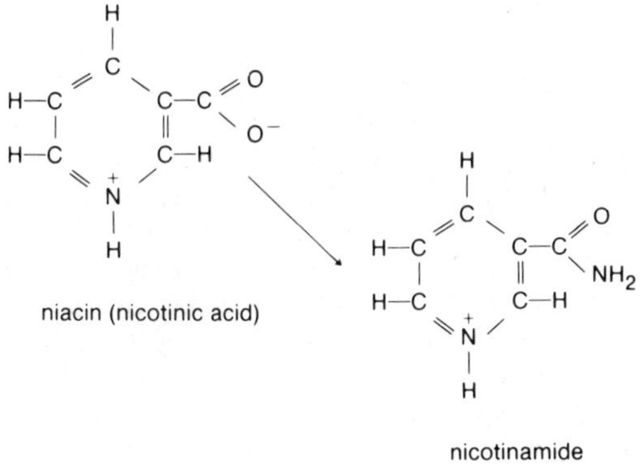

niacin (nicotinic acid)

nicotinamide

Conversion of niacin to nicotinamide

Like all water-soluble vitamins, niacin is not stored in significant amounts in the body and must be supplied regularly from food. The richest sources of niacin include cereals, legumes, and meats, as well as coffee and tea. In some cereals, such as corn, however, niacin is present in a bound form and is biologically unavailable. Unlike other vitamins, niacin has a precursor in the form of an amino acid, TRYPTOPHAN. Therefore, in calculating the niacin content of the diet, both the free niacin and the tryptophan content must be counted. Approximately 60 mg of tryptophan are considered to form 1 mg of niacin. Since these calculations are cumbersome, a rule of thumb is used: If the protein content of the diet is adequate, the niacin content will be adequate also.

Nicotinic acid and nicotinamide are absorbed within the stomach and proximal small intestine. Within the body, nicotinamide plays its most important role as a part of two ENZYMES, NAD^+ (nicotinamide adenine dinucleotide) and $NADP^+$ (nicotinamide adenine dinucleotide phosphate). These two coenzymes operate as transfer agents with the enzymes of metabolic pathways.

The transfer of hydrogens and electrons is involved in both catabolic and anabolic reactions. When fuel molecules are oxidized to produce ATP, hydrogens are transferred to carrier molecules. NADH (reduced NAD^+) is such a carrier in many catabolic reactions such as the decarboxylation of α-ketoglutarate to succinyl-CoA in the TCA CYCLE. When biomolecules are being synthesized, NADPH (reduced $NADP^+$) is often the electron donor, as it is in FATTY ACID SYNTHESIS or the conversion of the amino acid, PHENYLALANINE to another amino acid, TYROSINE.

The early symptoms of niacin deficiency are weakness, lassitude, and anorexia, as well as the mental symptoms of irritability and forgetfulness. Later symptoms of full-blown pellagra, the niacin deficiency disease, are known as the "3Ds"—Dermatitis, Diarrhea, and Dementia. These symptoms are related to a lack of energy for muscle control and lack of energy (GLUCOSE) for the neural tissues. This would be expected since niacin coenzymes are vital to enzymes that convert the fuel nutrients to ATP. A fourth D, Death, may also result from pellagra.

Pellagra is rarely seen in the United States today. This is attributed to the enrichment of bread and to federal programs that provide food for the poor. However, it is still recorded in heavy users of alcohol who are malnourished, and it is beginning to be seen among the elderly who live alone and often exist on an easily prepared single food item that is inadequate nutritionally.

During the early twentieth century, pellagra was prevalent among people of the southern United States; it was recorded from other parts of the world as early as 1720. Those individuals who developed pellagra in the South consumed a diet of salt pork with corn (maize) as their staple grain. Corn is low in the amino acid TRYPTOPHAN and high in LEUCINE.

It was suggested between 1913 and 1920 that pellagra was caused by a deficiency of tryptophan in maize; during the same time there was a more popular report that a yeast extract, which contained no tryptophan, could cure the disease. This confusion began to clear in 1937 when Elvehjem et al. showed that nicotinic acid would cure blacktongue, the pellagra analog seen in dogs. It was another eight years, however, before it was recognized that the vitamin could be made in the body if sufficient tryptophan were present.

Large doses of nicotinic acid and/or nicotinamide can alter central nervous system function as well as blood lipid and glucose concentrations. See also: B-VITAMIN TERMINOLOGY; NAD$^+$, NADP$^+$.

SUGGESTED READINGS

Bechgaard, H., and S. Jespersen. 1977. GI absorption of niacin in humans. *J. Pharm. Sci.* 66:871–872.

Mertz, W. 1975. Effects and metabolism of glucose tolerance factor. *Nutr. Rev.* 33:129–135.

Nakagawa, I., et al. 1969. Effect in man of the addition of tryptophan or niacin in the diet on the excretion of their metabolites. *J. Nutr.* 99:325–330.

Sydenstricker, V. P. 1958. The history of pellagra: Its recognition as a disorder of nutrition and its conquest. *Am. J. Clin. Nutr.* 6:409–414.

niacinamide. See NIACIN.

nicotinamide. See NIACIN.

nicotinamide adenine dinucleotide (NAD$^+$). See NAD$^+$, NADP$^+$.

nicotinamide adenine dinucleotide phosphate (NADP$^+$). See NAD$^+$, NADP$^+$.

nicotinic acid. See NIACIN.

Niemann-Pick disease. A hereditary disease of lipid metabolism caused by the lack of the catabolic ENZYMES responsible for degrading sphingolipids. As a result, sphingolipids accumulate in the brain and other tissues. Onset is in infancy and generally is fatal by the third year.

SUGGESTED READINGS

Brady, R. O. 1983. Sphingomyelin lipidosis: Niemann-Pick disease. In *The metabolic basis of inherited disease,* 5th ed., ed. J. B. Stanbury et al., 831–841. New York: McGraw-Hill.

nitrogen (N). The unique element in AMINO ACIDS, purines, pyrimidines, and other nitrogenous biomolecules, the major component of the atmosphere, and the element on which the human food supply is most dependent. The diatomic nitrogen gas, which makes up about 78 percent of the air, is unavailable to animals or plants for the building of amino acids until it has been "fixed," that is, changed into nitrogen-containing compounds that plants can use. Animals receive nitrogen by eating plants or other animals.

Fixation of nitrogen is accomplished in nature through an electrical discharge in the atmosphere (lightning), through blue-green algae, or through the action of bacteria located in root nodules of leguminous plants. The strong triple bonds that hold the two nitrogen atoms together in gaseous nitrogen must be broken before the nitrogen atoms can combine with hydrogen, carbon, or oxygen to form compounds that plants can use. The nitrogenase complex converts N_2 into NH_3 using ATP and a reductant.

Once the nitrogen of the air becomes "fixed nitrogen" in the soil, it can then be incorporated into the amino acids, purines, or other compounds in plants. The plants will be eaten by livestock that will break down the proteins into amino acids and rearrange them into their own species' proteins, or use the nitrogen to build other biomolecules. Humans eat both plants and animals and thus acquire the proteins that will be digested to the amino acids needed for the construction of human proteins. Gaseous nitrogen is returned to the atmosphere when fecal matter, urea, and dead plants and animals are acted upon by bacteria, thus completing the nitrogen cycle—the incorporation of gaseous nitrogen as nitrogen-containing compounds in plants and animals and the eventual return of gaseous nitrogen to the atmosphere.

With the present-day pressure of large human populations that must be fed from a declining number of acres of arable land, the natural process of revitalizing the soil is too slow. Chemical fertilizers are made from the nitrogen in the air combined with hydrogen to produce ammonia by a process invented by Fritz Haber and first used to produce explosives prior to World War I. The widespread use of these synthetic fertilizers has made it possible to increase the yield of crops and to feed the world's hungry.

However, a major ecological problem results from the runoff of soluble nitrogen-containing compounds from agricultural soils into wetlands where the growth of plants is greatly stimulated. When the plants die, they are oxidized. With this oxidation, there is not enough oxygen to support fish and other aquatic animals. Thus, the supply of animal foods is decreased while the fertilizer is increasing the plant life. Soon the pond, which was alive with aquatic life, becomes a swamp and eventually a meadow.

The evolution of a meadow from a pond is a natural aging process that in earlier times took many generations to accomplish. Now, however, with the push for more and more food to feed an increasing world population, the aging process is speeded up until ponds and lakes can be destroyed in less than a generation.   See also: AMINO ACIDS; PROTEIN BIOSYNTHESIS; PURINE, PYRIMIDINE BASES; UREA CYCLE.

nitrogen balance. The nutritional state of an individual in relation to his or her protein METABOLISM; it is a measure of the difference between ingested and excreted NITROGEN. During a period of rapid growth, a child would be in positive nitrogen balance since ingested nitrogen would be retained in the new tissues rather than be excreted. During an illness, a patient might be in negative nitrogen balance as muscle tissue is broken down for energy and its nitrogen excreted. Normal, healthy adults are in zero nitrogen balance—the nitrogen they ingest equals the nitrogen they excrete.

noncaloric sweeteners. See NONNUTRITIVE SWEETENERS.

nonessential amino acids (NEAA). Those AMINO ACIDS that a species is able to synthesize in sufficient quantity from materials already present in the cell. There is no implication in this designation that these amino acids are unnecessary or not important, only that it is not necessary for the species to obtain them preformed from food. An abundant supply of the nonessential amino acids is important for maintenance of healthy tissues so that, through transamination, any needed NEAA can be made instantly without dismantling an ESSENTIAL AMINO ACID for its amino group.

In humans, the nonessential amino acids include ALANINE, ASPARAGINE, ASPARTATE, CYSTEINE, GLUTAMATE, GLUTAMINE, GLYCINE, PROLINE, SERINE, and TYROSINE. ARGININE and HISTIDINE are sometimes included. See also: AMINO ACIDS; ESSENTIAL AMINO ACIDS.

nonnutritive sweeteners. Saccharin (noncaloric), sodium cyclamate (noncaloric), and aspartame (low calorie). These three are the best known of the synthetic molecules that are added to foods because they add a sweet taste without adding the calories of sucrose (table sugar) or stimulating an insulin response.

Saccharin has been in dietary use for nearly a hundred years by diabetics and other persons who wish to limit their intake of sugar. It is over 300 times as sweet as sucrose and is widely consumed in diet soft drinks. The carcinogenic potential of saccharin has been investigated intensively and some studies on rats have indicated an increase in the formation of tumors with large doses of saccharin. On the basis of the findings in some of these studies, the Food and Drug Administration (FDA) attempted to invoke the Delaney Clause of the Food, Drug, and Cosmetic Act, which prohibits the use of any chemical in foods that has

saccharin

sodium cyclamate

aspartame
(L-aspartyl-L-phenylalanine
methyl ester)

Nonnutritive sweeteners

203

been shown to cause cancer in animals or humans. However, pressure on the FDA by the public, legislators, and interest groups, as well as by industry, has kept saccharin on the market.

Sodium cyclamate, another artificial sweetener, attained great popularity in diet drinks and other food products prior to 1969. At that time it was found to produce cancer in rats when it was fed in large amounts. Under the rule of the Delaney Clause, the FDA removed the cyclamates from use in the United States.

Aspartame, aspartyl-phenylalanine methyl ester, is believed to be safe and has been approved by the FDA. It is made from two AMINO ACIDS, ASPARTATE and PHENYLALANINE, normally found in proteins. It is about 200 times as sweet as sucrose but loses its sweetness when heated; this precludes its being used widely in processed foods. When the two amino acids are metabolized in the body, they produce energy, but the amounts of aspartame needed to produce the desired sweetness is so small that, essentially, it is a noncaloric sweetener. Several studies suggest that ingestion of high doses of aspartame results in no harmful side effects. Products that contain aspartame carry a warning label directed at people with phenylketonuria (PKU), an inherited disorder of phenylalanine metabolism. See also: PHENYLALANINE.

SUGGESTED READINGS

Cohen, S. M. 1986. Saccharin: Past, present and future. *J. Am. Diet. Assoc.* 86:929–931.

Council on Scientific Affairs. 1985. Aspartame. *JAMA* 254:400–402.

Heller, A., and L. Jovanovic. 1985. Artificial sweeteners: Safety and utility in the treatment of diabetes mellitus. In *Nutrition and diabetes,* Ed. L. Jovanovic and C. M. Peterson, 37–50. New York: Alan R. Liss.

Stegnik, L. D., and L. J. Filer, Jr. 1984. Aspartame physiology and biochemistry. Food science and technology. A series of monographs and textbooks. Ed. S. R. Tannenbaum and P. Walstra. New York: Marcel Dekker, Inc.

norepinephrine. A CATECHOLAMINE that is a neurotransmitter produced in sympathetic nerves and released in response to nerve stimulation; it produces similar metabolic effects on peripheral tissues to those evoked by epinephrine.

nucleic acids. Chains of nucleotides, called polynucleotides, whose functions are to store and to transmit genetic information. A nucleotide contains one purine base (adenine or guanine) or one pyrimidine base (cytosine, thymine, or uracil) plus one molecule of a pentose sugar (D-ribose or D-deoxyribose) plus one, two, or three molecules of phosphate ($-PO_4^=$). See also: DNA; NUCLEOSIDES, NUCLE-OTIDES; PURINE, PYRIMIDINE BASES; RNA.

nucleosides, nucleotides. Structural components of many compounds, such as DNA, RNA, ATP, NAD$^+$, FAD, or COENZYME A, that are vital in biochemical processes.

A nucleoside is composed of a purine or pyrimidine base attached to a pentose. A nucleotide is a nucleoside that has condensed with one, two, or three phosphates.

In the structure of a nucleoside, the pentose is either ribose or deoxyribose and the base may be either a purine or a pyrimidine. The linkage is between the C-1 carbon of the pentose to either the N-1 nitrogen of the pyrimidine or the N-9 nitrogen of the purine. In the structure of ribonucleosides, ribose forms such a link with adenine (to yield adenosine), guanine (to yield guanosine), cytosine (to yield cytidine), and uracil (to yield uridine); however no such link is

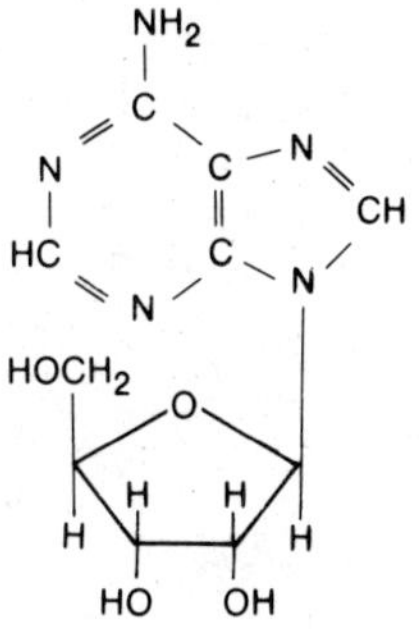

adenosine

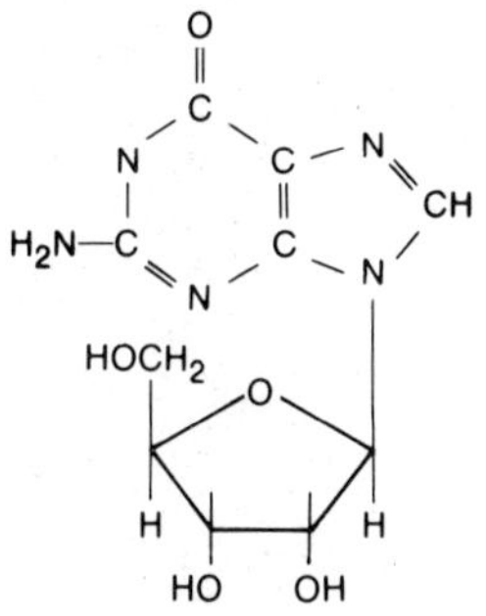

guanosine

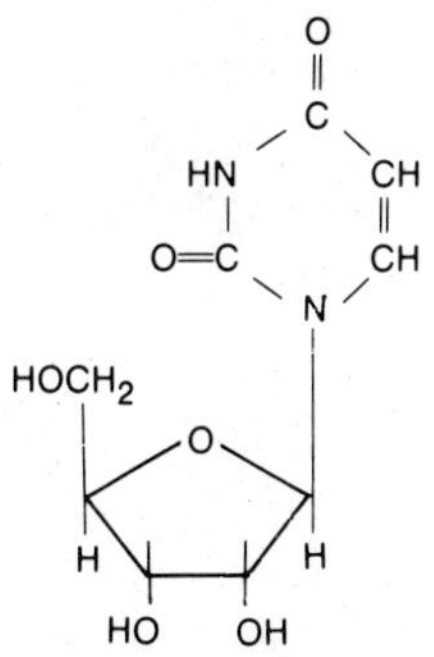

uridine

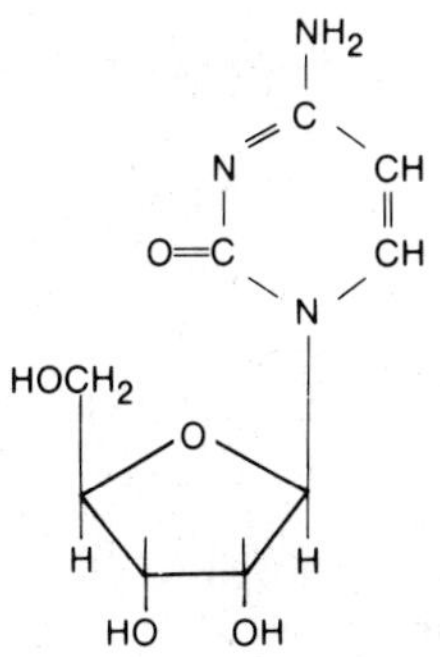

cytidine

Ribonucleosides (bases plus ribose)

205

formed with thymine. In the structure of deoxyribonucleo-sides, deoxyribose links with adenine (to yield deoxy-adenosine), guanine (to yield deoxyguanosine), cytosine (to yield deoxycytidine), and thymine (to yield deoxythymidine); however, no such link is formed with uracil.

deoxyadenosine

deoxyguanosine

deoxythymidine

deoxycytidine

Deoxyribonucleosides (bases plus deoxyribose)

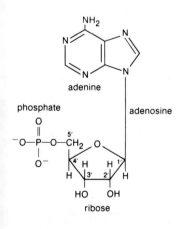

Adenosine 5′-monophosphate
(adenylate, AMP)

In the structure of a ribonucleotide, the phosphate is at-tached at the C-5′ carbon (read "five prime") of the pentose part of the ribonucleoside. For example, adenosine 5′-monophosphate, pictured at left, is also known as adenylate or most often by its initials, AMP. The other ribonucleotides are guanosine 5′-monophosphate (guany-late, GMP), uridine 5′-monophosphate (uridylate, UMP), and cytidine 5′-monophosphate (cytidylate, CMP).

If the pentose part of the nucleotide is deoxyribose, the phosphate again attaches at the C-5′ carbon, and these nucleotides are identified as deoxyribonucleotides. For example, deoxyadenosine 5′-monophosphate, also known as deoxyadenylate or dAMP, has the following structure:

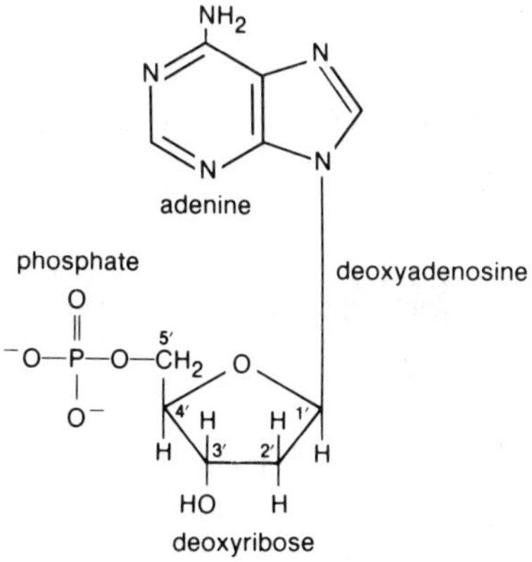

Deoxyadenosine 5′-monophosphate
(deoxyadenylate, dAMP)

The other deoxyribonucleotides are deoxyquanosine 5′-monophosphate (deoxyquanylate, dGMP), deoxythymidine 5′-monophosphate (deoxythymidylate, dTMP, or sometimes shortened to "thymidylate" since thymine is present only in deoxyribonucleotides, never in a ribonucleotide), and deoxycytidine 5′-monophosphate (deoxycytidylate, dCMP).

If there are two or three phosphates on the pentose of either the ribonucleotides or the deoxyribonucleotides, that fact is noted in the name. For example, AMP (monophosphate) becomes ADP (diphosphate) when two phosphates are attached, or it becomes ATP (triphosphate) when three phosphates are attached.

Along with ATP, ADP, and AMP, the high energy compounds that are thought of as the energy currency of the cells, the most widely known of the nucleotides are DNA and RNA (deoxyribonucleic acid and ribonucleic acid, respectively), the genetic material of the cells. DNA and RNA are polymers of repeating units of nucleotides. See also: ATP, ADP, AMP; DNA; PURINE, PYRIMIDINE BASES; RNA.

O

ornithine cycle. The series of reactions in the UREA CYCLE whereby ornithine combines with one molecule of ammonia and carbon dioxide to form citrulline. Citrulline then picks up another ammonia to form ARGININE. Urea is split off from arginine by hydrolysis, re-forming ornithine. See also: UREA CYCLE.

osteoblasts. Cells responsible for forming new bone tissue. See also: DYNAMIC STATE.

osteoclasts. Cells responsible for bone destruction by resorbing the calcium from bone. See also: DYNAMIC STATE.

oxalic acid. A substance found in high concentration in some plant foods, especially in spinach, rhubarb, parsley, cocoa, and tea. The biochemical function of oxalic acid has not been determined. The amount that is synthesized by humans is excreted in the urine and it is a constituent of some kinds of kidney stones. Oxalates in food may combine with some divalent metals to form insoluble compounds that cannot be absorbed, reducing the bioavailability of these minerals.

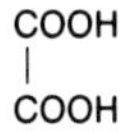

COOH
|
COOH

Oxalic acid

oxaloacetate (OAA). A carbohydrate intermediate of the TCA cycle. See also: GLUCONEOGENESIS; TCA CYCLE.

oxidase. A class of ENZYMES that are active in oxidation/reduction reactions which use oxygen as an electron acceptor.

oxidation. See BETA OXIDATION; FATTY ACID OXIDATION; RESPIRATORY CHAIN; TCA CYCLE.

oxidation/reduction. Reactions in which electrons are lost by one compound (it is oxidized) and electrons are gained simultaneously by another compound (it is reduced). The compound that loses electrons is the reducing agent, or the reductant; the compound that gains electrons is the oxidizing agent, or oxidant.   See also: FAD, FMN; RES-PIRATORY CHAIN.

oxidative deamination.   The removal of an amino group from a compound which results in the production of ammonia and a corresponding α-keto acid. This reaction may be accompanied by a transfer of hydrogens from the compound to a coenzyme, NAD^+ or FAD.

oxidative decarboxylation.   See DECARBOXYLATION.

oxidative phosphorylation (respiratory chain phosphorylation).   The mitochondrial process whereby the energy released during the passage of electrons along the RESPIRATORY CHAIN is partially conserved by the coupled synthesis of ATP from ADP and inorganic phosphate.

p

pantothenic acid. A vitamin that plays an important biological role as part of the structure of COENZYME A (CoA). In fact, the synthesis of CoA in animals starts with pantothenic acid.

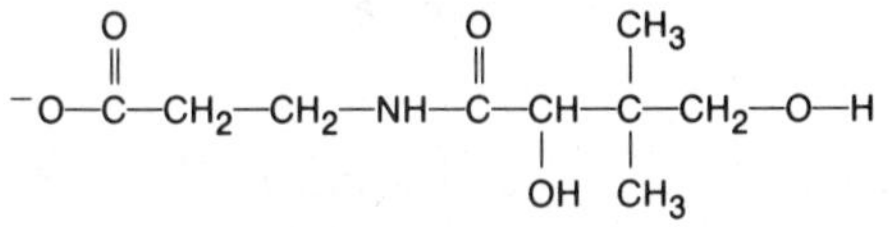

$$^-O-\overset{\overset{\displaystyle O}{\|}}{C}-CH_2-CH_2-NH-\overset{\overset{\displaystyle O}{\|}}{C}-\underset{\underset{\displaystyle OH}{|}}{CH}-\overset{\overset{\displaystyle CH_3}{|}}{\underset{\underset{\displaystyle CH_3}{|}}{C}}-CH_2-O-H$$

Pantothenic acid

In foods, pantothenic acid is found free and as coenzyme A and phosphopantetheine. The latter two compounds are digested within the gastrointestinal tract by *phosphatases* and *dipeptidases*. Absorption occurs by passive diffusion at pharmacologic doses and active transport at physiologic doses. Approximately 50 percent of pantothenic acid is absorbed from the intestine when consumed with food. From the blood pantothenic acid is actively absorbed into cells and then converted to coenzyme A.

CoA is a molecule that serves as an acyl group acceptor and donor, a transient carrier which activates a molecule so that it may enter into a reaction. These roles of CoA make pantothenic acid vital to the synthesis of FATTY ACIDS and to the oxidation of fatty acids, pyruvate, ACETALDEHYDE, α-ketoglutarate, and to many other metabolic reactions. Additionally, 4′-phosphopantetheine, made from pantothenic acid, binds to acyl carrier protein (ACP) and is important for the transport of acyl intermediates produced during FATTY ACID SYNTHESIS.

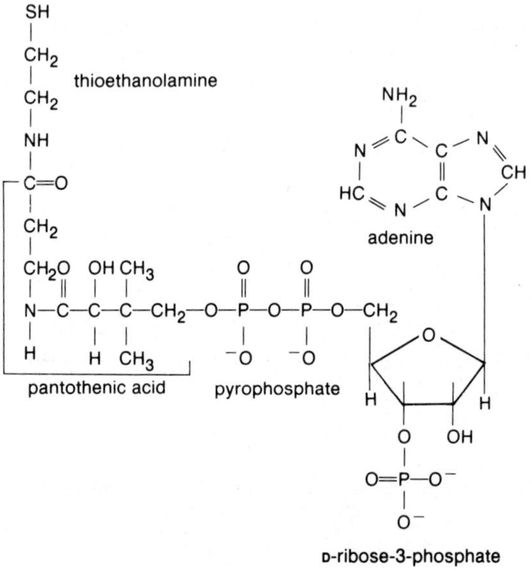

Structure of coenzyme A (CoA) showing the vitamin, pantothenic acid

Pantothenic acid is an essential nutrient for animals; however, it is synthesized by plants and microorganisms. A deficiency of it is rare because it is widespread in food—milk, meat, liver, egg yolk, and raw vegetables are good sources. It has been shown that the processing of foods, whether by cooking, canning, or freezing, destroys significant amounts of the vitamin.   See also: COENZYME A.

SUGGESTED READINGS

Fry, P. C., H. M. Fox, and H. G. Tao. 1976. Metabolic response to a pantothenic acid deficient diet in humans. *J. Nutr. Sci. Vitaminol.* 22:339–346.

Robishaw, J. D., and J. R. Neely. 1985. Coenzyme A metabolism. *Endocrinol. Metab.* 11:E1–9.

Tarr, J. B., T. Tamura, and E. L. R. Stokstad. 1981. Availability of Vitamin B$_6$ and pantothenate in an average American diet in man. *Am. J. Clin. Nutr.* 34:1328–1337.

pellagra.   A niacin-deficiency disease.   See also: NIACIN.

SUGGESTED READINGS

Sydenstricker, V. P. 1958. The history of pellagra: Its recognition as a disorder of nutrition and its conquest. *Am. J. Clin. Nutr.* 6:409–414.

pentose. A five-carbon sugar. D-ribose and 2-deoxy-D-ribose are two pentoses that are important in the structure of nucleosides and nucleotides, and, therefore, are important in the synthesis of DNA and RNA.

pentose phosphate pathway (pentose shunt, phosphogluconate pathway, hexose monophosphate shunt). A pathway by which a glycolytic intermediate, glucose 6-phosphate, can be degraded for the purpose of generating reducing power (NADPH) and pentoses for the synthesis of biomolecules.

The ENZYMES that catalyze the pathway are present in the cytoplasm of cells in the liver, adrenal cortex, mammary glands, and fat tissues. Skeletal muscle cells do not contain the enzymes for the pentose pathway.

Glucose 6-phosphate from the glycolytic path is oxidized to 6-phosphoglucono-δ-lactone by a dehydrogenase that uses $NADP^+$ as its prosthetic group. The next step is a hydrolysis followed by another dehydrogenation utilizing

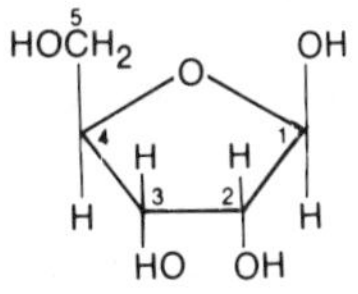

D-ribose

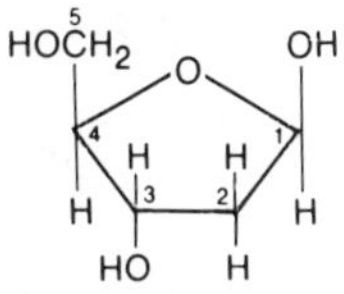

2-deoxy-D-ribose

D-ribose is the sugar component of RNA; 2-deoxy-D-ribose is the sugar component of DNA

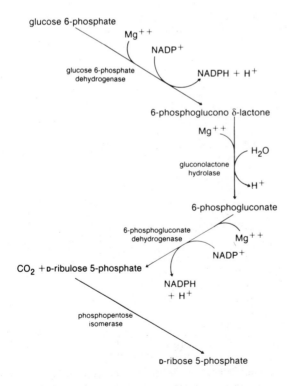

The synthesis of D-ribose 5-phosphate by the pentose phosphate pathway

$NADP^+$. The final step isomerizes D-ribulose 5-phosphate to D-ribose 5-phosphate. Two molecules of NADPH have been generated to this point and D-ribose 5-phosphate has been produced for its important work of synthesizing the ribonucleotides and deoxyribonucleotides. D-ribose 5-phosphate can also undergo some other conversions by *transketolase* and *aldolase* to produce 3-, 4-, 5-, 6-, or 7-carbon sugars. The transketolase-aldolase reactions, which require THIAMIN as THIAMIN PYROPHOSPHATE complete a cycle from GLYCOLYSIS to pentose phosphate pathway back to glycolysis.

pentose shunt.   See PENTOSE PHOSPHATE PATHWAY.

peptide bond.   The bond that unites the α-carboxyl group of one amino acid to the α-amino group of another amino acid to form a dipeptide with the loss of a water molecule. A more generalized term for this bond is "amide bond." See also: PROTEIN STRUCTURE.

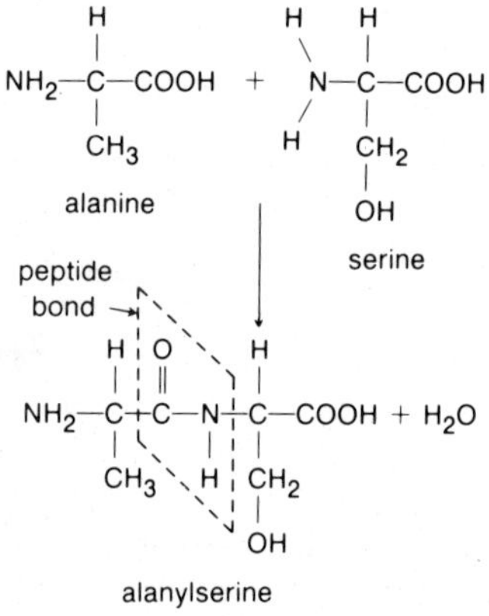

Formation of a peptide bond between the carboxyl carbon of one amino acid and the amino nitrogen of another amino acid

peptides.   See PROTEIN STRUCTURE.

pernicious anemia.   See VITAMIN B_{12}.

pH.   A numerical representation of the hydrogen ion concentration of a fluid that shows the acidity or alkalinity of the fluid. The pH scale ranges from 1, the most acidic, to 14, the least acidic. With a pH of 7, the hydrogen ion (H^+)

and hydroxyl ion (OH^-) concentrations are equal and a solution is neutral. A pH below 7 indicates a greater concentration of hydrogen ions (and a lesser concentration of hydroxyl ions) and an acidic solution. A pH above 7 indicates a higher concentration of hydroxyl ions (and a lower concentration of hydrogen ions) and an alkaline, or basic, solution.

The concentrations of ions in water are such small numbers that it is awkward to speak or write these concentrations, using ordinary nomenclature. For example, at 25°C water has a hydrogen ion concentration of 0.0000001 moles per liter. S. P. L. Sorenson suggested a way of expressing these concentrations in terms of the negative value of the logarithm of the concentration of the hydrogen ion:

$$pH = -\log[H^+]$$

By changing the decimal expression 0.0000001 (moles per liter) to its exponential form 1×10^{-7}, then substituting this value in the Sorenson equation, the answer becomes a simple 7 with no unit of measurement.

$$pH = -\log(1 \times 10^{-7}) = \log \frac{1}{1 \times 10^{-7}} = \log(1 \times 10^7) = 7$$

Some representative pH values are: stomach fluid, 1.2–3.0; lemon juice, 2.3; cola beverage, 2.8; tomato juice, 4.3; blood, 7.4; sea water, 7.0–7.5; baking soda, 8.5.

phenylalanine (Phe). An essential, nine-carbon, α-amino acid that, like TYROSINE and TRYPTOPHAN, has an aromatic side chain. Aromatic refers to a system of double bonds such as the phenyl ring. Compounds containing a phenyl ring have unusual chemical stability.

Upon degradation four of the carbons of phenylalanine enter the TCA CYCLE at fumarate and four enter through acetoacetyl-CoA; therefore, this amino acid is both ketogenic and glucogenic (glycogenic). The ninth carbon is lost as CO_2 in the step of tyrosine's degradation that leads to homogentisate.

The first step in the degradation of phenylalanine is catalyzed by *phenylalanine monooxygense* (also called *phenylalanine hydroxylase*) and uses $NADPH + H^+$. This reaction leads to the synthesis of the amino acid, tyrosine, and for this reason tyrosine, in normal persons, is considered a NONESSENTIAL AMINO ACID. After phenylalanine has been oxidized to tyrosine, the path of its degradation is that of tyrosine's degradation and will be examined in that topic.

phenyl ring

Phenylalanine (Phe)

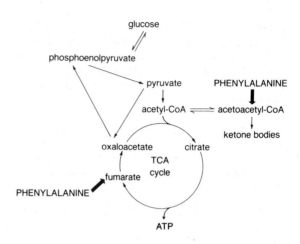

The carbons of phenylalanine, a ketogenic and glucogenic amino acid, enter metabolic pathways

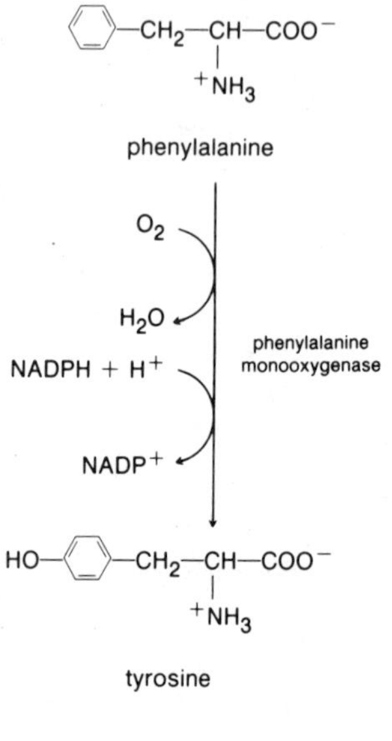

phenylalanine

O_2

H_2O

NADPH + H^+

phenylalanine monooxygenase

$NADP^+$

tyrosine

The conversion of phenylalanine to tyrosine

Of importance, however, are the many vitamins and minerals needed in the metabolism of phenylalanine. The enzyme that converts phenylalanine to tyrosine requires IRON, VITAMIN C, and NIACIN as NADPH.

The genetic absence or decreased production of the enzyme *phenylalanine monooxygenase* causes one of the best-known and most widely studied of the INBORN ERRORS OF METABOLISM, phenylketonuria (PKU). When this step is blocked, phenylalanine and other metabolites accumulate to toxic levels while tyrosine is not available for the synthesis of proteins that require it. The result of this imbalance is severe mental retardation.

Mass screening tests of newborn infants have revealed that about one in 10,000 babies has PKU. The molecular basis of the test is the elevation of a phenylketone, phenylpyruvate, in the urine. Early diagnosis and stringent dietary controls can minimize the mental retardation that accompanies the defect. Diet restrictions consist of careful monitoring and limiting of the phenylalanine content of the diet as well as supplementation of tyrosine to make up for its blocked synthesis. To the phenylketonuric, then, tyrosine is an ESSENTIAL AMINO ACID.

Classical PKU has been well researched and its symptoms and its medical and nutritional care are well understood. There are, however, other diseases that are caused, not by a defect in the enzyme, but by a genetic defect in the cofactor needed by the monooxygenase enzyme. When this cofactor, the electron carrier tetrahydrobiopterin, is defective, the hydroxylations of tyrosine and tryptophan are blocked as well as the hydroxylation of phenylalanine to tyrosine. These additional blocks produce severe neurological damage that is not responsive to dietary manipulation. These blocks result in deficiencies in the neurotransmitters dopamine, norepinephrine, and serotonin.

The enzyme that catalyzes the first step in the conversion of tyrosine to dopamine and epinephrine uses vitamin C, COPPER, iron, and niacin as cofactors. VITAMIN B$_6$ is required in the conversion from L-DOPA to dopamine. See also: TYROSINE.

SUGGESTED READINGS

Frimpter, G. W. 1973. Aminoacidurias due to inherited disorders of metabolism. Part 1. *N. Engl. J. Med.* 289:835–841.

Tourian, A., and J. B. Sidbury. 1983. Phenylketonuria and hyperphenylalaninemia. In *The metabolic basis of inherited disease*, 5th ed., ed. J. B. Stanbury et al., 270–286. New York: McGraw-Hill.

See suggested readings for INBORN ERRORS OF METABOLISM.

phenylketonuria (PKU). See PHENYLALANINE.

phosphatase. A class of ENZYMES that catalyzes the hydrolytic removal of a phosphoryl group from substrates. For example, in the liver, *glucose 6-phosphatase* removes the phosphate on carbon-6 of glucose 6-phosphate, making it possible for GLUCOSE to enter the general circulation.

phosphatidylcholine. A phospholipid commonly known as lecithin. See also: LIPIDS; MEMBRANES.

phosphocreatine. See CREATINE PHOSPHATE.

phosphoenolpyruvate (PEP). A high-energy phosphate compound that is an intermediate in both GLYCOLYSIS and GLUCONEOGENESIS. PEP has a much larger (more negative) standard free energy of hydrolysis ($\Delta G^{0'}$) than ATP. PEP's $\Delta G^{0'}$ is -14.8 kcal/mol while that of ATP is -7.3 kcal/mol.

phosphogluconate pathway (hexose monophosphate shunt). See PENTOSE PHOSPHATE PATHWAY.

phosphoglyceride. A lipid containing a glycerol backbone. The three hydroxyl groups of the glycerol are esterfied to one or two fatty acids and a phosphate group. See also: LIPIDS; MEMBRANES.

phospholipid. One of the family of lipid substances containing phosphate and either glycerol or sphingosine linked to long-chain fatty acids. See also: LIPIDS; MEMBRANES.

phosphoribosylpyrophosphate (PRPP). The donor of the ribose unit in the biosynthesis of purine and pyrimidine nucleotides. PRPP is also a key compound in the synthesis of HISTIDINE and TRYPTOPHAN.

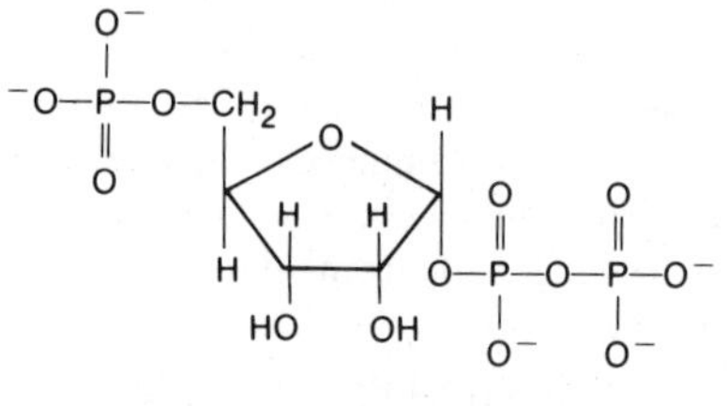

Phosphoribosylpyrophosphate (PRPP)

phosphorus (P). An element that is present in the body in both organic and inorganic compounds as phosphates. Approximately 85 percent of the body's phosphorus is in the skeleton with the rest distributed among components of muscles, nervous tissue, skin, and other organs. Most of the phosphorus in the soft tissues is in the form of organic esters, while that in the skeleton is mainly in the form of inorganic orthophosphate. In cells and extracellular fluids, phosphorus is found as organic phosphoric acid esters, phosphoproteins, phospholipids, and inorganic phosphate ions.

Phosphorus plays key roles throughout the systems of the body. The high-energy phosphate compounds are crucial in the metabolism of carbohydrate, fat, and protein, and in the delivery of the energy from the oxidation of these fuel nutrients to the cells. Also, phosphorus is important in the structure of genetic material as alternating phosphates and sugars form the "upright supports" for the double helix of DNA.

In the renal system, phosphorus functions in the excretion of hydrogen ions, thus aiding in maintaining the ACID-BASE BALANCE of the plasma and, consequently, of cells. In the skeletal system, it is part of the crystal, hydroxyapatite, $Ca_{10}(PO_4)_6(OH)_2$, which is laid down on COLLAGEN to form bone.

The absorption of phosphorus from the diet is as free phosphate and depends on how much is taken in and from what food sources it is derived. Organic forms of phosphorus in foods are hydrolyzed by intestinal phosphatases prior to absorption as inorganic phosphate. The best dietary sources of phosphorus are milk, meat, poultry, and fish, with about 70 percent of the mineral being absorbed if there is ample intake from these sources. With low dietary intake, absorption of phosphorus may be as high as 90 percent. A condition that may lower phosphorus absorption is the consumption of nonabsorbable antacids such as MAGNESIUM hydroxide and aluminum hydroxide.

SUGGESTED READINGS

DeLuca, H. F. 1979. The Vitamin D system in the regulation of calcium and phosphorus metabolism. *Nutr. Rev.* 37:161–193.

Schuette, S. A., and H. M. Linkswiler. 1982. Effects on Ca and P metabolism in humans by adding meat, meat plus milk, or purified proteins plus Ca and P to a low protein diet. *J. Nutr.* 112:338–349.

Spencer, H., L. Kramer, and D. Osis. 1984. Effect of calcium on phosphorus metabolism in man. *Am. J. Clin. Nutr.* 40:219–225.

phosphorylases. A class of ENZYMES that catalyze the degradation of glycogen. See also: GLYCOGENOLYSIS.

phosphorylation. The process whereby a phosphate group is attached to a substrate, for example, when fructose 1-phosphate becomes fructose 1-6, diphosphate during GLYCOLYSIS.

pK′. A constant that is the pH at which the protonated and unprotonated components are equal. Stated in other terms, pK′ is the pH at which an acid is one-half dissociated. The pK′ of each acid is unique.

PKU (phenylketonuria). An inborn error of amino acid metabolism. See also: PHENYLALANINE.

plasma. The liquid fraction of coagulated blood that still contains fibrinogen. Serum, on the other hand, is the liquid portion of blood from which the fibrinogen, as well as all cells, have been removed.

PLP (pyridoxal phosphate). See VITAMIN B_6.

polar. A substance having one region more negatively charged than another region.

polyunsaturated fatty acid (PUFA). A fatty acid that contains at least two carbon-carbon double bonds. See also: FATTY ACIDS.

Pompe's disease (glycogen storage disease: type II). A condition that results from the lack of the α-*1,4-glycosidase* enzyme. There is generalized storing of GLYCOGEN. Muscle weakness and wasting with minimal cardiac involvement are early symptoms; however, early cardiac death may occur.

SUGGESTED READINGS

Howel, R. R., and J. C. Williams. 1983. The glycogen storage diseases. In *The metabolic basis of inherited disease*, 5th ed., ed. J. B. Stanbury et al., 141–166. New York: McGraw-Hill.

potassium (K⁺). A positive ion (cation) that plays a key role in the maintenance of ACID-BASE BALANCE, cell volume, nerve transmission, muscle contraction, and PROTEIN BIOSYNTHESIS. A healthy level of potassium ions is maintained on the inside of cell MEMBRANES and of SODIUM ions on the outside of cell membranes by an enzyme, *sodium-potassium ATPase.* This active transport system is often simply called the SODIUM PUMP, even though it is responsible for "ushering" potassium into the cell in addition to pumping sodium out of the cell. While potassium is the principal cation on the inside of cells, it also plays an important role in the extracellular fluid where it influences muscle activity, especially that of the heart.

Transmission of signals along a neural axon is produced by the flow of ions across the plasma membrane. When a neuron is stimulated, the permeability of the membrane to sodium is changed, thus allowing sodium ions to flow in as though channels had opened through the membrane. The inward flow of sodium alters the ratio of potassium to sodium ions. This change in concentration of potassium ions travels along the axon, producing the signal in millionths of seconds. When a certain ionic potential is reached, the channels are closed and the resting potential of the cell is restored. The restoration of the resting potential involves *sodium-potassium ATPase* for the hydrolysis of ATP and is essential to the neuron's ability to transmit the next signal.

Potassium ions are needed in the cytoplasm of the cell because of their role in protein biosynthesis in the ribosomes. They also are important in GLYCOLYSIS for the activity of *pyruvate kinase,* as well as in transmission of neural signals along an axon.

Because potassium is widespread in foods, supplements are rarely needed and should never be used except on the advice of a physician who is aware of all other medications being taken by the patient. Chicken, beef liver, pork, dried apricots, orange juice, bananas, pineapple, yams, broccoli, and Brussels sprouts are good sources of potassium that do not, at the same time, increase the sodium intake. Potassium is absorbed in the small intestine; its normal excretion route is via the urine with a small amount exiting in the feces.

Serum or plasma concentrations of potassium are not good indicators for its status in the cells; therefore serum values are not generally used as a basis for treatment except at the far ends of the spectrum. For example, if the serum level is above 6 mEq/L (hyperkalemia), the medical team should be looking for the cause, whereas a value above 7 mEq/L constitutes a medical emergency. Such high levels in the plasma indicate that potassium is being drawn out of the cells into the extracellular spaces and, hence, into the bloodstream. If potassium is leaving the cells, sodium ions followed by water are entering; the integrity of the cells will be damaged if this direction of flow continues. Conditions that might produce such high-serum–low-cellular concentrations of potassium include renal insufficiency, diabetic ACIDOSIS, acute dehydration, shock, or the aftermath of a trauma such as major surgery, extensive burns, or anorexia nervosa.

If the potassium serum value is at the other end of the spectrum, perhaps below 3.5 mEq/L (hypokalemia), then smooth muscle operation may be impaired. Marked muscle weakness is observed, swallowing becomes difficult, and the muscles of respiration are affected. The most serious problem exists for heart patients since, frequently, digitalis toxicity occurs with low serum potassium concentrations. See also: ACID-BASE BALANCE; ACIDOSIS; ALKALOSIS; SODIUM PUMP.

SUGGESTED READINGS

Fregley, M. J. 1981. Sodium and potassium. *Ann. Rev. Nutr.* 1:69–94.

Mickelson, O., et al. 1977. Sodium and potassium intakes and excretions of normal men consuming sodium chloride or a 1:1 mixture of sodium and potassium chloride. *Am. J. Clin. Nutr.* 30:2033–2040.

prokaryotes. Simple cells having only a single membrane. They include bacteria and blue-green algae and are considered to be the first cells to arise in biological evolution. Prokaryotes have one molecule of double-helix DNA and lack the highly specialized organelles that characterize eukaryotic cells.

proline (Pro). A nonessential, glucogenic (glycogenic), five-carbon, α-amino acid whose side chain is bonded to both the α-amino group and the α-carbon, producing a ring. In reality, the amino group in proline is an imino group since it is NH— rather than NH$_2$—.

Proline is probably best known for its role in the triple helix of COLLAGEN, a strong connective tissue that binds groups of cells together. Proline, hydroxyproline (a derivative of proline), and GLYCINE are regularly spaced in the amino acid sequence of the collagen fiber.

$$COO^-$$
$$H_2N^+ - CH$$
$$H_2C \diagdown \diagup CH_2$$
$$C$$
$$H_2$$

Proline (Pro)

Proline is synthesized from GLUTAMATE whose carboxyl group on its side chain reacts first with NADH + H$^+$ and ATP to form glutamate γ-semialdehyde. The side chain bends back on itself to form pyrroline 5-carboxylate that is then reduced by another NADH to yield proline.

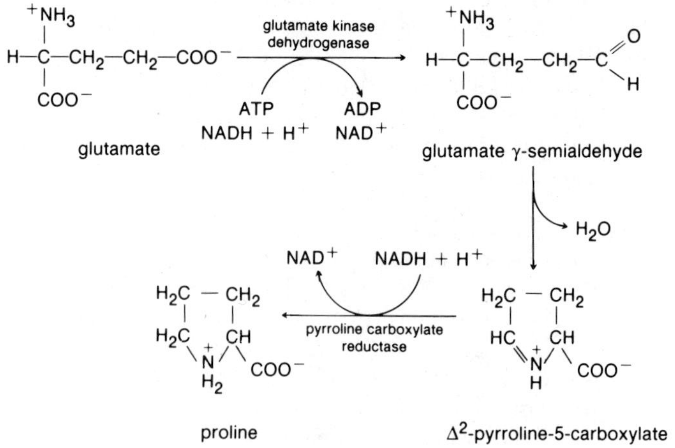

The synthesis of proline from glutamate

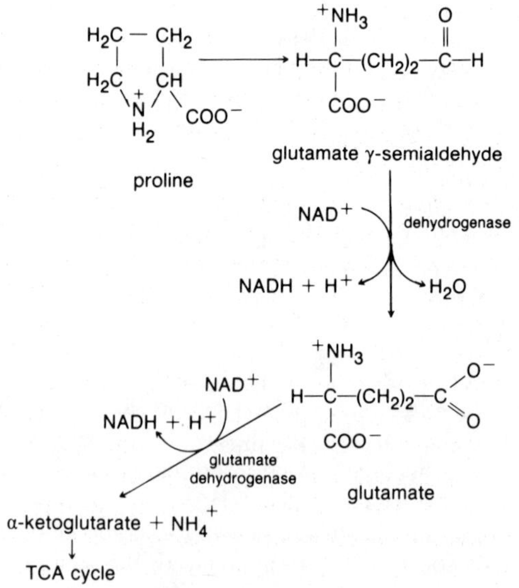

The degradation of proline so that its carbons may enter metabolic pathways

When proline is degraded, its carbon skeleton enters the TCA CYCLE at α-ketoglutarate. Its ring structure first opens to yield glutamate γ-semialdehyde, which is then reduced to glutamate. *Glutamate dehydrogenase* will deaminate glutamate to α-ketoglutarate, a process that requires either of two NIACIN coenzymes, NAD^+ or $NADP^+$.

prostaglandins (PG). A group of biologically active compounds derived from polyunsaturated FATTY ACIDS. Each prostaglandin is a twenty-carbon fatty acid that contains a five-carbon ring and differs structurally from another prostaglandin principally in the number of double bonds, as noted by the numerical subscript. An additional letter is added to indicate the type.

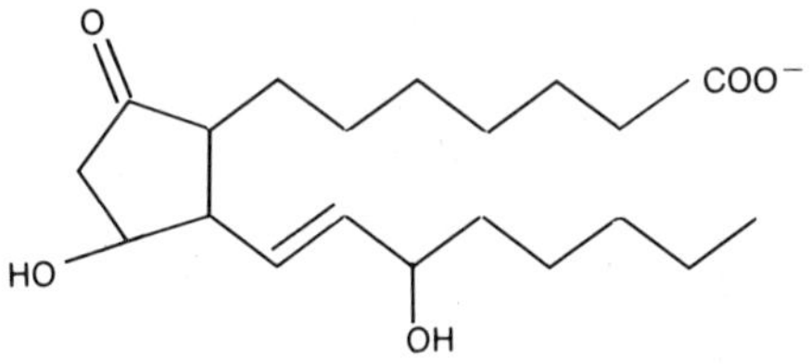

PGE_1 (prostaglandin type E_1)

Although prostaglandins are often referred to as "hormonelike" substances, they have a number of distinguishing characteristics. Unlike hormones, whose actions are the same for all their target cells, prostaglandins have different effects on different cells. Also, unlike hormones which can affect tissues all over the body, the consensus seems to be that prostaglandins only affect the cells in which they are synthesized. They appear to alter the actions of hormones rather than to act like hormones themselves.

While investigation into the nature of prostaglandins continues, some interactions and effects are now known. Aspirin has been shown to inhibit the synthesis of some prostaglandins by blocking the action of the enzyme, *cyclooxygenase*. The anti-inflammatory drug, indomethacin, prolongs the half-life of prostaglandins by interfering with their metabolism. Some general actions of prostaglandins include their effects on the function of the immune and nervous systems and on gastrointestinal secretions. In addition, some PG have the effect of lowering blood pressure and stimulating smooth muscles to contract or to relax.

Prostaglandins are widely distributed in animal tissue where they are synthesized from linoleic acid (18:2ω6), arachidonic acid (20:4ω6), and α-linolenic acid (18:3ω3). Linoleic acid gives rise to series 1, which have one double bond;

223

arachidonic acid yields series 2 which have two double bonds; and linolenic acid produces series 3 which have three double bonds. *Cyclooxygenase* is the enzyme catalyzing the production of all three series.

The PGGs are produced by the action of *cyclooxygenase* and then are acted upon by a peroxidase to form the PGHs which, in turn, yield the PGEs, PGDs, PGFs, and the PGIs.

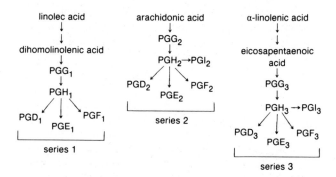

The production of three series of prostaglandins

The actions of the various prostaglandins are under continuing investigation and are producing interesting results. For example, PGE_2 and PGF_2 are metabolically active and their actions are antagonistic. PGE_2 causes smooth muscle relaxation and bronchial and vascular dilation, whereas PGF_2 causes smooth muscle contraction and bronchial and vascular constriction. PGI_2 also causes vascular dilation. PGE_2 retards the attraction or repulsion of leukocytes to chemicals (chemotaxis), while PGF_2 enhances chemotaxis. It is thought that some of the actions of some prostaglandins are mediated through cAMP and/or CALCIUM.

Possible therapeutic uses of prostaglandins include the prevention of conception, the termination of pregnancy, prevention of gastric ulcers and promotion of their healing, and the control of blood pressure, inflammation, and asthma.

SUGGESTED READINGS

Adam, O., and G. Wolfram. 1984. Effect of different linoleic acid intakes on prostaglandin biosynthesis and kidney function in man. *Am. J. Clin. Nutr.* 40:763–770.

Dyerberg, J., and H. O. Bang. 1979. Haemostatic function and platelet polyunsaturated fatty acids in Eskimos. *Lancet* 2:433–435.

Hammarstrom, S. 1983. Leukotrienes. *Ann. Rev. Biochem.* 52:355–377.

Harris, R. H., P. W. Ramwell, and P. J. Gilmer. 1979. Cellular mechanics of prostaglandin action. *Ann. Rev. Physiol.* 41: 653–668.

Harris, W. S., S. H. Goodnight, Jr., and W. E. Connor. 1983. Dietary fats, platelets, prostaglandins, and plasma lipids. In *Nutrition and heart disease,* ed. E. B. Feldman, 59–82. New York: Churchill Livingstone.

Herold, P. M., and J. E. Kinsella. 1986. Fish oil consumption and decreased risk of cardiovascular disease: A comparison of findings from animal and human feeding trials. *Am. J. Clin. Nutr.* 43:566–598.

Nelson, N. A., R. C. Kelly, and R. A. Johnson. 1982. Prostaglandins and the arachidonic acid cascade. C. & EN. August 16, 30–44.

Olley, P. M., and F. Coccani. 1980. The prostaglandins. *Am. J. Dis. Child* 134:688–696.

Piper, P. J. 1984. Formation and actions of leukotrienes. *Physiol. Rev.* 64:744–761.

Samuelsson, B. 1981. Leukotrienes: A novel group of compounds including SRS-A. *Prog. Lipid Res.* 20:23–30.

prosthetic group. A nonprotein component attached to a protein that is generally necessary for the protein's biologic activity. Without the prosthetic group, the molecule is referred to as the "apoprotein." For example, *pyruvate carboxylase,* the enzyme that attaches a carboxyl group to pyruvate forming oxaloacetate in GLUCONEOGENESIS, is inactive unless BIOTIN, its prosthetic group, is attached. Prosthetic groups may be considered the same as coenzymes, but some authorities make a distinction between the two. "Prosthetic groups" such as biotin, they say, are covalently bound, whereas "coenzymes" such as pyridoxal phosphate are not, and, for this reason, coenzymes can be removed more easily.

protein. A molecule composed of α-amino acids joined together by peptide bonds. A protein may consist of one or more "strings" of AMINO ACIDS. The amino acids are made of common elements: carbon, hydrogen, oxygen, nitrogen, and sometimes sulfur. Proteins are distinguished from other proteins made of the same elements by the sequence of their amino acids.

Protein is found in the structure of all living organisms. It forms the bone, muscle, skin, brain, red blood cells, and all the other organs and tissues of the human body. Proteins also play many roles in the body. There are proteins—ENZYMES—that are responsible for the chemical events in the cells. These enzymes not only control what reactions take place but also the speed with which they happen.

There are proteins in the body—immunoglobulins, also called antibodies—that can recognize and destroy foreign substances. Other proteins—hormones—are messengers that are secreted in response to altered conditions in the body. In the blood, some proteins help maintain ACID-BASE BALANCE by binding and releasing hydrogen ions while others maintain osmotic pressure.

Proteins act as carriers to transport various ions or molecules across cell membranes or in the blood. Lipoproteins, for example, encase hydrophobic fats so they can be transported in the blood. A protein in the blood—albumin—carries minerals such as ZINC or CALCIUM throughout the body. Another protein—hemoglobin—transports oxygen from the lungs to the cells. Other transport proteins are required for absorption of nutrients from the intestinal cells. See also: AMINO ACIDS; PROTEIN BIOSYNTHESIS; PROTEIN DIGESTION; PROTEIN STRUCTURE.

protein biosynthesis. The bonding of AMINO ACIDS one to another in a specific sequence to build a peptide chain; then, if the protein has more than one chain, to complete the biosynthesis by binding the chains together. All this activity is under the instructions contained in the DNA of a cell.

DNA→RNA→protein

All genetic instructions are carried out by proteins. The central dogma for normal cells is that genetic information goes from DNA in the nucleus to RNA, which can enter the cytosol, to protein, which is constructed on the ribosomes from materials present in the cytosol. In terms of processes, the dogma is replication → transcription → translation.

A variety of substances must be present for the peptide chain to be synthesized. All the ESSENTIAL AMINO ACIDS must be present in adequate amounts. They enter the body either from the digestion and absorption of complete protein foods, such as meat, milk, egg, fish, or poultry, or from incomplete protein foods, such as whole wheat bread and peanut butter, whose amino acid profiles complement each other. If one essential amino acid is absent or becomes limited at the time a protein is being built, synthesis will cease and the unfinished chain will be dismantled.

In addition, many of the NONESSENTIAL AMINO ACIDS or the materials to synthesize them must be present as well as mRNA, rRNA, various factors, a mixture of tRNAs, and the *aminoacyl-tRNA synthetases.* These synthetases are the ENZYMES that activate the amino acids and attach them to the correct tRNA, thus ensuring that each amino acid is put in its proper place in the chain. The energy to drive the attachment of the amino acid to the tRNA demands a ready supply of ATP and MAGNESIUM; other steps of the synthesis require GTP.

When the cell needs a particular protein, the DNA of the gene for that protein is "unzipped" and a complementary copy is made of one of the strands. The resulting molecule is messenger RNA (mRNA) that leaves the nucleus, enters the cytosol, and, with the help of various factors, attaches itself to the smaller of the two subunits of a ribosome. After both subunits become attached, mRNA directs the construction of the protein.

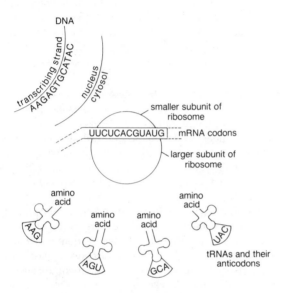

Amino acid segment of a protein being
translated: Phe-Ser-Arg-Met

The mRNAs contain codons—a group of three nucleotides that designates a single amino acid. The order of the codons represents the sequence in which the amino acids will be brought together to form a protein.

As each codon is "read," there is at least one transfer RNA (tRNA) that will bring its activated amino acid to the construction site on the ribosome. The amino acids are activated at their carboxyl end by the attachment of a highly reactive molecule, aminoacyl adenylate, which holds the energy from ATP. Through the action of *synthetases*, the activated amino acid is attached to the tRNA. The tRNA is able to interact with mRNA through the anticodon on one of its arms. The anticodon is a complementary copy of the codon on mRNA and can readily form hydrogen bonds.

When everything in the cytosol is ready, that is, the mRNA is attached to the small subunit of the ribosome and the large subunit of the ribosome joins with the small subunit to make an intact ribosome. Then each amino acid is brought to the ribosomes by the tRNAs and is attached in a peptide bond to the growing protein chain. Once the amino acid is attached, the tRNAs return to the cytoplasm to carry another amino acid to the ribosome. When all the amino acids have been attached, the protein chain is completed and disconnected from the ribosome.

Each peptide bond will have cost four high-energy phosphate bonds: two bonds come from ATP to activate the amino acid, and two come from GTP, one for the elongation process and one for the interaction of various factors. See also: DNA; GENETIC CODE; RNA; TRANSCRIPTION; TRANSLATION.

protein digestion. The hydrolysis of the peptide bonds of large, complex protein molecules, breaking them into smaller sizes and resulting in freed AMINO ACIDS, dipeptides, and tripeptides, which can be absorbed into the intestinal cells. This progressive action of the proteolytic enzymes begins in the stomach, continues in the lumen of the small intestine, and then is completed in the mucosa of the small intestine.

The first act of protein digestion occurs in the acidic environment of the stomach where small pieces of protein-containing food, resulting from mastication in the mouth, are denatured by hydrochloric acid secreted by gastric parietal cells. Once the small fragments of protein are uncoiled, their bonds can be attacked by the gastric protease, *pepsin*. *Pepsin* is produced by the mucosa cells (called the "chief" cells) of the stomach as the zymogen *pepsinogen*, which is converted to its active form by hydrochloric acid and free *pepsin*. *Pepsin* hydrolysis results in a fragmenting of the protein chain into oligopeptides of varying lengths.

The ENZYMES, proteases, that catalyze this breaking apart are specific for certain bonds. For example, one of the first proteases encountered, *pepsin*, attacks only the bonds on the carboxyl side of amino acids that have an aromatic side chain. Because the tissues that synthesize and secrete these enzymes are themselves made of protein, the proteolytic enzymes generally are released in an inactive form, a ZYMOGEN. Once released, the zymogen will be altered so that it may hydrolyze its intended target substrate.

This digestive action is time consuming as the strong muscles of the stomach continually churn the contents to allow the enzyme and acid to be positioned closer to the bonds. As the stomach contents become liquified, small amounts of chyme leave the stomach and enter the duodenum where the bicarbonate ions from the pancreas neutralize the acid in the mixture.

The pancreas also secretes into the duodenum the zymogens, *trypsinogen, chymotrypsinogen,* and *procarboxypeptidase. Enterokinase,* which is synthesized in the intestinal cells, "frees" the enzyme *trypsin* from *trypsinogen.* Then *trypsin,* in turn, acts on the zymogen from which it came to free more *trypsin. Trypsin* also activates *chymotrypsin* and the *carboxypeptidase.*

Trypsin attacks peptide bonds on the carboxyl side of those amino acids that have basic side chains, *chymotrypsin* cleaves the peptide bond on the carboxyl side of amino acids that have aromatic side chains, and *carboxypeptidase* frees amino acids that are at the carboxyl end of the chain. An additional enzyme, among others that also hydrolyze protein, is *aminopeptidase,* which frees an amino acid at the amino terminal of the protein chain. The shorter and shorter peptide chains resulting from these actions include tripeptides,

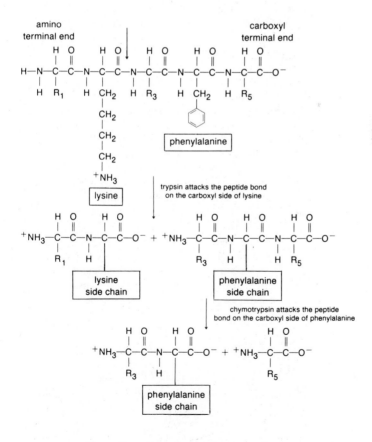

The action of trypsin and chymotrypsin

R_1, R_3, R_5 = side chains of other amino acid residues

dipeptides, and free amino acids that will be taken into the mucosal cells of the small intestine by active transport.

The small peptides are quickly hydrolyzed into free amino acids and these, along with the other free amino acids, are transported from the mucosal cells into the portal vein. This vein will carry them to the liver where they will be redistributed or chemically altered according to the demands of the body. See also: GLUCONEOGENESIS; PROTEIN BIOSYNTHESIS; ZYMOGEN; individual amino acids.

SUGGESTED READINGS

Silk, D. B. A., G. K. Grimble, and R. G. Rees. 1985. Protein digestion and amino acid and peptide absorption. *Proc. Nutr. Soc.* 44:63–72.

protein structure. A complex molecule composed of α-amino acids joined in peptide linkages. A protein is built of one or more strings of amino acids, each string containing a prescribed, unique sequence of amino acids.

While the structure of a protein molecule appears complex, the principles which govern it—the laws of mass, energy, electrical charge, and chemical bonding—govern the entire universe.

There are about 20 amino acids each containing carbon, hydrogen, oxygen and nitrogen atoms. (Some amino acids also contain sulfur.) Part of the structure of α-amino acids is identical to that of all other α-amino acids; however, a side chain on each of the amino acids differs. Thus, the side chains make each amino acid unique.

Protein's primary structure consists of a chain of amino acids joined by peptide bonds. The peptide bond is formed between the α-carboxy group of one amino acid and the α-amino group of another amino acid. The hydroxy (OH^-) ion removed from the carboxy group and the hydrogen (H^+) ion removed from the amino group form water.

The genetic code in DNA specifies the exact sequence of the amino acids in the protein chain. A single variation in the inherited instructions often has lethal results. For example, in the disease, SICKLE CELL ANEMIA, the code for VALINE is given in place of the code for GLUTAMATE in normal DNA for hemoglobin. This slight difference confers on the person inheriting it this often fatal disease as well as immunity from another disease, malaria.

When many amino acids are joined in peptide bonds, the backbone is a string of N—C—C—N—C—C ... The completed protein chain begins with the α-amino group of the first amino acid (which is called the N-terminus) and ends with the α-carboxyl group of the last amino acid

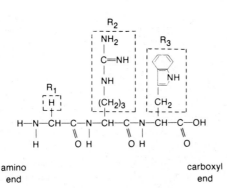

$$\begin{array}{c}
CH_3 \\
| \\
OH—CH
\end{array}
\qquad
\begin{array}{c}
H_3C \quad CH_3 \\
\backslash \; / \\
CH
\end{array}$$

H—N—C—C+OH + H+N—C—C—OH→

threonine   valine

threonylvaline, a dipeptide

peptide bond

**Formation of peptide bonds create the
primary structure of a protein**

H—N—CH—C—N—CH—C—N—CH—C—OH

amino   carboxyl
end   end

Glycylarginyltryptophan, a tripeptide

R_1, R_2, R_3 enclosed in dotted portion of drawing
represent the side chains of amino acids.

H—N—CH—C—N—CH—C—N—CH—C—OH

The backbone of a protein
N—C—C—N—C—C—N—C—C

231

(which is called the C-terminus). The side chains protruding from the protein backbone affect the conformation of the protein and, thus, its physical and chemical characteristics.

The secondary structure of the protein results from interactions between the side chains to cause a coiling of the single protein chain where about every fourth amino acid interacts to produce a coil. However, if the side groups of the two amino acids in these spots repel each other, there may be a "kink" at that point. This adds to the individuality of the protein.

The tertiary structure of a protein is determined by the attraction or repulsion of the side chains of amino acids. These side chains may be at a great distance from each other in the sequence along the straightened out chain. The tertiary level of organization results in the twisting and turning of the chains back on themselves and produces shapes that are crucial for specific work. For example, globular proteins may be needed for carrying substances through the blood whereas, the long, thin, fibrous proteins may be used for strength in such related structures as hair, nails, and skin.

The quaternary structure is not present in all proteins but it is important in the conformation of some. At the quarternary level of organization, two or more protein chains interact. However, they also function somewhat independently. Hemoglobin, a good example, has four chains, each of which binds one molecule of oxygen. Each chain acts independently in giving up its oxygen; however, when one chain has released its oxygen, the remaining ones release theirs more readily.

In its most favorable environment of temperature and pH, the natural conformation of the protein is surprisingly stable. This stability is accounted for by the types of bonds that hold the parts together in a particular conformation. The peptide bond has about 50 percent double bond characteristics, which means that its atoms are not very free to rotate. In a primary chain of amino acids, about a third of the bonds, then, are rigid. This stabilizes the shape and allows other parts of the molecule to interact with minimal energy spent on disruption.

Another type of bond that is important in determining protein conformation is the hydrogen bond that can occur between atoms in side chains or in the main peptide chain. The hydrogen bond is a weak bond formed when a hydrogen atom is shared by two other atoms. The hydrogen is linked more strongly to one atom than to the other; the one to which it is strongly linked is thought of as the hydrogen "donor" and the other is considered the hydrogen "acceptor." The most important characteristic of this bond is that it has direction, as though the bond were "pointing" from the donor atom through the hydrogen to the acceptor atom. The more nearly this pointing is in a straight line, the stronger the bond.

The strongest bond in a protein is the covalent bond between two cysteine residues. When two cysteines are oxidized and their sulfurs bond to each other, a "disulfide bridge" is formed within cystine. If the cysteines are at some distance from each other on the same amino acid chain, the bridge will form a loop in the chain. If the cysteines are on different chains, the bridge will connect the two chains.

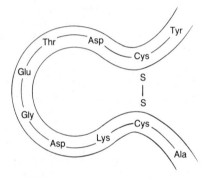

Formation of a disulfide bridge forms
a loop in a protein chain

Two environmental factors influencing protein conformation are temperature and pH. A bond requires a certain amount of energy for stability. When temperature increases, more energy is available to break the bond. A shift in pH in either direction would tend to disrupt hydrogen bonds. Sometimes these shifts are useful; for example, if the product of an enzyme's action in a cell contributes hydrogen ions to the cytoplasm, then an accumulation of that product would cause a lowering of the pH. At some point, the pH shift will be great enough to change the conformation of the enzyme, thus "turning it off." As the product is used up and more is needed, the pH would rise to the level most favorable to the enzyme. The enzyme would then reassume its natural conformation and be back in business, making more product. Such a feedback mechanism is very economical. It does not involve another compound as a messenger, stimulator, or inhibitor; rather it is just a simple turning on and turning off of the conformation of the enzyme.

An increase in temperature, a shift in either direction of the pH, as well as other factors can denature a protein, that is, disrupt the bonds so that the chains will uncoil and the conformation will be lost. When conformation is altered, biological activity is lost. The cooking of egg white is a good visual example of denaturation. See also: AMINO ACIDS; ENZYMES; PROTEIN; PROTEIN DIGESTION.

protophoryrin IX. A compound found in cytochromes, hemoglobin, and myoglobin. See also: HEME.

PRPP. See PHOSPHORIBOSYLPYROPHOSPHATE.

PUFA. See POLYUNSATURATED FATTY ACID.

purine, pyrimidine bases. The nitrogenous bases that are fundamental structural units of nucleotides. The nucleotides play a role in almost every chemical process in living organisms including being the precursors of the genetic material, DNA. The base adenine, for example, is present in the vital nucleotides ATP, ADP, AMP, NAD^+, FAD, and COENZYME A.

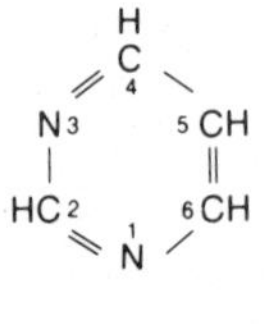

Pyrimidine 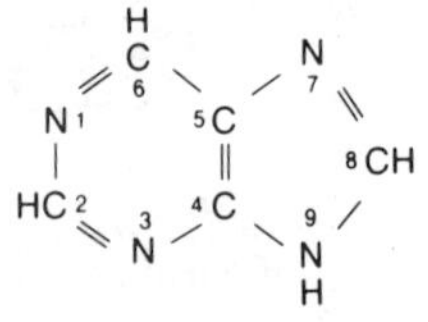   Purine

There are two major purine bases, adenine and guanine. Xanthine and hypoxanthine may also be included. There are three major pyrimidine bases: cytosine, thymine, and uracil. These bases are of major importance in DNA replication.

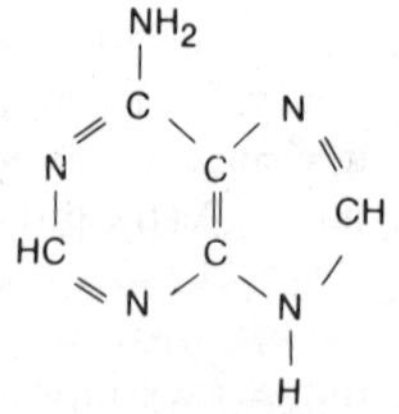

adenine 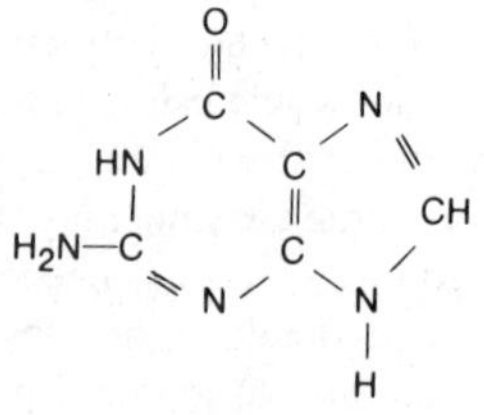   guanine

Purine bases

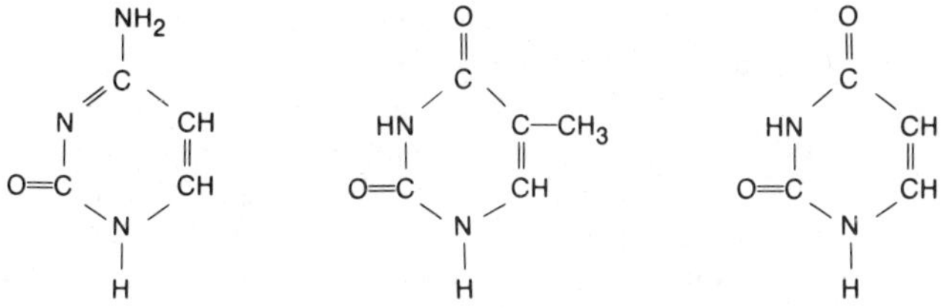

cytosine

thymine

uracil

Pyrimidine bases

In the double strands of DNA, a purine base on one strand is paired with a pyrimidine base on the opposing strand. An adenine (A) is opposite a thymine (T), and a guanine (G) is opposite a cytosine (C). When the DNA double strands separate during replication, a complementary strand can be constructed opposite each original strand. When completed, the two new double strands will be identical to each other and to the original double strand.

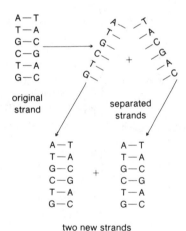

original strand

separated strands

two new strands

Replication of double-stranded DNA

The composition of the diet seems to have little influence on the synthesis of these bases. Metabolites from protein and carbohydrate METABOLISM seem to be sufficient for the synthesis of the nitrogen ring structures if the vitamins FOL-ACIN, B_6, and NIACIN are present.

The pyrimidine ring is made in the liver from two plentiful compounds, the amino acid, ASPARTATE, and carbamoyl

$$H_2N-\underset{\underset{O^-}{\overset{O^-}{|}}}{\overset{O}{\overset{\|}{C}}}-O-\underset{\overset{O}{\overset{\|}{P}}}{\overset{O}{\overset{\|}{}}}-O^-$$

Carbamoyl phosphate

$$^-OOC-CH_2-\underset{\overset{+}{NH_3}}{CH}-COO^-$$

Aspartate

(also spelled "carbamyl") phosphate. Carbamoyl phosphate, the same compound important in the urea cycle, is made from CO_2, NH_3 from GLUTAMINE, and two molecules of ATP. The enzyme for the synthesis of carbamoyl phosphate of the UREA CYCLE is in the mitochondrion and the enzyme needed for the synthesis of the pyrimidine ring is in the cytosol, thus the two syntheses can take place at the same time. Another difference between the two reactions is that the urea cycle carbamoyl phosphate can utilize NITROGEN from the deamination of AMINO ACIDS in general, whereas the amino group for the pyrimidine ring carbamoyl comes specifically from the amino acid glutamine. By the action of a *transcarbamoylase* and several other ENZYMES, the compound orotic acid is formed from carbamoyl phosphate and aspartate. Orotic acid may then combine with 5-phosphoribosyl-1-pyrophosphate (PRPP), derived from ribose, to form OMP (orotidylic acid), which may then be used to form the pyrimidine nucleotides.

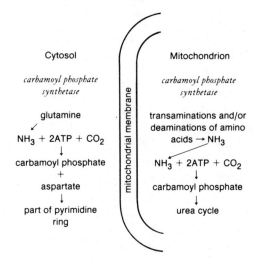

Distinct reactions involving carbamoyl phosphate are separated by the mitochondrial membrane

The synthesis of the purine ring is much more complex than that of the pyrimidine ring. A purine ring is built in a stepwise process. The origin of the nitrogens and carbons of the purine ring is as follows: N-1 from aspartate, N-3 and N-9 from glutamine, N-7, C-4, and C-5 from glycine, C-2 and C-8 from folacin, and C-6 from carbon dioxide.

Purine nucleotides (AMP, GMP) are degraded by a series of reactions. AMP degradation yields hypoxanthine that, by the action of *xanthine oxidase* which requires MOLYBDENUM and IRON, forms xanthine; GMP degradation also yields xanthine. Xanthine is further degraded by *xanthine oxidase* to form uric acid, which is then excreted in the urine. In the reaction, oxygen is reduced to hydrogen peroxide.

The salvage pathway, however, is able to recover free purines before they are degraded to uric acid and remake new nucleotides. The free purines (adenine and guanine) react with 5-phosphoribosyl-1-pyrophosphate (PRPP) to form the respective nucleotide (AMP or GMP) plus pyrophosphate. Hypoxanthine may also react with PRPP to form IMP (inosinic acid) in a reaction catalyzed by *hypoxanthine-guanine phosphoribosyl transferase*. This enzyme is also responsible for the salvage of guanine and is the enzyme that is missing in Lesch-Nyhan syndrome, a genetic disorder. Uridine, cytidine, and thymidine (pyrimidines) may be salvaged by reacting with ATP and thus re-form their respective nucleotides. See also: ATP, ADP, AMP; DNA; LESCH-NYHAN SYNDROME; PHOSPHORIBOSYLPYRO-PHOSPHATE; PROTEIN BIOSYNTHESIS; RNA.

pyridoxal. See VITAMIN B_6.

pyridoxal phosphate (PLP). A coenzyme form of vitamin B_6. See also: VITAMIN B_6.

pyridoxamine. See VITAMIN B_6.

pyridoxine. See VITAMIN B_6.

pyridoxol. See VITAMIN B_6.

pyruvate. A key intermediate in the extraction of energy from glucose, some amino acids, and glycerol. See also: GLYCOLYSIS; GLUCONEOGENESIS.

reducing equivalents. A more generalized term for the electrons that are transferred from one compound to another in oxidation/reduction reactions. Reducing equivalents refer to electron transfer without regard to the form of the electron—whether it is a hydrogen atom that is transferred as in NADH when it collects the electrons from glycolysis, or whether it is an electron that is transferred along the electron transport chain. See also: RESPIRATORY CHAIN.

replication. In genetics, replication refers to duplication of the DNA in the nucleus of cells. This take place only in dividing cells where the entire DNA in the nucleus is duplicated. The DNA of daughter cells is identical to that of the parent cell. In the development of some cells, replication ceases at a prescribed point; for example, by the time red blood cells are mature, they have lost all their DNA and therefore cannot replicate. In general scientific parlance, "replication" refers to the successful repetition of an experiment.

respiratory chain (electron transport chain). A series of oxidation-reduction reactions that transport electrons from NADH or $FADH_2$ to oxygen. The respiratory chain is the last process in reclaiming the energy in the chemical bonds of fuel nutrients. Through digestion and METABOLISM, most nutrients become ACETYL-COA; acetyl-CoA enters the TCA cycle after which the released hydrogens, along with their electrons, are picked up by NAD^+ and FAD which become $NADH + H^+$ and $FADH_2$. At three points along the respiratory chain, the energy will be used to phosphorylate ADP to ATP.

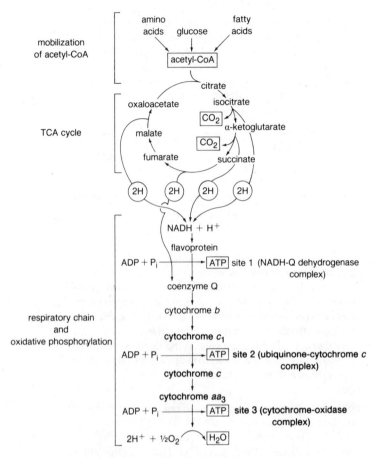

Pathway of energy production from acetyl-CoA to ATP

Like the TCA CYCLE, the respiratory chain is located in the MITOCHONDRION, the "power house" of the cell. The substances that receive electrons and transfer them to the next carrier are located in the inner membrane of the mitochondria. Along this inner membrane are knoblike structures, called "inner membrane spheres," which house the *ATP synthase* that will convert ADP to ATP. The inner membrane is relatively impermeable, allowing one ADP in for every molecule of ATP that leaves.

The substances that make up the chain are called electron "carriers" because they have prosthetic groups which have the ability to be both electron acceptors and donors: for the moment that they pick up and deliver, they are carriers of electrons. Actually, the chain is a series of oxidations and reductions with the donor being the reducing agent and the acceptor being the oxidizing agent. The flow of electrons is from NADH, which has a relatively high tendency to lose electrons, to water, which has a relatively low tendency to lose electrons. Stated in other terms, the conjugate pair of $NAD^+:NADH + H^+$, has a negative standard reduction potential of -0.11, and the conjugate pair water:oxygen has a positive standard reduction potential of $+0.82$, so the flow of electrons is from NADH to oxygen.

The dehydrogenases that use the NIACIN coenzymes NAD^+ and $NADP^+$ as prosthetic groups catalyze the transfer of two hydrogens from the substrate to form NADH + H^+ and NADPH + H^+ (the reduced forms), which are linked to the dehydrogenases. One hydrogen and two electrons are bound as NADH and a hydrogen ion is set free in the medium: NADH + H^+. Hydrogen ions are not carried along the respiratory chain; however, they are later picked up by oxygen from the medium to form water.

The dehydrogenases that use the RIBOFLAVIN coenzymes FAD and FMN as prosthetic groups transfer a pair of hydrogens from the substrate to form the reduced forms, $FADH_2$ and $FMNH_2$, which are linked to the dehydrogenases.

Coenzyme Q collects these reducing equivalents and transfers them to the cytochromes, which then "hand" them down the chain to oxygen. Cytochromes are in the same class of compounds as hemoglobin and myoglobin, the HEME proteins. All the cytochromes, except cytochrome c, are tightly bound to the mitochondrial membrane.

At three places along the chain, the oxidation-reduction energy of the electrons is great enough to oxidatively phosphorylate ADP to ATP. The first site is at the NADH-Q dehydrogenase complex where a pair of reducing equivalents is transferred from NADH to the prosthetic group (FMN) of *NADH dehydrogenase*, forming $FMNH_2$. By shifting IRON from a valence of $+2$ to $+3$, the iron-sulfur centers of the complex transfer the reducing equivalents to the next carrier in the chain, coenzyme Q. Coenzyme Q not only collects reducing equivalents from NADH or NADPH but also from *succinate dehydrogenase* and *fatty acyl-CoA dehydrogenase* and transfers these to the first of the cytochromes, cytochrome b.

The second energy-conserving site is the ubiquinone-cytochrome c site where transfers are made from cytochrome b to c_1 and then to cytochrome c. The third site is the cytochrome-oxidase site where the reducing equivalents that were transferred from cytochrome c to cytochrome aa_3 are transferred to oxygen. One ATP is generated at each of the three sites.

If electrons are carried from NADH to oxygen, three ATPs are formed since these reducing equivalents pass through all three sites. But if the electrons entering the chain are carried by $FADH_2$, only two ATPs are formed since $FADH_2$ equivalents enter the chain at coenzyme Q and pass through only two sites.

If the muscles of the body are at rest, the ATP level will be high at these sites and the level of ADP will be low since there is little requirement for energy. Even though there will be plenty of substrate to donate electrons and an excess of oxygen to receive the electrons, there is such a tight coupling with phosphorylation that, if the ATP is not being used (thus producing ADP), few electrons will flow down the chain. This condition—a low level of ADP—slows the respiratory chain. When activity resumes, the ADP level will be raised as ATP is used and electrons will again flow down the chain. See also: NAD^+, $NADP^+$ and FAD, FMN for the mechanics of the molecular action of NADH, NADPH, $FADH_2$, and $FMNH_2$ in receiving and transferring electrons; COENZYME Q; CYTOCHROMES; HEME.

SUGGESTED READINGS

Hatefi, Y. 1985. The mitochondrial electron transport and oxidative phosphorylation system. *Ann. Rev. Biochem.* 54:1015–1070.

Wikstrom, M., K. Krab, and M. Saraste. 1981. Proton-translocating cytochrome complexes. *Ann. Rev. Biochem.* 50:623–655.

retinal. See VITAMIN A.

retinol. See VITAMIN A.

riboflavin (vitamin B$_2$). A unique B-complex vitamin that is irreversibly altered by light and irradiation. The yellow-green fluorescent pigment in milk whey was known as early as 1879, but it was not until 1933 that the substance was recognized as part of the B-complex of VITAMINS. Riboflavin consists of an isoalloxazine ring attached to a ribityl side chain.

The importance of riboflavin to good health lies in its role of reclaiming the energy in the bonds of fuel nutrients. Riboflavin is the reactive group for two important coenzymes, flavin mononucleotide (FMN) and flavin adenine dinucleotide (FAD). These flavin coenzymes, synthesized from riboflavin, are essential parts of enzyme complexes that transfer hydrogens and electrons during the stepwise oxidation of energy nutrients.

Riboflavin is absorbed from the small intestine. Dietary FMN and FAD are hydrolyzed in the gastrointestinal tract prior to absorption. In the blood, riboflavin is transported

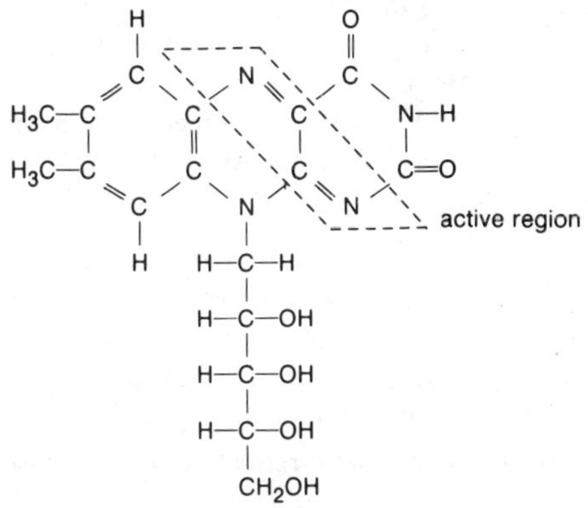

Riboflavin

free or bound to plasma proteins, principally albumin. Riboflavin is excreted mainly via the kidney; however, small amounts are excreted via sweat and bile.

Milk, milk products, and meats are the best food sources of riboflavin. Cereal grains generally are a poor source; however, in the United States, enrichment of bread and flour has made this group of foods a donor of perhaps as much as 10 percent of the Recommended Dietary Allowance (RDA). Precautions must be taken not to destroy riboflavin in milk during the addition of vitamin D by irradiation; also, milk and milk products must be packaged in opaque containers to exclude light. However, riboflavin is heat stable and therefore is not destroyed by ordinary cooking.

The primary effect of riboflavin deficiency is the halting of growth. Unlike the situation with some other vitamin deficiencies, there is no one disease associated with a riboflavin deficiency. In experimental animals a riboflavin-deficient diet results in severe ophthalmia, various disorders of the skin, delayed growth, and eventual death. No behavioral or neurologic symptoms have been observed such as seen in THIAMIN deficiency.   See also: FAD, FMN.

SUGGESTED READINGS

Belko, A. Z., et al. 1983. Effects of exercise on riboflavin requirements of young women. *Am. J. Clin. Nutr.* 37:509–517.

Lewis, C. M., and J. C. King. 1980. Effect of oral contraceptive agents on thiamin, riboflavin, and pantothenic acid status in young women. *Am. J. Clin. Nutr.* 33:832–838.

Roe, D. A., et al. 1982. Factors affecting riboflavin requirements of oral contraceptive users and nonusers. *Am. J. Clin. Nutr.* 35:495–501.

Spector, R. 1980. Riboflavin homeostatis in the central nervous system. *J. Neurochem.* 35:202–209.

ribonucleic acid. See RNA.

ribose. A five-carbon sugar produced by the PENTOSE PHOSPHATE PATHWAY. See also: PENTOSE.

ribosome. A highly organized assembly of RNA and protein molecules present in the cytosol. Ribosomes may be found unbound ("free") in the cytosol or may be found attached to the endoplasmic reticulum of the cytosol. Ribosomes are important in the production of protein within cells. Specifically, ribosomes function in the translation of sequences of nucleotides in mRNA into sequences of amino acids in protein—that is, ribosomes translate the language of DNA and RNA into the language of protein. See also: DNA; GENETIC CODE; RNA; TRANSCRIPTION; TRANSLATION.

SUGGESTED READINGS

Wool, I. G. 1979. The structure and function of eukaryotic ribosomes. *Ann. Rev. Biochem.* 48:719–754.

RNA (ribonucleic acid). Single-stranded molecules that are complementary copies of a segment of DNA. Some RNAs are in the information-carrying business and some are in the protein-building business.

RNA molecules differ from DNA in several ways. One way is obvious from their names: the sugar in the sugar-phosphate backbone of RNA is 2-ribose, not 2'-deoxyribose as in DNA. Another difference is that the base uracil in RNA replaces thymine in DNA; both bases, however, pair with adenine.

There are three kinds of RNA: messenger RNA (mRNA), ribosomal RNA (rRNA), and transfer RNA (tRNA). These differ from each other in molecular weight as well as in function. All three are synthesized in the nucleus and can be found in the nucleus, in the cytoplasm, and associated with the organelles of the cytoplasm.

Messenger RNA (mRNA) is transcribed from a segment of one strand of the DNA. The complementary copy enters the cytosol where it acts as a template for the ordering of the sequence of AMINO ACIDS in the building of a protein. Several ribosomes attach along its single chain and at these sites the amino acids will be bonded to each other in a specific sequence to form the protein.

The copying of a segment of DNA to make mRNA is called "transcription" and occurs throughout life at the dictate of the needs of the cells for specific proteins. This is in

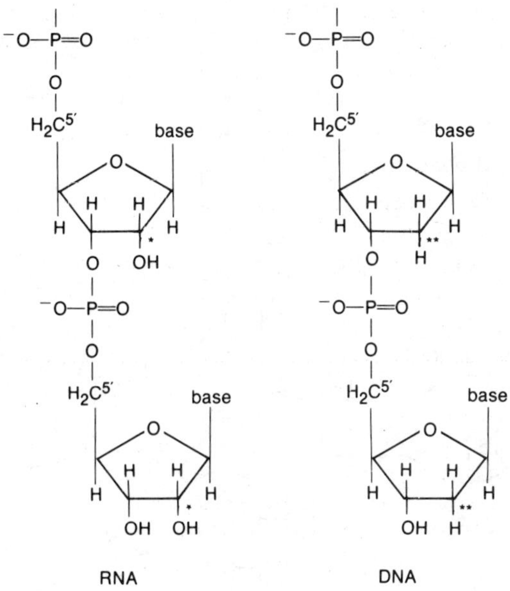

The sugar-phosphate backbone of ribonucleic acid (RNA) contains 2-ribose*; that of deoxyribonucleic acid (DNA) contains 2'-deoxyribose**

contrast to "replication," which is a process that copies the entire strand of DNA and occurs only during times when cells are dividing.

Transfer RNA (tRNA) is present in the cytosol and functions to transport activated amino acids to the ribosomes for incorporation into the growing protein chain. There is at least one tRNA for each of the 20 amino acids. In addition to the four major bases, tRNAs also contain many minor bases. Guanylic acid always forms one end of the tRNAs while the other end is always formed by an A—C—C— (adenylate-cytidylate-cytidylate) nucleotide sequence.

The 3'-hydroxyl group of the terminal adenylic acid is the acceptor of the amino acid that is carried by the tRNA. Moreover, tRNA has a specific sequence of three nucleotides that constitutes the "anticodon." The anticodon is the complementary copy of the "codon," a group of three nucleotides on the mRNA. The anticodon identifies which amino acid is to be carried to the ribosome for incorporation into the protein. Thus, mRNA plays a supervisory role as it holds the information for the sequence of amino acids in an entire gene whereas tRNA is the actual carrier and has the information for only one amino acid.

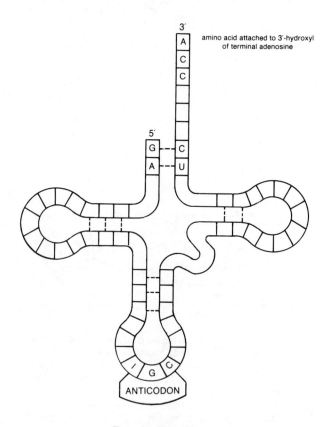

Transfer RNA (tRNA)

Ribosomal RNA (rRNA) makes up the largest percentage of the RNA in the cell and represents about 65 percent of the weight of the ribosomes. The ribosomes, found either free or attached to the endoplasmic reticulum in the cytosol, are the site of PROTEIN BIOSYNTHESIS. See also: DNA; GENETIC CODE; NUCLEOSIDES, NUCLEOTIDES; PROTEIN BIOSYNTHESIS.

S

saturated fatty acids.   Fatty acids that contain only single carbon-carbon bonds.   See also: LIPIDS.

scurvy.   A disease resulting from a deficiency of vitamin C.   See also: VITAMIN C.

selenium (Se).   An essential trace element with many of the same properties as SULFUR. Selenium is usually present in METHIONINE, a sulfur-containing amino acid, where it is inserted in place of sulfur. The selenium content of food depends on the soil from which the food is produced and the protein content of the food. Meats and other animal products are generally better sources of selenium than plant foods. In humans, selenium is at the highest concentration in liver, kidney, heart, and spleen; the excretion route is via the kidneys to urine.

Through animal studies it has been determined that selenium spares or decreases the need for VITAMIN E by (1) helping maintain normal pancreatic function required for normal LIPID DIGESTION and absorption, (2) acting as a component of *glutathione peroxidase* which reacts with hydrogen peroxide before it destroys the cell membrane, and (3) aiding in the retention of vitamin E in the plasma LIPOPROTEINS.

Selenium deficiency results in muscle pain and heart failure; selenium toxicity results in production of dimethylselenide, which is excreted via the lungs and gives the breath the odor of garlic.

SUGGESTED READINGS

Burk, R. F. 1976. Selenium in man. In *Trace elements in human health and disease,* ed. A. S. Prasad, 105–133. New York: Academic Press.

Burk, R. F. 1978. Selenium in nutrition. *World. Rev. Nutr. Diet.* 30:88–106.

Johnson, R., et al. 1981. An accidental case of cardiomyopathy and selenium deficiency. *N. Engl. J. Med.* 304:1210–1213.

Kien, C. L., and H. E. Ganther. 1983. Manifestations of chronic selenium deficiency in a child receiving total parenteral nutrition. *Am. J. Clin. Nutr.* 37:319–328.

Lane, H. W., S. Dudrick, and D. C. Warren. 1981. Blood selenium levels and glutathione-peroxidase activities in university and chronic intravenous hyperalimentation subjects. *Proc. Soc. Exper. Biol. Med.* 167:383–390.

Levander, O., et al. 1981. Selenium balance in young men during selenium depletion and repletion. *Am. J. Clin. Nutr.* 34:2662–2669.

Stadtman, T. C. 1980. Selenium-dependent enzymes. *Ann. Rev. Biochem.* 49:93–110.

Van Rij, A. M., et al. 1979. Selenium deficiency in total parenteral nutrition. *Am. J. Clin. Nutr.* 32:2076–2085.

Yang, G., et al. 1983. Endemic selenium intoxication of humans in China. *Am. J. Clin. Nutr.* 37:872–881.

Young, V. R. 1981. Selenium: A case for its essentiality in man. *N. Engl. J. Med.* 304:1228–1230.

serine (Ser). A three-carbon, dietarily nonessential, glucogenic (glycogenic) α-amino acid that, along with THREONINE, has a hydroxyl group (—OH) on its side chain. Because of this hydroxyl group, serine can be deaminated directly to yield pyruvate and an ammonium ion in a reaction requiring VITAMIN B_6 as a coenzyme. The enzyme that catalyzes this deamination is *serine dehydratase,* so-called because water is extruded before deamination occurs. It is not misleading to speak of serine as being converted "directly" to pyruvate because the intermediate compound, aminoacrylate, is highly unstable.

The major pathway in the synthesis of serine starts from 3-phosphoglycerate which is an intermediate in GLYCOLYSIS.

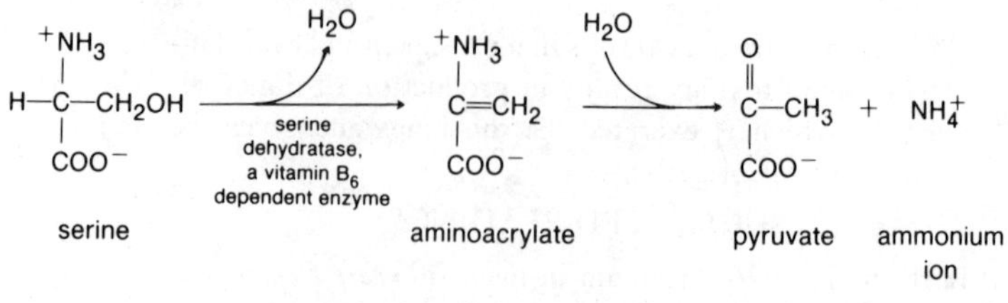

$$HO-CH_2-\overset{\overset{\displaystyle H}{|}}{\underset{\underset{\displaystyle +NH_3}{|}}{C}}-COO^-$$

Serine (Ser)

The degradation of serine to pyruvate

First, the α-hydroxyl group on the α-carbon of 3-phosphoglycerate is converted to a single oxygen double bond. This reaction requires NAD^+ and forms the compound 3-phosphohydroxypyruvate. Next the amino group from GLUTAMATE is transferred to phosphohydroxypyruvate to form phosphoserine, resulting in an amino group replacing the oxygen. The phosphate group then is split off by hydrolysis, forming serine.

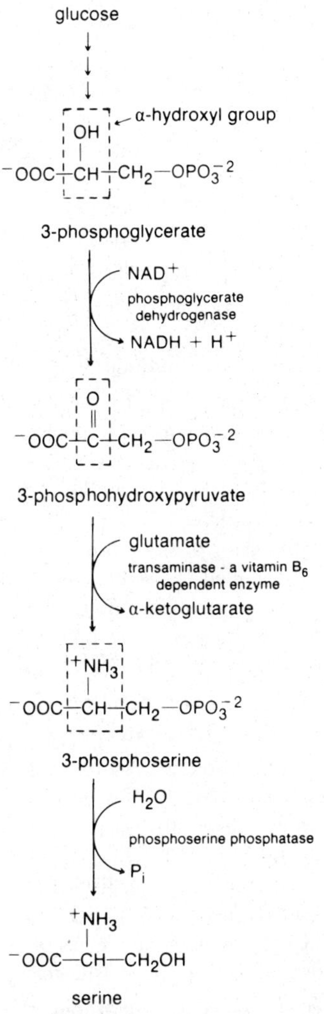

glucose

↓
↓
↓

α-hydroxyl group

$$^-OOC-CH(OH)-CH_2-OPO_3^{-2}$$

3-phosphoglycerate

NAD^+

phosphoglycerate
dehydrogenase

$NADH + H^+$

$$^-OOC-C(=O)-CH_2-OPO_3^{-2}$$

3-phosphohydroxypyruvate

glutamate

transaminase - a vitamin B_6
dependent enzyme

α-ketoglutarate

$$^-OOC-CH(^+NH_3)-CH_2-OPO_3^{-2}$$

3-phosphoserine

H_2O

phosphoserine phosphatase

P_i

$$^-OOC-CH(^+NH_3)-CH_2OH$$

serine

The synthesis of serine
from 3-phosphoglycerate

Serine can also be synthesized from GLYCINE by way of a reversible reaction with a FOLACIN-containing compound, N^5,N^{10}-methylenetetrahydrofolate. This reaction is catalyzed by a vitamin B_6 enzyme, *serine hydroxymethyltransferase.*

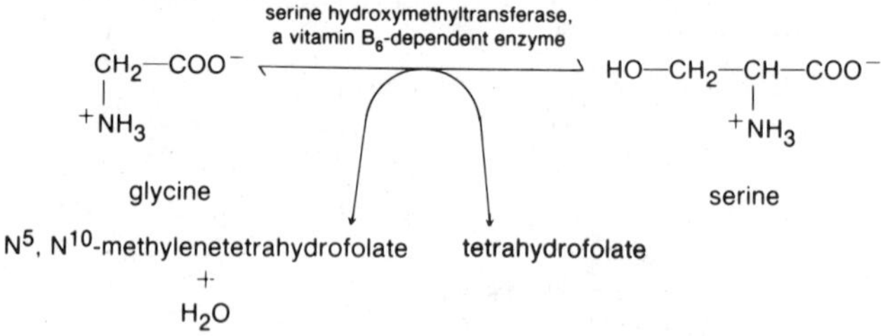

The synthesis of serine from glycine

Serine, along with METHIONINE, is responsible for the synthesis of CYSTEINE, an amino acid that is crucial to the conformation of many proteins. Serine contributes the carbon backbone of cysteine and methionine provides the sulfur.

serotonin (5-hydroxytryptamine). A neurotransmitter synthesized in the central nervous system from TRYPTOPHAN by hydroxylation followed by decarboxylations. VITAMIN B_6 (PLP) is required for serotonin synthesis. Serotonin, also found in the intestinal tract and lungs, is a potent vasoconstrictor and a stimulator of smooth muscle contraction.

Serotonin is degraded by *monoamine oxidase* (MAO). Thus, drugs known as monoamine oxidase inhibitors (MAOI) produce an increase in serotonin concentrations in the nervous system.   See also: CATECHOLAMINES.

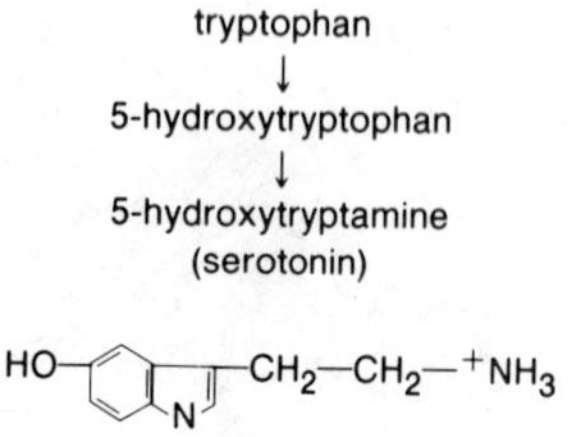

tryptophan
↓
5-hydroxytryptophan
↓
5-hydroxytryptamine
(serotonin)

The synthesis of serotonin from tryptophan

serum. The liquid portion of coagulated blood from which all cells and fibrinogen have been removed.

SGOT (serum glutamate-oxaloacetate transaminase). A VITAMIN B_6-dependent enzyme whose level in the serum is a valuable indicator of heart or liver damage. SGOT and SGPT are ENZYMES whose level is increased in the blood when there is a myocardial infarction or liver damage, for example, from alcohol or industrial chemicals, such as carbon tetrachloride. The increase in serum levels of these enzymes shows the extent of heart or liver damage.

SGPT (serum glutamate-pyruvate transaminase). A VITAMIN B_6-dependent enzyme whose level in the serum is a valuable indicator of heart or liver damage.   See also: SGOT.

sickle-cell anemia.   An inherited disease, caused by an alteration in the beta chains of hemoglobin, that results in a decreased ability of red blood cells to carry oxygen. The disease, named after the altered shape of the red blood cells that resemble sickles, or crescents, is characterized by a low hemoglobin content, fatigue, cardiac enlargement, kidney damage, jaundice, and a generalized swelling of lymph nodes.

There are four chains which make up hemoglobin, the oxygen-carrying protein in the red blood cells: two α-chains and two β-chains. In a person afflicted with sickle-cell anemia, the hemoglobin contains one substituted amino acid; VALINE displaces GLUTAMATE at position 6 on the β-chains. This alteration is due to a mutation in DNA.

normal hemoglobin	Val—His—Leu—Thr—Pro—Glu—Glu
	(1) (2) (3) (4) (5) (6) (7)
sickle-cell hemoglobin	Val—His—Leu—Thr—Pro—Val—Glu
	(1) (2) (3) (4) (5) (6) (7)

Substitution of valine for glutamate in the
6th position on β-chains of
hemoglobin results in sickle-cell anemia

This type of mutation is called a "point mutation" because the mutation occurs in only one base of a DNA triplet: thymine is changed to adenine. The DNA triplet for position 6 of β-chains of normal hemoglobin is CTT (deoxycytidylate, deoxythymidylate, deoxythymidylate) that becomes the complementary base sequence for the mRNA codon of GAA (guanylate, adenylate, adenylate), which translates as glutamate. The position 6 DNA triplet of the person with sickle-cell anemia reads CAT (deoxycytidylate, deoxyadenylate, deoxythymidylate) that transcribes as GUA (guanylate, uridylate, adenylate) in the mRNA codon, which in turn translates as the amino acid valine. Because glutamate is replaced by valine in the completed hemoglobin protein, hemoglobin's ability to carry oxygen to the cells is impaired.

If the sickle-cell base sequence is inherited from one parent, only one β-chain will be affected and the person will be said to have the "sickle-cell trait." Such a person may be symptom-free unless that person encounters a low-oxygen environment. If, however, the person receives the sickle-cell base sequence from both parents, both β-chains will be affected and the person will have sickle-cell anemia, which is often fatal.

Mutations that are expressed in a fatal disease are usually diluted out of a population because death occurs before reproductive age is reached. In the case of this substitution, however, those who are heterozygotes (have only one gene for sickle cells) are protected from the most virulent form of malaria. At the same time, they do not suffer the severe consequences of the homozygote (a person who receives the abnormal gene from both parents). This double benefit provides strong selective pressures to keep the mutation in the population.

The heterozygote is not entirely without health problems: anesthesia, air travel in unpressurized planes, or vigorous activity at high altitudes may be hazardous. There is also the possibility that union with another heterozygote will produce an offspring with sickle-cell anemia. In some African populations, the incidence of the sickle-cell trait is as high as 40 percent, while Africans who have migrated to the United States have a much lower incidence, about 8 percent. The incidence of the disease is about four per thousand among American blacks. The mortality rate from complications produced by sickle-cell anemia is much higher among poor blacks. The disease is often fatal before age thirty, usually as a result of untreated infections or from heart or renal failure.   See also: GENETIC CODE.

SUGGESTED READINGS

Winslow, R. M., and W. F. Anderson. 1983. The hemoglobinopathies. In *The metabolic basis of inherited disease*, 5th ed., ed. J. B. Stanbury et al., 1666–1710. New York: McGraw-Hill.

sodium (Na⁺).   The principal positive ion (cation) in the extracellular fluids of the body. This ion is critical to the maintenance of fluid balance, neural transmissions, and muscle contraction.

In almost all animal cells, sodium ions are in high concentration outside cells and POTASSIUM ions are in high concentration inside cells. This state is maintained against a concentration gradient and thus requires energy (ATP) and a transport mechanism (the Na^+, K^+-ATPase system). The process, known as the SODIUM PUMP, is the most widely distributed of the active transport systems.

Sodium chloride, or table salt, is the principal dietary source of sodium, animal foods containing more than plant foods. Salt is used extensively in food preparation and in the manufacture of snack foods, such as pretzels and potato chips.

Sodium is absorbed from the small intestine. The kidneys maintain a balance of sodium over a wide range of intakes. Serious loss of sodium may occur in profuse sweating. This sodium along with the water must be replaced. Toxic effects of excess sodium, when ingested as table salt or sodium bicarbonate, include gastrointestinal distress and irritation, hemorrhaging, and kidney damage, as well as depression of the respiratory and circulatory systems.

SUGGESTED READINGS

Bostad, R., W. Blystad, and O. Knutrud. 1964. Sodium chloride intoxication in newborn infants. *Clin. Pediatr.* 3:1–4.

Fregley, M. J. 1981. Sodium and potassium. *Ann. Rev. Nutr.* 1:69–94.

Mickelson, O., et al. 1977. Sodium and potassium intakes and excretions of normal men consuming sodium chloride or a 1:1 mixture of sodium and potassium chloride. *Am. J. Clin. Nutr.* 30:2033–2040.

Schlierf, G., et al. 1980. Salt and hypertension: Data from the Heidelberg study. *Am. J. Clin. Nutr.* 33:872–875.

sodium pump (Na^+-K^+ pump). The energy-requiring process by which a high concentration of POTASSIUM ions (K^+) and a low concentration of SODIUM ions (Na^+) are maintained inside nearly all animal cells. The high and low designations are comparisons between the internal and external concentrations of each ion, not high and low in relation to each other. It is estimated that kidney and brain cells use 70 percent of their ATP for maintaining these concentrations.

Normally, when a solute is able to pass through a MEMBRANE, the particles diffuse back and forth until the concentration on one side equals the concentration on the other. In the case of the concentrations of Na^+ and K^+ in cells, however, the integrity of the cell demands that a higher concentration of Na^+ be maintained outside the plasma membrane than inside and that a higher concentration of K^+ be maintained inside than outside the cell. This requires energy and a mechanism for pumping the ions back to their proper side.

The enzyme responsible for transporting sodium and potassium ions across the plasma membrane is *Na^+-K^+ ATPase*, which has an absolute requirement for MAGNESIUM. The presence of sodium inside the cell and potassium outside is responsible for activating *ATPase*. The enzyme functions unidirectionally, that is, the sodium ion is only pumped out of the cell while the potassium ion is only pumped in. The hydrolysis of ATP in a tightly coupled reaction provides the energy to transport these ions across the plasma membrane. Three sodium ions and two potassium ions are transported across for every molecule of ATP that is hydrolyzed.

In addition, the sodium pump is responsible for the active transport of sugars and AMINO ACIDS into cells and of CALCIUM ions back into the sarcoplasmic reticulum after a muscle contraction.

sphingomyelin. A major group of PHOSPHORUS-containing sphingolipids found primarily in the myelin sheath surrounding nerves and in cell MEMBRANES. Sphingomyelin is derived from CHOLINE, phosphate, and a ceramide. See also: MEMBRANES.

sphingosine. A complex alcohol that forms the backbone of the phospholipids known as "sphingomyelin." See also: MEMBRANES.

starch. A complex carbohydrate composed of glucose units linked together by α-1,4-glycosidic bonds. See also: CARBOHYDRATE STRUCTURE.

starvation. A lack of sufficient fuel nutrients to support life. Because the body cannot discern the reason for the lack of food, it cannot alter its reaction based on a "good" reason for its absence. In addition to natural disasters that may eliminate a group's food supply, the body perceives as starvation the following: fasting for any reason including weight reduction, religion, or medical tests; anorexia nervosa; any other disease or medical procedure that results in an abhorence of food or inability to eat.

When the food supply is stopped, the first priority of METABOLISM is to provide GLUCOSE for the brain. Initially, glucose can be supplied from GLYCOGEN stored in the liver from earlier feeding. When blood glucose levels drop, glycogen is promptly broken down to glucose, which is secreted into the blood. Unless replaced, this glycogen will not supply more than a day's demand for glucose. Another source of glucose is glycerol released during the oxidation of TRIACYLGLYCEROLS.

Still another source of glucose is body PROTEIN. Some glucogenic AMINO ACIDS incorporated in body proteins can be degraded to pyruvate or to TCA CYCLE intermediates that can lead to the production of glucose. Muscle protein breakdown is a supplier of glucose in the early stages of starvation. Later, as muscles shift to FATTY ACIDS for fuel, muscle wasting is lessened. The source of fatty acids is from the catabolism of the body's fat stores.

The rapid breakdown of protein to amino acids in order to supply glucose must not continue because these amino acids are necessary to build certain vital proteins, such as antibodies for fighting infection, hemoglobin to carry oxygen to the tissues, ENZYMES for many life-sustaining reactions, and constant muscle repair, particularly of the heart.

As starvation or fasting continues, the second priority of the body is to spare valuable protein. One of the earliest protein-sparing actions is lethargy where slowed activity reduces the body's demand for calories. Another protein-conserving action is a fuel shift from glucose to fatty acids by tissues such as muscles and heart. Furthermore, production and release of KETONE BODIES by the liver provide a potential source of energy for peripheral tissues. The brain, for example, which cannot use the fatty acids from the body's stored fat, begins to shift from the use of glucose to use of ketone bodies for fuel—a remarkable survival process.

The shift to the use of ketone bodies and fatty acids for fuel lessens the drain on the scarce glucose and protein supply. Ultimately, survival time depends on how much fat the person had accumulated prior to starvation. See also: GLUCONEOGENESIS; FATTY ACID OXIDATION; KETONE BODIES; KETOSIS.

SUGGESTED READINGS

Cahill, G. F., Jr. 1970. Starvation in man. *N. Engl. J. Med.* 282:668–675.

Lowry, S. F., et al. 1985. Whole-body protein breakdown and 3-methylhistidine excretion during brief fasting, starvation, and intravenous repletion in man. *Ann. Surg.* 202:21–27.

stereoisomer.   Isomers that are physically and chemically identical to each other but which rotate the plane of plane-polarized light oppositely.   See also: AMINO ACIDS for the discussion of D- and L-amino acids.

sterols.   A group of alcohol derivatives with a steroid ring structure.   See also: LIPIDS.

succinate.   An intermediate in the TCA CYCLE synthesized from succinyl-CoA.   See also: TCA CYCLE.

succinyl-CoA.   An intermediate in the TCA CYCLE synthesized from α-ketoglutarate.   See also: TCA CYCLE.

sucrose.   A disaccharide composed of GLUCOSE and FRUCTOSE joined in a glycosidic bond.   See also: CARBOHYDRATE STRUCTURE.

sulfur (S).   A mineral present in body tissues as part of the AMINO ACIDS, METHIONINE and CYSTEINE, as well as of TAURINE.

Because most sulfur is absorbed as part of these compounds, the primary sources of sulfur are protein-containing foods. Small amounts of sulfur may be derived from inorganic sulfates, sulfides, and THIAMIN. Oxidation of sulfur-containing amino acids in the kidney yields sulfate, which is normally excreted in the urine.

The sulfur atoms in cysteine are responsible for the major covalent cross-links in PROTEIN STRUCTURES where the disulfide bridge formed between two cysteine molecules is important in stabilizing protein conformation. Tissues, such as hair and fingernails, that require strength and rigidity of shape have a high percentage of the amino acid cysteine.

Sulfur has a structural function as part of mucopolysaccharides and sulfolipids. It occurs in the iron-sulfur proteins of the coenzyme Q/cytochrome c reductase complex of the RESPIRATORY CHAIN. Sulfur atoms are also important in the iron-containing flavoenzymes, such as *succinate dehydrogenase* and NADH *dehydrogenase*. Sulfur, as part of the sulfhydryl groups, forms thioester linkages that are necessary for the activation of molecules such as acetate.

Interconversions between disulfide and sulfhydryl groups in oxidation-reduction reactions are used to eliminate hydrogen peroxide from the cell before it can cause cellular destruction. These interconversions occur as the sulfur-containing compound glutathione is reduced and oxidized.

$$\text{GSSG (oxidized glutathione)} + \text{NADPH} + \text{H}^+ \xrightarrow[\substack{\text{glutathione} \\ \text{reductase}}]{} 2\,\text{GSH} + \text{NADP}^+$$

$$2\,\text{GSH (reduced glutathione)} + \text{H}_2\text{O}_2 \xrightarrow[\substack{\text{glutathione} \\ \text{peroxidase,} \\ \text{requiring selenium} \\ \text{as cofactor}}]{} \text{GSSG} + 2\text{H}_2\text{O}$$

NADPH provided by the pentose phosphate pathway reduces glutathione which removes the hydrogen peroxide that could destroy red blood cells if allowed to accumulate

SUGGESTED READINGS

Cooper, A. J. L. 1983. Biochemistry of sulfur-containing amino acids. *Ann. Rev. Biochem.* 52:187–222.

Zlotkin, S. H., and G. H. Anderson. 1982. Sulfur balances in intravenously fed infants: Effects of cysteine supplementation. *Am. J. Clin. Nutr.* 36:862–867.

sulfur-containing amino acids. See CYSTEINE; METHIONINE.

t

Tangier disease (familial HDL deficiency). A rare familial disorder in which there is a very low plasma CHOLESTEROL level, an accumulation of cholesterol esters in the tissues, a low HDL level, and peculiar, yellow-orange colored tonsils.

SUGGESTED READINGS

Herbert, P. N., et al. 1983. Familial lipoprotein deficiency: Abetalipoproteinemia, hypobetalipoproteinemia, and Tangier disease. In *The metabolic basis of inherited disease,* 5th ed., ed. J. B. Stanbury et al., 589–621. New York: McGraw-Hill.

taurine. An amino acid involved in a variety of metabolic activities. These activities are thought to include the following: (1) functions as a neurotransmitter or an inhibitory neuromodulator of nervous excitability (a variant of neurotransmitter); (2) functions in the photoreceptors of the retina and in the heart to effect CALCIUM ion movement; (3) involved in glucose uptake; (4) operates in association with several hormones; and (5) functions as a BILE SALT when conjugated to cholyl-CoA to form taurocholate.

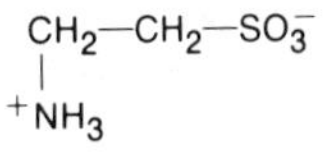

In humans, the major pathway for taurine biosynthesis originates from METHIONINE and proceeds through a series of reactions requiring VITAMIN B_6 to yield taurine. Taurine is excreted by the kidneys.

$$CH_2\!-\!CH_2\!-\!SO_3^-$$
$$|$$
$$^+NH_3$$

Taurine
(2-aminoethylsulfonic acid)

SUGGESTED READINGS

Garbutt, J. T., L. Lack, and M. I. Tyor. 1971. Physiological basis of alterations in the relative conjugation of bile acids with glycine and taurine. *Am. J. Clin. Nutr.* 24:218–228.

Gaull, G. E. 1982. Taurine in the nutrition of the human infant. *Acta* Paediatr. Scand. (Suppl.) 296:38–40.

Hardison, W. G. M., and S. M. Grundy. 1983. Effect of bile acid conjugation pattern on bile acid metabolism in normal humans. *Gastroenterology* 84:617–620.

Hayes, K. C., and J. A. Sturman. 1981. Taurine in metabolism. *Ann. Rev. Nutr.* 1:401–424.

Posantes-Morales, H., and C. Cruz. 1985. Taurine and hypotaurine inhibit light induced lipid peroxidation and protect rod outer segment structure. *Brain Res.* 330:154–157.

Rassin, D. K., et al. 1983. Feeding the low-birth-weight infant. II. Effects of taurine and cholesterol supplementation on amino acids and cholesterol. *Pediatrics* 71:179–186.

Vinton, H. S., and M. E. Geggell. 1985. Taurine deficiency in a child on total parenteral nutrition. *Nutr. Rev.* 43:81–83.

Tauri's disease (glycogen storage disease: type VII). Characterized by GLYCOGEN storage in muscles and erythrocytes and deficient *phosphofructokinase* activity in muscle.

SUGGESTED READINGS

Howell, R. R., and J. C. Williams. 1983. The glycogen storage diseases. In *The metabolic basis of inherited disease*, 5th ed., ed. J. B. Stanbury et al., 141–166. New York: McGraw-Hill.

taurocholate. A biosalt derived from TAURINE. See also: BILE SALTS.

Tay-Sachs disease. An inherited disease transmitted as a recessive trait. The condition is characterized by the absence of the enzyme *hexosamidase A* that is involved in the normal degradation of certain gangliosides in the brain. The prognosis is poor: signs and symptoms include enlargement of the head that begins about age 4 to 6 months, poor muscle tone and paralysis developing about the first year. Death usually results by the third year.

A high incidence of this disease is found among the American Jewish population, especially those of Ashkenazi descent whose ancestors came from the Balkan provinces of Poland. Amniocentesis can reveal the presence of Tay-Sachs in a fetus in time for an early abortion. Mass screening tests, which are set up in many cities where there is a large Jewish population, can reveal heterozygotes in time for genetic counseling.

SUGGESTED READINGS

O'Brien, J. S. 1983. The gangliosidoses. In *The metabolic basis of inherited disease*, 5th ed., ed. J. B. Stanbury et al., 945–969. New York: McGraw-Hill.

TCA cycle (tricarboxylic acid cycle, citric acid cycle, Krebs cycle). A series of catabolic reactions taking place in the mitochondrial matrix. The primary purpose of these reactions is the transfer of energy carried in the bonds of ACETYL-COA to electron-carrier molecules. The molecules receiving the hydrogens and electrons are the coenzymes NAD$^+$ and FAD, which transfer the hydrogens and electrons to the RESPIRATORY CHAIN for the phosphorylation of ADP to ATP.

The series is called a "cycle" because a four-carbon compound (oxaloacetate) joins with a two-carbon compound (acetyl-CoA) to form a six-carbon compound (citrate), with the ultimate regeneration of the four-carbon compound. Oxaloacetate is re-formed after a number of precisely orchestrated molecular rearrangements during which two carbons exit as carbon dioxide (but not the same two carbons that just entered as acetyl-CoA) and hydrogens and electrons exit as NADH + H$^+$ and FADH$_2$. Oxaloacetate can now combine with another acetyl-CoA to begin the process again.

It is a mistake, however, to picture the TCA cycle as an independent merry-go-round of reactions that runs continuously while taking in a two-carbon compound and producing carbon dioxide, hydrogens, and electrons. A better analogy is that of a monorail continuously circling a busy airport, picking up disembarking passengers, and letting them off at their connecting flights or at the airport exit.

This is a valid analogy because the TCA cycle not only receives the two-carbon remains of the degradation of fuel nutrients, but also receives other multiples of carbons at

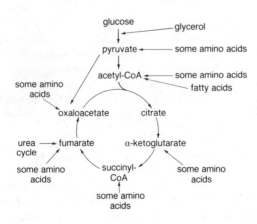

Arrivals at the TCA cycle

259

various "stations" around the cycle. For instance, the carbon skeletons of amino acids may enter at α-ketoglutarate, succinyl-CoA, fumarate, or oxaloacetate. The carbons may exit at any of the following: in carbon dioxide for excretion via the lungs or kidneys; in oxaloacetate for the synthesis of GLUCOSE and some AMINO ACIDS; in ASPARTATE for the synthesis of purines and pyrimidines; in aspartate for the synthesis of urea; in citrate for transport to the cytosol; in succinyl-CoA for the synthesis of HEME; and in α-ketoglutarate for the synthesis of some amino acids and GABA (an inhibitory neurotransmitter). The TCA cycle is thus a busy transfer point for carbons that will be used to build biomolecules, as well as for the transfer of energy from food into a form the body can use.

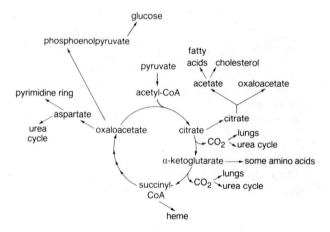

Departures from the TCA cycle

The TCA cycle, examined below in five stages, considers (A) what happens to each intermediate to transform it into the next intermediate, (B) what arrivals and departures occur during each stage and what biosynthetic and degradative pathways are involved, (C) what are the control points—or sites—at which the rate of the cycle is stimulated or inhibited.

Stage 1 (Oxaloacetate to Citrate): Oxaloacetate condenses with acetyl-CoA to form citryl-CoA, which is then hydrolyzed to citrate and COENZYME A (which leaves the cycle). The enzyme for the formation of citrate is *citrate synthetase*. This step is the first control point. *Citrate synthetase* activity is controlled by the concentration of acetyl-CoA, as well as succinyl-CoA. Citrate itself and NADH may also regulate *citrate synthetase* activity.

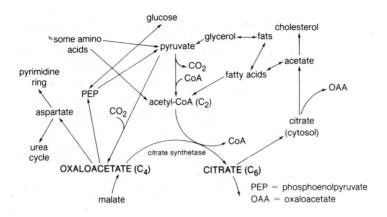

Oxaloacetate to citrate

Where did the oxaloacetate and acetyl-CoA come from? The acetyl-CoA was formed in the mitochondria from pyruvate which arose from the beta oxidation of fatty acids, and/or from the oxidation of the carbon skeletons of some amino acids. The oxaloacetate was re-formed in the final stage of the TCA cycle from succinate through fumarate and malate or was formed from transamination of aspartate. If there is an abundance of acetyl-CoA relative to the amount of oxaloacetate to condense with it, additional oxaloacetate may be made by the carboxylation of pyruvate.

In the mitochondria the carboxylation of pyruvate is cata- lyzed by a BIOTIN-dependent enzyme, *pyruvate carboxylase,* which is active only in the presence of acetyl-CoA. The production of oxaloacetate from pyruvate ensures the con- tinuation of the TCA cycle when acetyl-CoA must be oxidized.

Oxaloacetate and acetyl-CoA can leave the cycle and be used in other ways. Oxaloacetate can exit the cycle in cit- rate and become the carbon skeleton of amino acids, or it can leave through phosphoenolpyruvate and resynthesize glucose. Acetyl-CoA is routed out of the cycle when ATP levels are high; that is, when sufficient food has been eaten to meet energy needs. Acetyl-CoA can then be used to syn- thesize FATTY ACIDS or other lipids, such as CHOLESTEROL. The fatty acids may be incorporated into body fat (mostly as TRIACYLGLYCEROLS) which stores the energy that origi- nally came from excess food consumption.

Both oxaloacetate and acetyl-CoA can leave the mito- chondria as part of citrate which has the ability to cross the mitochondrial membrane and enter the cytosol. Once in the

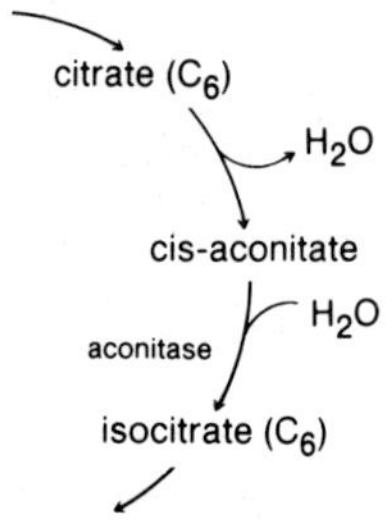

citate (C_6)

H_2O

cis-aconitate

aconitase H_2O

isocitrate (C_6)

Rearrangement of citrate
to isocitrate

cytosol, *citrate lyase* breaks the bonds of citrate, regenerating acetyl-CoA and oxaloacetate.

Stage 2 (Citrate to α-Ketoglutarate): The rearrangement of citrate to isocitrate is catalyzed by *aconitase*, an IRON-containing enzyme that first dehydrates citrate to cis-aconitate and then hydrates it to isocitrate. This isomerization is necessary so that decarboxylation can take place next.

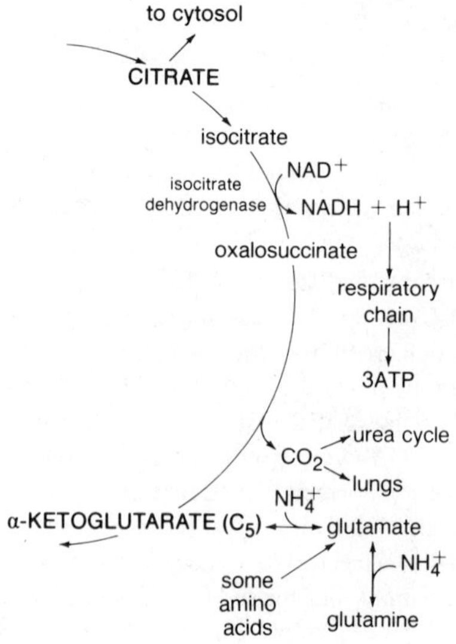

to cytosol

CITRATE

isocitrate

isocitrate
dehydrogenase

NAD^+

$NADH + H^+$

oxalosuccinate

respiratory
chain

3ATP

CO_2

urea cycle

lungs

NH_4^+

α-KETOGLUTARATE (C_5) ← glutamate

NH_4^+

some
amino
acids

glutamine

Decarboxylation of citrate to α-ketoglutarate
A high level of ADP and NAD^+ stimulates
isocitrate dehydrogenase. A high level of ATP and NADH
inhibits the enzyme.

The reactions from isocitrate to α-ketoglutarate contain the first oxidation-reduction encountered and comprise the second control point of the TCA cycle. A high level of ADP and NAD^+ pushes this step toward completion and thus increases the rate of the cycle. These reactions require the enzyme *isocitrate dehydrogenase*, NAD^+ as the coenzyme, and both Mg^{++} and Mn^{++}. NADH transfers the electrons to the respiratory chain where their energy will be conserved in three molecules of ATP. Oxalosuccinate is formed temporarily. When it picks up the freed hydrogen ion and releases a carbon dioxide, the transformation to α-ketoglutarate, the important five-carbon intermediate, is complete.

Several amino acids can enter the TCA cycle by their conversion to α-ketoglutarate. The carbon skeletons of ARGININE, GLUTAMINE, HISTIDINE, and PROLINE are first transformed to glutamate, then deaminated to become α-ketoglutarate. If not needed to replenish the carbohydrate intermediates of the cycle, these carbons can exit upon their conversion to oxaloacetate. Through the gluconeogenic pathway, the carbons may be incorporated into glucose; this is a valuable method for maintaining the BLOOD GLUCOSE LEVEL during fasting.

The exit of α-ketoglutarate from the cycle through the reverse of the glutamate-to-α-ketoglutarate reaction provides an important route by which ammonia is quickly detoxified. α-Ketoglutarate protects the brain from ammonia where it is most toxic. In the brain, one molecule of ammonia combines with α-ketoglutarate to form the amino acid glutamate, thus putting one ammonia molecule where it can be carried safely. Glutamate, however, does not diffuse from the brain easily. Therefore, in times of an elevated level of ammonia, another molecule of ammonia is used to transform glutamate into glutamine, which is able to diffuse into the blood stream and takes with it two molecules of ammonia. The toxicity of ammonia is thought to be due to the depletion of α-ketoglutarate, which blocks the TCA cycle and consequently robs the brain of ATP.

Stage 3 (α-Ketoglutarate to Succinyl-CoA): This is the second oxidative decarboxylation of the cycle and the third control point. This stage is inhibited by its products: succinyl-CoA and NADH. A highly organized complex of three enzymes organized as the α-ketoglutarate dehydrogenase complex catalyzes these reactions. The cofactors involved are NAD^+, CoA, TPP, lipoamide, and FAD. NAD^+ picks up one hydrogen ion and releases one into the medium, then transfers the electrons to the respiratory chain where they will provide the energy for phosphorylating three molecules of ADP to ATP. The long arm of lipoamide picks up and delivers parts from one enzyme to the next within the complex.

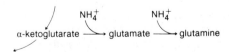

α-Ketoglutarate in the TCA cycle may be depleted by synthesis of glutamine when ammonia level is high

263

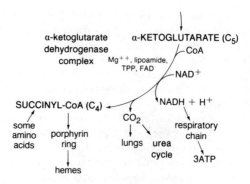

Decarboxylation of α-ketoglutarate to succinyl-CoA
A high level of succinyl-CoA and NADH inhibits
the α-ketoglutarate dehydrogenase complex

Succinyl-CoA may leave the cycle to participate in the first step in the synthesis of the porphyrin ring present in heme. This is another avenue by which the carbohydrate intermediates of the TCA cycle could become depleted.

The carbon skeletons of several amino acids, ISOLEUCINE, THREONINE, METHIONINE, and VALINE, can be converted to succinyl-CoA and thereby replenish the carbohydrate intermediates of the cycle. If not needed to resupply the carbohydrate intermediates, these amino acid carbons could be routed out at oxaloacetate and, through phosphoenolpyruvate, used to resynthesize glucose.

Stage 4 (Succinyl-CoA to Succinate): The TCA cycle is known for its high energy output. This step from succinyl-CoA to succinate, however, is the only one that directly generates a high-energy compound, GTP. The energy to phosphorylate GDP to GTP comes from the breaking of the thioester bond of succinyl-CoA by the enzyme, succinate thiokinase (*succinyl-CoA synthetase*).

SUCCINATE (C_4)

CoA

ATP ← GTP

succinate
thiokinase

MG

GDP

P_i H_2O

SUCCINYL-
CoA (C_4)

Succinyl-CoA to succinate

The high ATP output usually attributed to the cycle is actually generated by the respiratory chain through the oxidation of the hydrogens carried out of the cycle by NADH + H^+ and $FADH_2$.

Stage 5 (Succinate to Oxaloacetate): There are two oxidations and a hydration taking place in this group of reactions. In the first oxidation, *succinate dehydrogenase* transfers two hydrogens to FAD, forming fumarate that is hydrated by *fumarase* to form malate. Then, with the oxidation of malate by *malate dehydrogenase* and NAD^+, the reforming of oxaloacetate is complete.

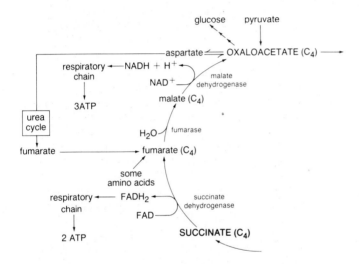

Succinate to oxaloacetate

New arrivals at this stage may be the carbon skeletons of the amino acids, aspartate, phenylalanine, and TYROSINE, which enter the TCA cycle at fumarate, and ASPARAGINE and aspartate, which can enter at oxaloacetate.

A departure from the cycle involves the conversion of oxaloacetate to glucose or aspartate. This conversion to aspartate is more important than might first appear. Aspartate participates in the formation of urea by condensing with citrulline to form argininosuccinate, which is then cleaved to form fumarate and arginine. Fumarate re-enters the TCA cycle and is converted to oxaloacetate. This revolving-door series of oxaloacetate-to-aspartate-to-fumarate-to-oxaloacetate connects the intermediates of the

TCA and UREA CYCLES. Also, the need of the urea cycle for the ATP and CO_2 produced by the TCA cycle creates an interdependence.

In summary, oxaloacetate may follow many paths: to citrate to keep the TCA cycle moving; to phosphoenolpyruvate for the synthesis of glucose; to aspartate that will lead either to the urea cycle or to the synthesis of the pyrimidine ring.

In this final stage of the TCA cycle, one molecule each of $FADH_2$ and $NADH + H^+$ are formed. When their electrons go through the respiratory chain, 5 ATPs are produced from this one stage. Earlier in the TCA cycle, 6 ATPs resulted from $2\ NADH + H^+$. One ATP was generated from the GTP formed, making a total of 12 ATPs gleaned from one molecule of acetyl-CoA oxidized through the TCA cycle and the respiratory chain.   See also: GLUCONEOGENESIS, for the synthesis of glucose from oxaloacetate.

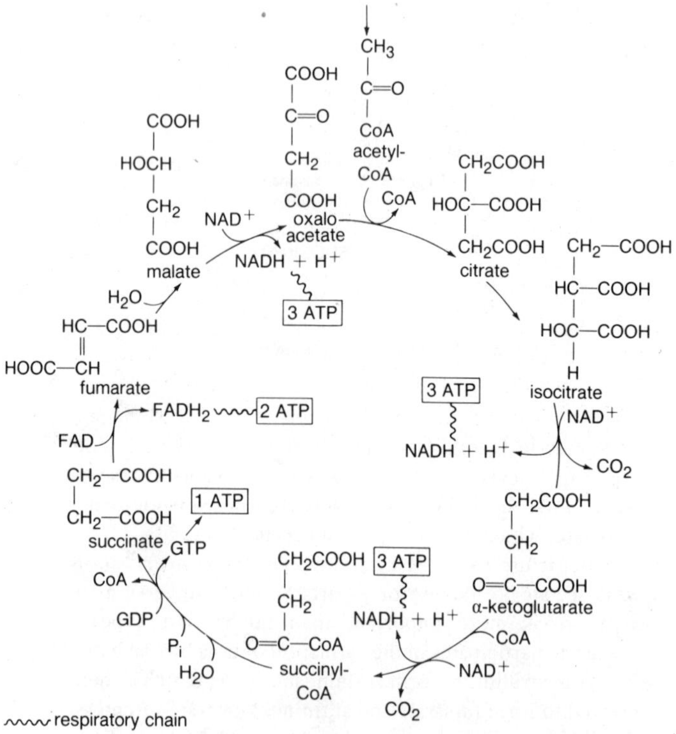

TCA cycle

TDP. See THIAMIN DIPHOSPHATE.

tetrahydrofolate (FH₄). The coenzyme form of the vitamin FOLACIN and a carrier of one-carbon units. See also: FOLACIN; GLYCINE; SERINE.

thalassemia. A group of anemias occurring in populations bordering the Mediterranean and in Southeast Asia. The anemia results from a defect in the alpha or beta chain of hemoglobin. See also: HEMOGLOBIN; HEME.

SUGGESTED READINGS

Kan, Y. W. 1983. The thalassemias. In *The metabolic basis of inherited disease,* 5th ed., ed. J. B. Stanbury, et al., 1711–1728. New York: McGraw-Hill.

thiamin (vitamin B₁). A water-soluble vitamin, made up of a pyrimidine ring and a thiazole ring, with limited body stores in muscle, heart, liver, kidney, and brain.

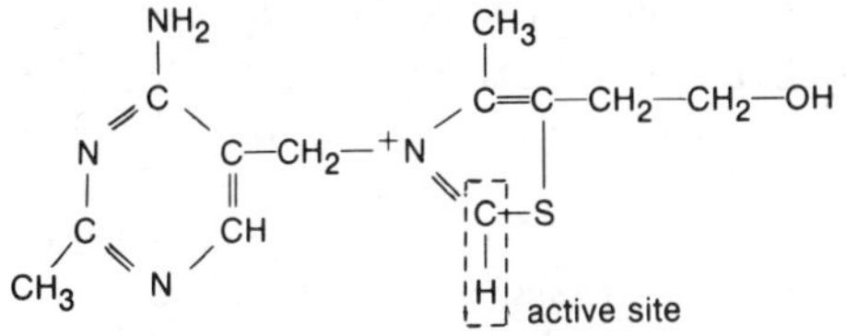

Thiamin

Food sources of thiamin include lean pork, ham, oysters, whole grains, green peas, beef liver, and lima beans. It occurs in smaller quantities in some other foods. In the United States, thiamin is added to enriched breads and cereals.

During cooking, thiamin dissolves in meat drippings or cooking water. The alkaline medium, created when sodium bicarbonate is added to the cooking water of green vegetables to make them a brighter green, destroys thiamin; however, it is fairly stable over a wide range of temperatures in an acid medium.

Thiamin is absorbed from the small intestine by passive diffusion when present in high concentrations and by active absorption when present in low concentrations. In the intestinal and liver cells, thiamin is phosphorylated. It is excreted primarily in the urine.

Thiamin was discovered when it was observed that chickens, eating the scraps from a prison mess table, developed symptoms similar to those of the prisoners who had the disease beriberi. Further investigation revealed that the vitamin was contained in the rice hulls that the kitchen workers discarded as unfit for consumption by humans or birds.

A dietary deficiency of thiamin in humans affects the cardiovascular and gastrointestinal systems; however, its most overt effects are on the nervous system. Mental confusion is often the first symptom noticed in a mild deficiency; paralysis of the extremities is one of a cluster of symptoms seen in the thiamin deficiency disease beriberi.

The vitamin's active form is the coenzyme, THIAMIN PYROPHOSPHATE (TPP), also called THIAMIN DIPHOSPHATE (TDP). TPP is required for the oxidative decarboxylation of α-keto acids, such as pyruvate and α-ketoglutarate, and of the keto-analogs of leucine, isoleucine, and valine, and for the transketolation reactions in the pentose phosphate pathway. See also: THIAMIN PYROPHOSPHATE.

SUGGESTED READINGS

Elsas, L. J., and D. J. Danner. 1982. The role of thiamin in maple syrup urine disease. *Ann. N.Y. Acad. Sci.* 378:404–421.

Scriver, C. R. 1973. Vitamin-responsive inborn errors of metabolism. *Metabolism* 22:1319–1344.

Shaw, S., B. D. Gorkin, and C. S. Lieber. 1981. Effects of chronic alcohol feeding on thiamin status: Biochemical and neurological correlates. *Am. J. Clin. Nutr.* 34:856–860.

Wood, B., and K. J. Breen. 1980. Clinical thiamin deficiency in Australia: The size of the problem and approaches to prevention. *Med. J. Aust.* 1:461–464.

thiamin diphosphate (TDP). The coenzyme form of the vitamin THIAMIN. Also called thiamin pyrophosphate (TPP). See also: THIAMIN PYROPHOSPHATE.

thiamin pyrophosphate (TPP, thiamin diphosphate, TDP). The coenzyme form of the B-vitamin THIAMIN. When a thiamin molecule, made up of a pyrimidine ring and a thiazole ring, attaches to two phosphate groups, it functions as the coenzyme thiamin pyrophosphate (TPP). The action of TPP is thought to occur at a chemically active site on the thiazole ring where a carbon bears a negative charge. While attention centers on the thiazole ring, it should be remembered that the pyrimidine ring and the phosphates are just as necessary for TPP to be active as a coenzyme.

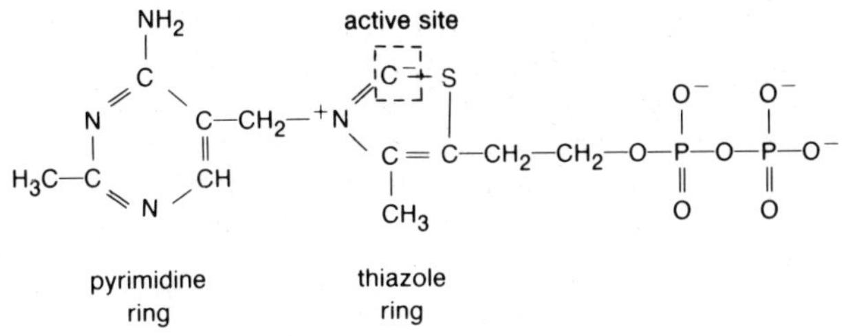

Thiamin pyrophosphate (TPP),
thiamin diphosphate (TDP)

TPP is the coenzyme for the decarboxylases, the group of ENZYMES that remove a carboxyl group. *Pyruvate decarboxylase, α-ketoglutarate decarboxylase, branched-chain decarboxylase,* and the enzyme *transketolase* are considered here.

Pyruvate decarboxylase is the first enzyme in a complex of three enzymes critical to the extraction of energy from foods. (The other two enzymes in the pyruvate dehydrogenase complex are *dihydrolipoyl transacetylase* and *dihydrolipoyl dehydrogenase*.) Pyruvate, a three-carbon compound, is formed in the cytosol during GLYCOLYSIS, the anaerobic stage of GLUCOSE degradation. To enter the aerobic stage of the degradation (the TCA CYCLE in the mitochondria) pyruvate must lose a carbon and undergo other rearrangements to form ACETYL-CoA, a two-carbon compound.

In the first step of this action, *pyruvate decarboxylase* removes carbon dioxide from pyruvate to form a two-carbon molecule that becomes attached to TPP. The removal of CO_2 is followed rapidly by reactions catalyzed by the other two enzymes of the complex. The overall reaction requires lipoic acid, FAD, NAD^+, and, finally, COENZYME A to which the two carbons become attached to form acetyl-CoA. The two-carbon fragment from the breakdown of the fuel nutrients is now activated and can enter the TCA cycle.

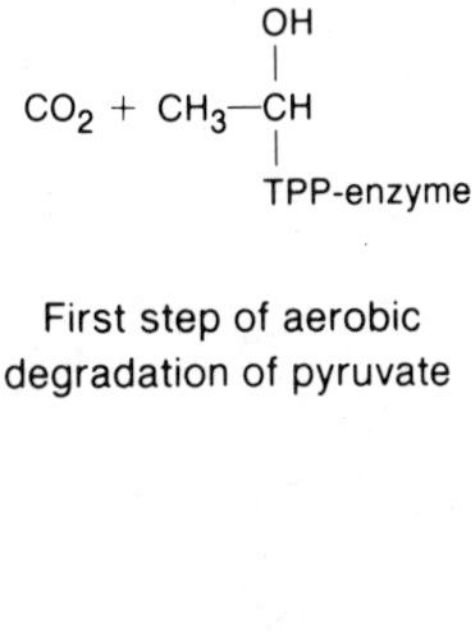

To understand how the enzyme effects the removal of carbon dioxide, note that carbon-2 of pyruvate in the figure on the next page has four bonds, two with oxygen and two with adjacent carbons, and that this carbon is held close to the electron-rich carbon in the active site of the thiazole ring of TPP. To make room for the electrons of the thiazole carbon, electrons move in pyruvate, resulting in a change of bonding so that only one bond between carbon-2 and oxy-

First step of aerobic
degradation of pyruvate

269

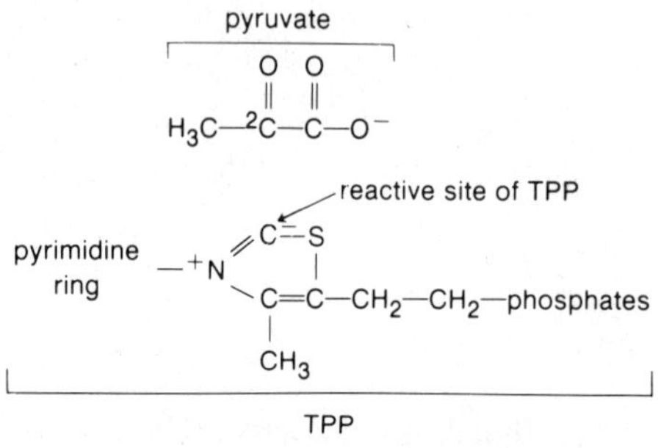

pyruvate

$$H_3C-{}^2C-C-O^-$$

with the O, O double bonds (both carbonyls).

pyrimidine ring — ${}^+N$ ... reactive site of TPP

$$C=S$$
$$C=C-CH_2-CH_2-phosphates$$
$$CH_3$$

TPP

Note the bonding of carbon 2 of pyruvate and its position in relation to the active site of TPP

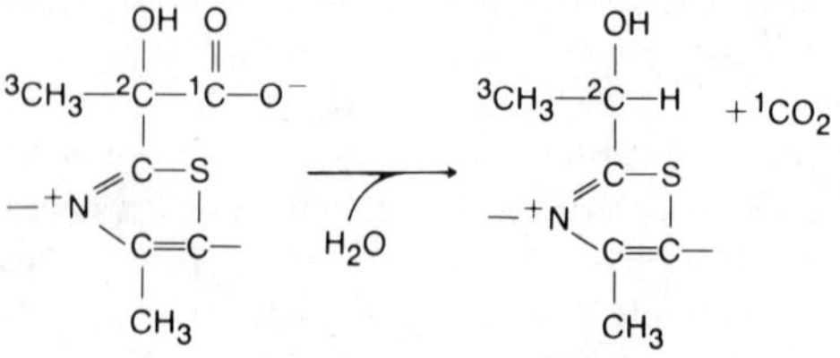

$$^3CH_3-{}^2C-{}^1C-O^-$$
OH   O

$$-{}^+N \begin{matrix} C-S \\ C=C- \end{matrix}$$
$$CH_3$$

$H_2O \longrightarrow$

$$^3CH_3-{}^2C-H \quad +{}^1CO_2$$
OH

$$-{}^+N \begin{matrix} C-S \\ C=C- \end{matrix}$$
$$CH_3$$

Carbon dioxide is released when pyruvate bonds at the active site of TPP

gen remains and a new bond forms between carbon-2 of pyruvate and the thiazole carbon. The substrate bonds are weakened by this shift of the electrons to the point that the one between carbon-1 and carbon-2 of pyruvate breaks and a carbon dioxide molecule is released.

Another TPP enzyme, *α-ketoglutarate decarboxylase,* acts within the TCA cycle to convert α-ketoglutarate to succinyl-CoA. This enzyme functions similarly to *pyruvate decarboxylase* and removes a carbon from the five-carbon compound, α-ketoglutarate. The other two enzymes of the complex complete the conversion to succinyl-CoA.

TPP is also needed as the coenzyme for *glyoxylate carboligase* which catalyzes the condensation of glyoxylate and α-ketoglutarate to form 2-hydroxy 3-ketoadipate. This enzyme is important in the METABOLISM of the AMINO ACIDS GLYCINE, HYDROXYPROLINE, and SERINE.

Branched-chain α-ketoacid decarboxylase prepares selected amino acids for synthesis of fatty acids if there is a surplus of amino acids or for use as energy if there is a scarcity of calories. After the branched-chain amino acids, ISOLEUCINE, LEUCINE, and VALINE, are converted to α-ketoacids, *branched-chain α-ketoacid decarboxylase,* a TPP-dependent enzyme, converts them to carbon dioxide and their acyl-CoA thioesters, α-methylbutyryl-CoA, isovaleryl-CoA, and isobutyryl-CoA, respectively. The ultimate fates of the carbons from the branched-chain amino acids is as follows: those from isoleucine enter the TCA cycle in acetyl-CoA and succinyl-CoA; those from leucine enter in acetyl-CoA; those from valine enter in succinyl-CoA.

A genetically defective version of branched-chain α-ketoacid dehydrogenase complex is associated with maple syrup urine disease, named for the odor of the branched-chain α-ketoacids that accumulate. Sometimes this condition can be helped by supplements of thiamin since the binding of TPP appears to change the shape of the complex and increase its stability.

Transketolase, a TPP-dependent enzyme, is one of two enzymes that forms a reversible link between glycolysis and the PENTOSE PHOSPHATE PATHWAY. (*Transaldolase,* the other enzyme, is not TPP-dependent.) The action of TPP with *transketolase* is similar to that of the other enzymes discussed here except that instead of a single carbon being released as carbon dioxide, a large three-carbon fragment of the molecule separates. The large residue is a high-energy compound, glyceraldehyde 3-phosphate, an intermediate in glycolysis, which has been released from xylulose 5-phosphate, an intermediate in the pentose phosphate

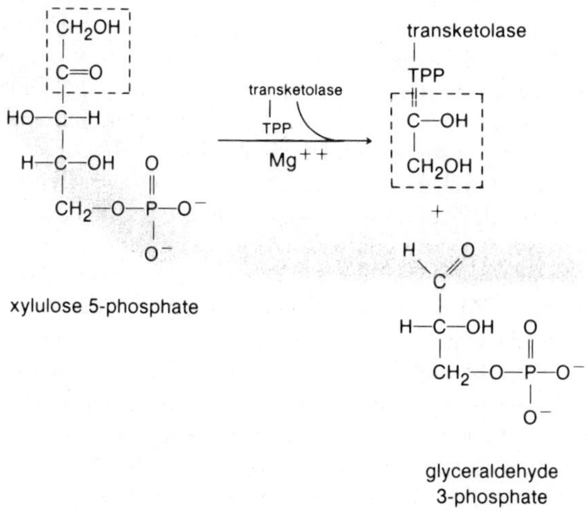

A TPP-dependent enzyme, transketolase, participates in the pentose phosphate pathway and releases a high-energy 3-carbon intermediate of glycolysis

271

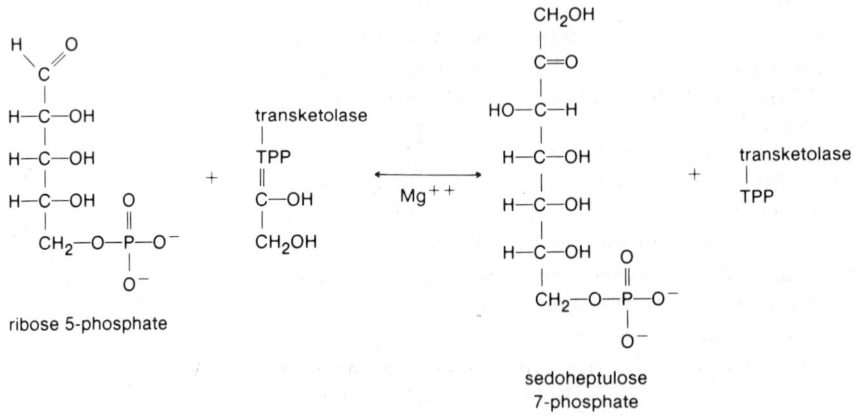

A reaction catalyzed by transketolase in the pentose phosphate pathway

pathway. The fragment still attached to the enzyme reacts with a second pentose, ribose 5-phosphate, producing sedoheptulose 7-phosphate. Thus glyceraldehyde 3-phosphate (an intermediate in the glycolytic path) and sedoheptulose 7-phosphate have been produced from two pentoses of the pentose phosphate pathway.

One neuropsychiatric disorder, Wernicke-Korsakoff syndrome, deserves mention for it illustrates how much damage can occur when just one enzyme fails to work properly. In this syndrome, usually thought to be caused by alcoholism, TPP does not bind properly to *transketolase*. Because of this, the person suffers mental confusion, poor memory, spastic gait, and poor eye movements. The failure to bind TPP to *transketolase* is a genetic trait, hence not every person who is deficient in thiamin develops the syndrome; also, contrary to popular belief, not every person who develops the disorder is a heavy user of alcohol.

It is now clear why a deficiency of thiamin in the diet can have grave consequences for energy-producing reactions in the body. At several key points, especially at the link between glycolysis and the TCA cycle (the conversion of pyruvate to acetyl-CoA) and in one step of the TCA cycle (the conversion of α-ketoglutarate to succinyl-CoA), thiamin is crucial to the production of energy from foods. Since the nervous system relies almost solely on the METABOLISM of glucose through glycolysis and the TCA cycle for its energy, it is not surprising that neural disorders occur with thiamin deficiency.

The energy from carbohydrates that is produced without thiamin can come only from reactions preceding the pyruvate-to-acetyl-CoA reaction. Such reactions produce relatively small amounts of energy and so are driven very hard as the body tries to produce enough energy to sustain itself. Unless this situation is remedied, an accumulation of pyruvic and lactic acids will lower the pH of the fluid in the cells—this condition will develop into metabolic ACIDOSIS, a serious medical problem. See also: PENTOSE PHOSPHATE PATHWAY; TRANSALDOLASE; TRANSKETOLASE.

thioester bond. An energy-rich bond of the general formula R—S—C—R. See also: COENZYME A.

threonine (Thr). An essential, four-carbon α-amino acid that, like SERINE, contains a hydroxyl group on its side chain. Threonine is considered glucogenic (glycogenic) because two of its carbons form pyruvate that could lead to their incorporation in GLUCOSE.

Threonine is thought to be degraded by two pathways. In one, two of threonine's carbons can be converted to GLYCINE and the other two to ACETALDEHYDE. *Threonine aldolase,* a VITAMIN B$_6$-dependent enzyme, catalyzes this reaction. The glycine from this reaction can be metabolized by either of two pathways: in one to serine, which can be deaminated to pyruvate, and in a second to carbon dioxide and ammonia. The acetaldehyde from this degradation can be converted to ACETYL-COA.

In the second degradative pathway, threonine can be degraded by a vitamin B$_6$-dependent enzyme, *threonine dehydratase,* to yield ammonia plus α-ketobutyrate (also

$$CH_3-\overset{\displaystyle H}{\underset{\displaystyle OH}{C}}-\overset{\displaystyle}{\underset{\displaystyle {}^+NH_3}{C}}-COO^-$$

Threonine (Thr)

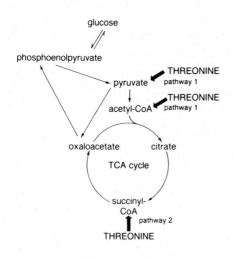

The carbons of threonine
enter metabolic pathways

called 2-oxobutyrate). The latter compound may be decarboxylated to propionyl-CoA, which, through a series of reactions requiring VITAMIN B_{12} and BIOTIN, forms succinyl-CoA.   See also: GLYCINE; SERINE.

thymidine.   A nucleoside composed of thymine (a pyrimidine base) and deoxyribose (a five-carbon sugar).   See also: NUCLEOSIDES, NUCLEOTIDES.

thymidine diphosphate (TDP).   A nucleotide composed of thymine (a pyrimidine base), deoxyribose (a five-carbon sugar), and two phosphates.   See also: NUCLEOSIDES, NUCLEOTIDES.

thymidine monophosphate (TMP, thymidylate).   A nucleotide composed of thymine (a pyrimidine base), deoxyribose, (a five-carbon sugar), and one phosphate.   See also: NUCLEOSIDES, NUCLEOTIDES.

thymidine triphosphate (TTP).   A nucleotide composed of thymine (a pyrimidine base), deoxyribose (a five-carbon sugar), and three phosphates.   See also: NUCLEOSIDES, NUCLEOTIDES.

thymidylate (dTMP).   A shortened way of saying deoxythymidylate. Since the base thymine bonds only to deoxyribose, it is often considered redundant to use the prefix deoxy-.   See also: DEOXYTHYMIDYLATE; NUCLEOSIDES, NUCLEOTIDES.

thymine.   A pyrimidine base found primarily in DNA.   See also: PURINE, PYRIMIDINE BASES; NUCLEIC ACIDS.

thyroid-stimulating hormone (TSH).   See IODIDE.

thyroxine.   A hormone secreted by the thyroid gland.   See also: IODIDE.

TMP.   See THYMIDINE MONOPHOSPHATE; DEOXYTHYMIDYLATE.

tocopherol.   See VITAMIN E.

TPP.   See THIAMIN PYROPHOSPHATE.

transaldolase.   An enzyme in carbohydrate METABOLISM that catalyzes the transfer of three-carbon units in reversible reactions which link GLYCOLYSIS and the PENTOSE PHOSPHATE PATHWAY. From three pentoses derived from the pentose phosphate pathway, *transaldolase* works with *transketolase* in a series of reactions to produce two hexoses and one triose, which can enter the glycolytic path. When the pentose phosphate pathway is activated because there is a need for NADPH to synthesize biomolecules, excess pentoses are produced. These can be funneled back to glycolysis to produce ATP through the actions of *transaldolase* and *transketolase*.

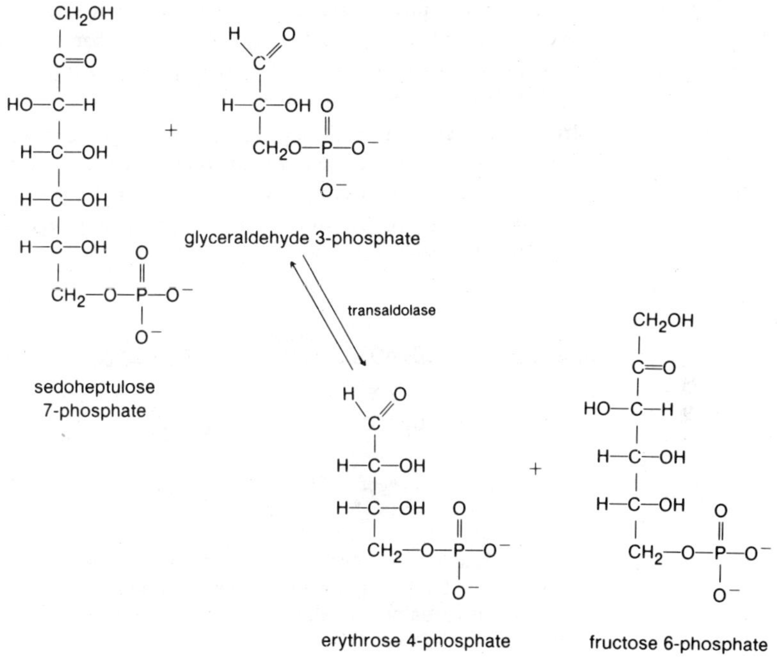

A reversible reaction catalyzed by transaldolase in the
pentose phosphate pathway forms fructose 6-phosphate or
glyceraldehyde 3-phosphate which can enter glycolytic path

Specifically, *transaldolase* catalyzes the reversible reaction between sedoheptulose 7-phosphate and glyceraldehyde 3-phosphate which produces erythrose 4-phosphate and fructose 6-phosphate.   See also: PENTOSE PHOSPHATE PATHWAY; TRANSKETOLASE.

transamination.   The transfer of an amino group (NH_2) from one amino acid to an α-ketoacid, producing a new amino acid and a new α-keto acid.   See also: VITAMIN B_6.

transcription.   The process, occurring in the nucleus, whereby the genetic information in a segment of DNA is copied in RNA.   See also: DNA; GENETIC CODE; PROTEIN BIOSYNTHESIS; RNA.

trans fatty acids.   See CIS-, TRANS-BONDS.

transfer RNA (tRNA, transfer ribonucleic acid).   A molecule that carries a specific amino acid during PROTEIN BIOSYNTHESIS. Each amino acid has at least one transfer RNA. One of the "arms" of the cloverleaf-shaped tRNA molecule contains an anticodon, a specific sequence of three bases that is complementary to a codon on mRNA. The anticodon identifies the specific amino acid that is to be picked up and delivered to the growing protein chain.   See also: PROTEIN BIOSYNTHESIS; RNA.

transketolase.   A TPP-dependent enzyme in carbohydrate *metabolism* that catalyzes the transfer of two-carbon units in reversible reactions which link GLYCOLYSIS and the PENTOSE PHOSPHATE PATHWAY.   See also: PENTOSE PHOSPHATE PATHWAY; THIAMIN PYROPHOSPHATE; TRANSALDOLASE.

$$C_5 + C_5 \xrightleftharpoons{\text{transketolase}} C_3 + C_7$$

$$C_7 + C_3 \xrightleftharpoons{\text{transadolase}} C_4 + C_6$$

$$C_5 + C_4 \xrightleftharpoons{\text{transketolase}} C_3 + C_6$$

Reactions in which three pentoses produced by the pentose phosphate pathway produce two hexoses and a triose for the glycolytic path

translation.   The process whereby the genetic message picked up from nuclear DNA by messenger RNA is transformed into the action of protein synthesis on the ribosomes. The "language" of messenger RNA is that of a polynucleotide sequence (GENETIC CODE); it is "translated" into the "language" of the protein, which is its amino acid sequence.   See also: PROTEIN BIOSYNTHESIS; RNA.

triacylglycerols (triglycerides).   A highly concentrated form of energy. Most body fat is in the form of triacylglycerols stored in adipose cells. Triacylglycerols also furnish glycerol and FATTY ACIDS as building blocks of glycolipids and phospholipids, which are important components of MEMBRANES.

A triacylglycerol is composed of a glycerol molecule joined in an ester bond to three fatty acids replacing the three hydroxyl groups with the liberation of three molecules of water. Most naturally occurring triacylglycerols contain even-numbered fatty acid chains, from 4 to 20 carbons in length. The fatty acids attached to glycerol are not necessarily identical; each may be a different length and may be either saturated or unsaturated.

Fat-rich foods provide more energy per gram than carbohydrate and protein foods. The reason that fat provides approximately 9 calories per gram while carbohydrate and

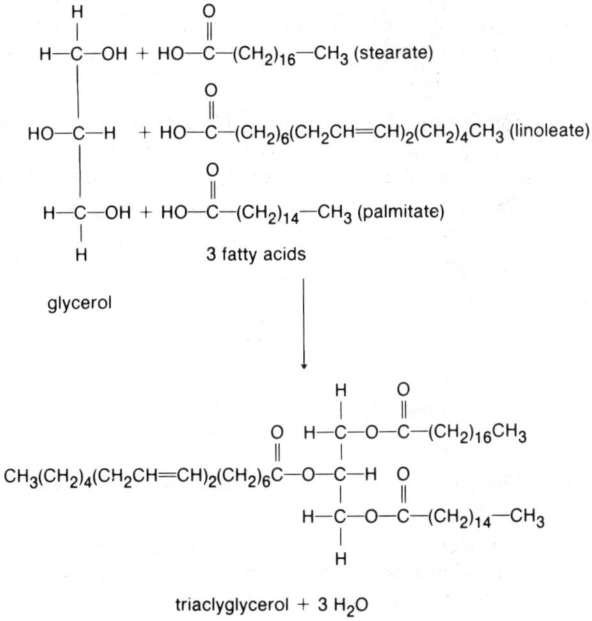

$$
\begin{array}{l}
\text{H} \qquad\qquad \text{O} \\
| \qquad\qquad\quad \| \\
\text{H—C—OH + HO—C—(CH}_2)_{16}\text{—CH}_3 \text{ (stearate)} \\
| \qquad\qquad\quad \text{O} \\
\qquad\qquad\qquad \| \\
\text{HO—C—H + HO—C—(CH}_2)_6(\text{CH}_2\text{CH}{=}\text{CH})_2(\text{CH}_2)_4\text{CH}_3 \text{ (linoleate)} \\
| \qquad\qquad\quad \text{O} \\
\qquad\qquad\qquad \| \\
\text{H—C—OH + HO—C—(CH}_2)_{14}\text{—CH}_3 \text{ (palmitate)} \\
| \\
\text{H} \qquad\qquad\quad \text{3 fatty acids}
\end{array}
$$

glycerol

triaclyglycerol + 3 H_2O

Formation of triacylglycerol

protein provide approximately 4 calories per gram is that triglycerides are highly reduced, that is, they contain a larger percentage of hydrogens than the other nutrients.

The glycerol portion of a triacylglycerol is the portion that can replenish the BLOOD GLUCOSE LEVEL. When triacylglycerols are degraded by *lipases,* glycerol is separated (hydrolyzed) from the fatty acids. The fatty acids, in turn, are degraded by beta oxidation to ACETYL-COA, which is oxidized through the TCA CYCLE. On the other hand, glycerol enters the glycolytic path at dihydroxyacetone phosphate. Upon conversion to glyceraldehyde 3-phosphate, the glycerol carbons can be used to synthesize GLUCOSE if they are not metabolized through the TCA cycle for energy.

In a triacylglycerol with three 18-carbon fatty acids attached to the 3-carbon glycerol, only three of the 57 total carbons are available for conversion to glucose. Thus, the mathematics of the METABOLISM of triacylglycerols for the production of ATP or the resynthesis of glucose has important implications. During fasting or STARVATION, the breakdown of body fat provides energy, but little glucose for use by neural tissues.

Another pathway exists by which some of the carbons resulting from fatty acid oxidation find their way into glucose. During the first turn of the TCA cycle, some of these carbons will become incorporated in succinate, a symmetric compound, and eventually in oxaloacetate. If, during the second turn of the cycle, oxaloacetate should be routed through phosphoenolpyruvate to glucose, some of these carbons may find their way into glucose. While this pathway is insignificant under normal conditions, it may be lifesaving during starvation. See also: FATTY ACIDS; STARVATION.

tricarboxylic acid cycle. See TCA CYCLE.

triglycerides. See TRIACYLGLYCEROLS.

triiodothyronine. See IODIDE.

tRNA. See TRANSFER RNA; RNA.

troponin system. A group of three regulating proteins, found in striated muscles, which mediate muscle contraction. These include troponin T (TpT), troponin I (TpI), and troponin C (TpC). TpC is a calcium-binding protein. See also: CALCIUM.

tryptophan (Trp). An essential, 11-carbon, α-amino acid with an aromatic side chain. Aromatic refers to a system of double bonds such as the ones in the phenyl ring in tryptophan; compounds with this system have unusual chemical

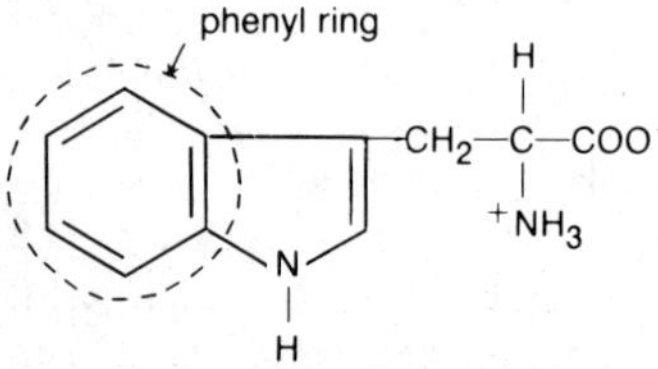

Tryptophan (Trp)

stability. When tryptophan is degraded for energy, some of its carbons are incorporated in ALANINE and some in acetoacetyl-CoA; tryptophan can be said, then, to be both glucogenic and ketogenic.

Tryptophan is a precursor of a number of significant compounds. It is estimated that about half the NIACIN requirements of the body are provided from the metabolism

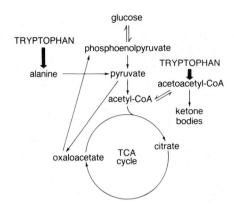

The carbons of tryptophan
enter metabolic pathways

of tryptophan, which involves a series of reactions requiring IRON, COPPER and VITAMIN B_6. Serotonin, a neurotransmitter and vasoconstrictor is also synthesized by the degradation of tryptophan.

An excellent example of the interdependence of nutrients is provided by the study of tryptophan degradation. Kynureninase, which catalyzes the cleavage of 3-hydroxykynurenine, must have vitamin B_6 as its coenzyme; otherwise, it cannot form 3-hydroxyanthranilate, the compound that forms the pyridine ring of niacin. Thus, a patient's symptoms may indicate a niacin deficiency when in fact the dietary deficiency is that of vitamin B_6, without which the production of niacin from tryptophan is blocked.

The degradative paths open to tryptophan are varied and complex. The first step of one of tryptophan's degradative paths, oxygen and *tryptophan oxygenase* (also called *tryptophan pyrrolase*), which requires IRON and COPPER as cofactors, break open the pyrrole ring forming N-formylkynurenine. N-formylkynurenine is used to synthesize kynurenine by the action of *kynurenine formylase*. Through a series of reactions, three carbons are split off forming the amino acid, alanine, which can form pyruvate and enter the TCA CYCLE. This leaves 3-hydroxyanthranilate that is degraded into CO_2 and acetoacetyl-CoA, which can be converted to ACETYL-CoA and enter the TCA cycle or to acetoacetate, a ketone body. 3-Hydroxyanthranilate can also lead to the formation of the pyridine ring of niacin.

The degradation of tryptophan scheme:

tryptophan $\xrightarrow[\text{tryptophan oxygenase, Fe, Cu}]{O_2}$ N-formylkynurenine

$\xrightarrow[\text{kynurenine formamidase}]{H_2O}$ formate

kynurenine $\xleftarrow[\text{kynurenine 3-monooxygenase}]{}$

3-hydroxykynurenine $\xrightarrow[\text{kynureninase, vitamin B}_6\text{ dependent}]{H_2O}$

alanine: $CH_3-CH-COO^- \rightarrow \rightarrow \rightarrow$ glucose with $^+NH_3$

3-hydroxyanthranilate $\rightarrow$ acetoacetyl-CoA, $3CO_2$, nicotinamide

Degradation of tryptophan

TSH (thyroid stimulating hormone). See IODIDE.

TTP. See THYMIDINE TRIPHOSPHATE.

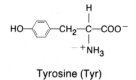

Tyrosine (Tyr)

tyrosine (Tyr). A nonessential, 9-carbon, α-amino acid that, like TRYPTOPHAN and PHENYLALANINE, has an aromatic side chain. Aromatic refers to a system of double bonds such as the ones in the phenyl ring of tyrosine; compounds with this system have unusual chemical stability.

Tyrosine is synthesized from the ESSENTIAL AMINO ACID phenylalanine in a reaction catalyzed by *phenylalanine monooxygenase* (also called *phenylalanine hydroxylase*), an enzyme that requires IRON, VITAMIN C, and NIACIN. In cases where phenylalanine monooxygenase is genetically defective (about 1 in 10,000), there is a buildup of phenylalanine and its abnormal metabolites in the blood and urine following ingestion of phenylalanine-containing foods (any complete protein). At the same time, tyrosine is not synthesized

$$\text{phenylalanine} + O_2 + \text{tetrahydrobiopterin}$$

phenylalanine

NADPH + H$^+$

phenylalanine
monooxygenase

NADP$^+$

$$\text{tyrosine} + H_2O + \text{dihydrobiopterin}$$

tyrosine

Synthesis of tyrosine from phenylalanine

and becomes an essential amino acid. The inability of the enzyme to degrade phenylalanine to tyrosine results in the disease phenylketonuria (PKU), which is marked by severe mental retardation.

Tyrosine is the precursor of a number of small, important biomolecules including the CATECHOLAMINES dopamine, norepinephrine, and epinephrine. These are

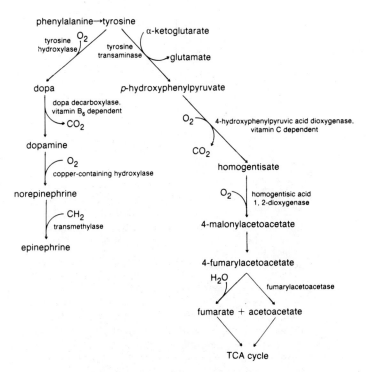

Degradation of tyrosine and phenylalanine

neurotransmitters synthesized from tyrosine at sympathetic nerve terminals and in the adrenal gland. The synthesis of dopamine requires VITAMIN B$_6$, iron, and vitamin C; norepinephrine synthesis also requires vitamin C. The hormone thyroxine and the pigment melanin are also derived from tyrosine. Thus it can be seen that a deficiency of tyrosine or the inability to metabolize tyrosine could have a profound effect on many functions of the body.

When tyrosine's skeleton is degraded, four of its nine carbons enter the TCA CYCLE as fumarate, four enter by way of acetoacetyl-CoA, and one is incorporated in CO$_2$ in the step that produces homogentisate. Tyrosine, then, is both ketogenic and glucogenic.

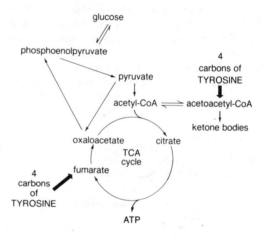

The carbons of tyrosine
enter metabolic pathways

The first step in the degradation removes the amino group and converts tyrosine into its α-keto acid. The next steps add oxygen, which will open up the phenyl ring. The resulting compound is isomerized and hydrolyzed to fumarate, an intermediate in the TCA cycle, and to acetoacetyl-CoA, which can be converted into acetoacetate, a ketone body. See also: PHENYLALANINE, for a discussion of PKU.

SUGGESTED READINGS

Frimpter, G. W. 1973. Aminoacidemias due to inherited disorders of metabolism. Part 1. *N. Engl. J. Med.* 289:835–841.

Furukawa, N. 1984. The enzyme defects in hereditary tyrosinemia type 1. *J. Inherit. Metab. Dis.* 2:137–138.

Goldsmith, L. A. 1983. Tyrosinemia and related disorders. In *The metabolic basis of inherited disease*, 5th ed., ed. J. B. Stanbury et al., 287–299. New York: McGraw-Hill.

u

ubiquinone. See COENZYME Q.

UDP. See URIDINE DIPHOSPHATE.

UDP-glucose. A nucleotide containing uracil, ribose, and two phosphates plus GLUCOSE. UDP-glucose is used, for example, in the synthesis of GLYCOGEN from glucose and in galactose METABOLISM. It is formed by *UDP-glucose pyrophosphorylase* that catalyzes UTP plus glucose 1-phosphate to yield UDP-glucose plus pyrophosphate. See also: GALACTOSE; GLYCOGENESIS.

UMP. See URIDINE MONOPHOSPHATE.

unsaturated fatty acids. Fatty acids that have at least one double bond between two of the carbons. See also: FATTY ACIDS.

uracil. A pyrimidine base that is a constituent of nucleic acids. See also: DNA; NUCLEIC ACIDS; PURINE, PYRIMIDINE BASES; RNA.

urea cycle. A metabolic cycle, taking place in the liver, which prepares toxic ammonia for safe travel through the blood and then excretion by the kidney. It was the first such chemical cycle discovered and it is chemically meshed with another famous cycle, the TCA CYCLE. Another name for the TCA cycle is the "Krebs Cycle" after Hans Krebs who first elucidated it and who, with Kurt Henseleit, worked out the details of the urea cycle. (Punsters frequently speak of the two cycles, both credited to Krebs, as the "Krebs Bi-Cycles.")

Urea was the first natural compound to be synthesized in the laboratory. This accomplishment led to a redefinition of "organic" compounds because it had been generally thought that only living organisms could produce organic

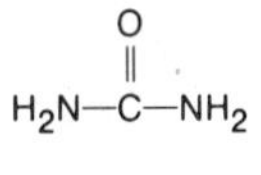

$$H_2N-\overset{\displaystyle O}{\overset{\displaystyle \|}{C}}-NH_2$$

Urea

compounds. In the biological synthesis of urea, the carbon atom comes from one of the two CO_2 molecules released during a revolution of the TCA cycle, one nitrogen atom comes from the amino acid ASPARTATE, and the other nitrogen atom comes from ammonia, generated from the deamination of AMINO ACIDS. The products of the combination of CO_2, ammonia, aspartate, and 3 ATP are urea, fumarate, 2 ADP, $2P_i$, AMP, and PP_i.

Following is a stepwise discussion of the five main reactions that comprise the urea cycle and detail its relationship to the TCA cycle.

The first reaction of the urea cycle involves the synthesis in the MITOCHONDRION of carbamoyl phosphate from ammonia and carbon dioxide. The carbon dioxide was derived from the TCA cycle. This reaction, catalyzed by *carbamoyl phosphate synthetase I* and requiring N-acetyl glutamate, is essentially irreversible since it requires 2 ATP.

In the second reaction, carbamoyl phosphate, carrying a carbon and a nitrogen that will become part of urea, unites

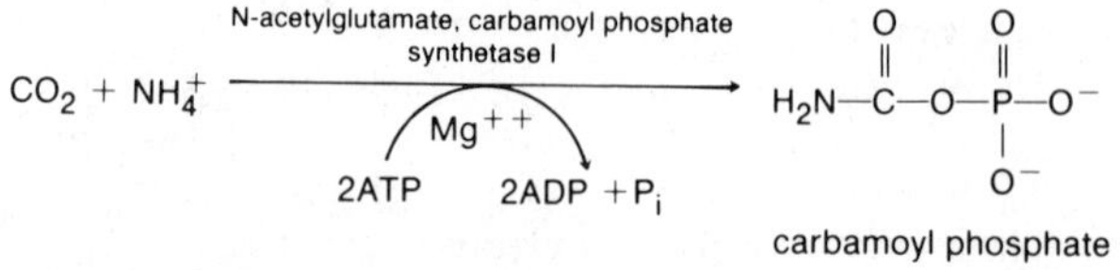

First reaction of urea cycle takes place in the mitochondria

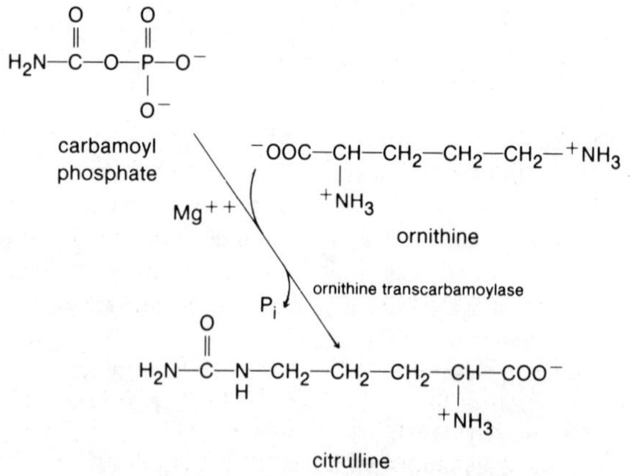

Second reaction of urea cycle
takes place in mitochondria

with ornithine to become citrulline in a reaction catalyzed by MAGNESIUM-dependent *ornithine transcarbamoylase.* (The ornithine was re-formed during the degradation of ARGININE, a reaction that occurs with each full turn of the urea cycle.)

In the third reaction citrulline leaves the mitochondrion and enters the cytosol where it is bonded to aspartate, which is carrying the second amino group that will become incorporated in urea. (This second amino group was acquired by aspartate by transamination from glutamate that, in turn, acquired it from the deaminations of all the other amino acids; or, aspartate could have been derived from the amination of oxaloacetate, a TCA cycle intermediate.) The resulting compound is argininosuccinate. ATP is hydrolyzed to AMP and pyrophosphate in this reaction, which is catalyzed by *argininosuccinate synthetase.*

$$
\underset{\text{citrulline}}{H_2N-\overset{\overset{\displaystyle O}{\|}}{C}-\underset{H}{N}-CH_2-CH_2-CH_2-\underset{\underset{+NH_3}{|}}{CH}-COO^-}
$$

$$
\underset{\text{aspartate}}{^-OOC-CH_2-\underset{\underset{+NH_3}{|}}{CH}-COO^-}
$$

ATP

Mg^{++}

argininosuccinate
synthetase

AMP + PP$_i$

$$
^-OOC-CH_2-\underset{\underset{\displaystyle NH}{|}}{CH}-COO^-
$$

$$
\underset{\text{argininosuccinate}}{HN=\overset{}{C}-\underset{H}{N}-CH_2-CH_2-CH_2-\underset{\underset{+NH_3}{|}}{CH}-COO^-}
$$

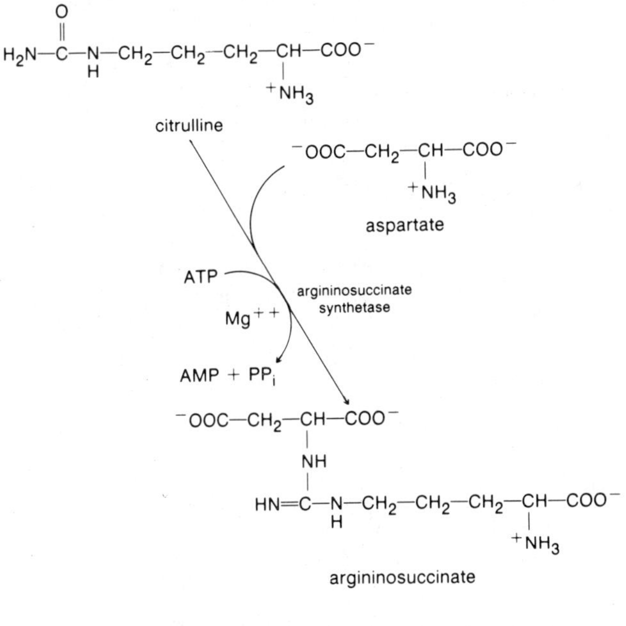

Third reaction of urea cycle takes place in cytosol

In the fourth reaction, catalyzed by *argininosuccinase,* argininosuccinate breaks (is hydrolyzed) into arginine and fumarate. The fumarate leaves the urea cycle and returns to the TCA cycle where it is oxidized to oxaloacetate through malate. *Malate dehydrogenase* will generate NADH + H$^+$. When the electrons from NADH are funneled through the

287

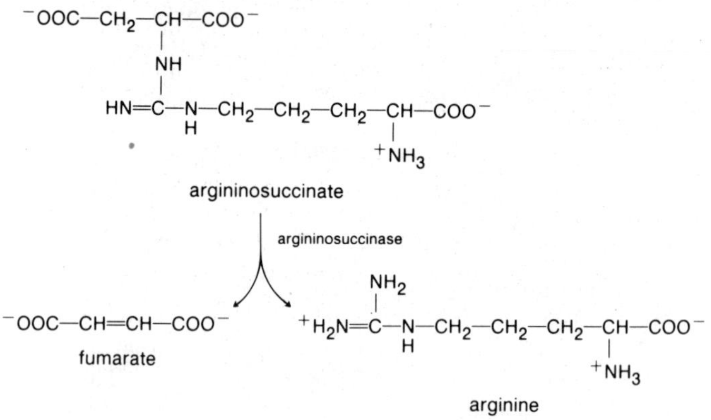

$$^-OOC-CH_2-CH-COO^-$$

NH

$$HN=C-N-CH_2-CH_2-CH_2-CH-COO^-$$
$$\quad\quad\quad H$$
$$\quad\quad\quad\quad\quad\quad\quad\quad\quad\quad\quad\quad ^+NH_3$$

argininosuccinate

argininosuccinase

$$NH_2$$

$$^-OOC-CH=CH-COO^- \quad\quad ^+H_2N=C-N-CH_2-CH_2-CH_2-CH-COO^-$$
$$\quad\quad\quad H$$
fumarate
$$\quad\quad\quad\quad\quad\quad\quad\quad\quad\quad\quad\quad\quad\quad\quad\quad ^+NH_3$$

arginine

Fourth reaction of urea cycle

RESPIRATORY CHAIN, 3 ADP will be phosphorylated to 3 ATP. (Significantly, 3 ATP is the exact amount of energy needed by the urea cycle—2 ATP for the synthesis of carbamoyl phosphate and 1 ATP for the entry of aspartate into the urea cycle.) Oxaloacetate can be aminated to aspartate, which can return to the urea cycle.

In the fifth and final reaction of the urea cycle, *arginase*, an enzyme that is dependent on cobalt and MANGANESE, hydrolyzes arginine to form urea and ornithine. Ornithine may then reenter the mitochondrion and combine with more carbamoyl phosphate to start the cycle again. The

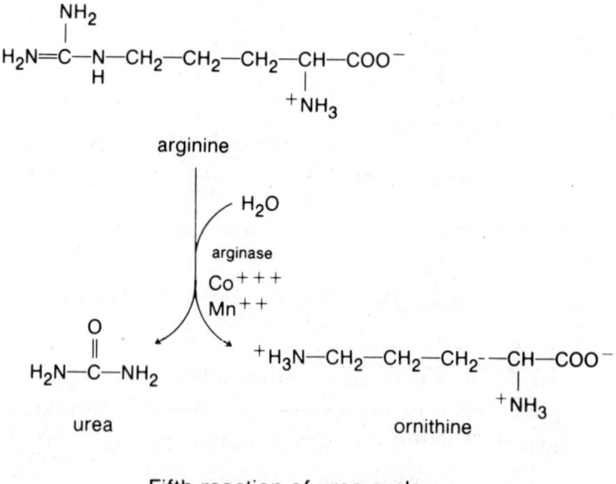

$$NH_2$$
$$H_2N=C-N-CH_2-CH_2-CH_2-CH-COO^-$$
$$\quad\quad\quad H$$
$$\quad\quad\quad\quad\quad\quad\quad\quad\quad\quad ^+NH_3$$

arginine

$$H_2O$$

arginase
$$Co^{+++}$$
$$Mn^{++}$$

$$O$$
$$\|$$
$$H_2N-C-NH_2 \quad\quad\quad\quad ^+H_3N-CH_2-CH_2-CH_2-CH-COO^-$$
$$\quad\quad\quad\quad\quad\quad\quad\quad\quad\quad\quad\quad\quad\quad\quad\quad ^+NH_3$$

urea
ornithine

Fifth reaction of urea cycle
Urea is excreted,
ornithine returns to mitochondria

urea enters the blood stream where it is removed by the kidneys and sent to the bladder for excretion. Some urea cycle reactions take place in the cytosol and some in the mitochondria. Ornithine and citrulline are able to cross the membrane.

Interference with any of the reactions of the urea cycle will cause serious health effects. Urea is the body's way of detoxifying and disposing of ammonia. The toxicity of ammonia is thought to be due to the slowdown of the TCA cycle in the brain as α-ketoglutarate is siphoned out of the cycle to combine with one molecule of ammonia to form glutamate. Glutamate does not readily exit the brain. Glutamate can, however, pick up another molecule of ammonia to become glutamine that is able to diffuse through the brain's membrane and enter the bloodstream. If ammonia continues to be produced above normal levels, the supply of α-ketoglutarate will be exhausted, thus interfering with the production of ATP from the TCA cycle in the brain and having tragic consequences.

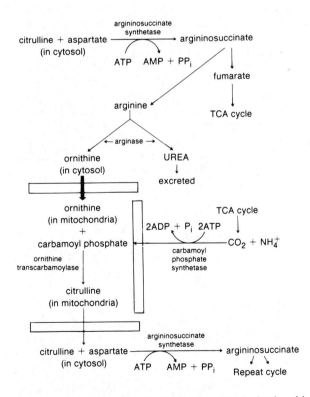

The urea cycle takes place in both the cytosol and mitochondria

Some genetic disorders are caused by a low production level of urea cycle enzymes. These have the same symptoms as ammonia toxicity—vomiting, lethargy, and, in infants, mental retardation and possibly death.

ureotelic. Organisms that excrete nitrogen as urea. Humans are ureotelic.

uricotelic. Organisms, with limited water intake, that excrete nitrogen as a solid uric acid. Birds are uricotelic.

uridine. A nucleoside consisting of uracil (a pyrimidine) and ribose. It is usually found as part of RNA. See also: NUCLEOSIDES, NUCLEOTIDES; RNA.

uridine diphosphate (UDP). A nucleotide containing uracil (a pyrimidine), ribose, and two phosphates.

uridine monophosphate (UMP, uridylate). A nucleotide containing uracil (a pyrimidine), ribose, and one phosphate.

uridine triphosphate (UTP). A nucleotide containing uracil (a pyrimidine), ribose, and three phosphates.

UTP. See URIDINE TRIPHOSPHATE.

valine (Val). An essential, glucogenic (glycogenic), 5-carbon, α-amino acid with a hydrocarbon side chain.

The degradation of valine takes place primarily in skeletal muscle and is especially active during fasting and in uncontrolled diabetes mellitus when protein is being catabolized for energy. Three of valine's carbons form succinyl-CoA, an intermediate of the TCA CYCLE. The path from valine to succinyl-CoA begins with transamination of valine to its corresponding α-keto acid, followed by oxidative decarboxylation requiring THIAMIN PYROPHOSPHATE. Further reactions produce propionyl-CoA, and through

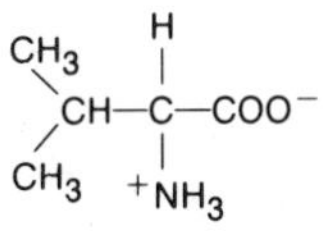

Valine (Val)

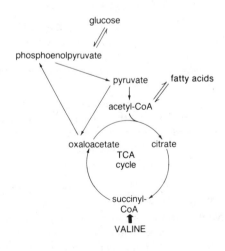

The carbons of valine enter
metabolic pathways

291

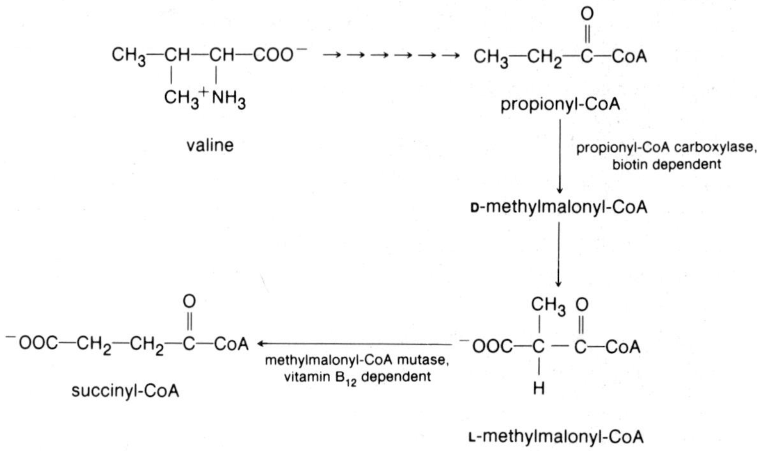

$$CH_3-CH-CH-COO^- \rightarrow \rightarrow \rightarrow \rightarrow \rightarrow \rightarrow CH_3-CH_2-\overset{\overset{O}{\|}}{C}-CoA$$

$$\underset{CH_3\ ^+NH_3}{\underset{|\qquad|}{}}$$

valine · propionyl-CoA

propionyl-CoA carboxylase,
biotin dependent

D-methylmalonyl-CoA

$$^-OOC-CH_2-CH_2-\overset{\overset{O}{\|}}{C}-CoA \longleftarrow \underset{\substack{\text{methylmalonyl-CoA mutase,} \\ \text{vitamin B}_{12} \text{ dependent}}}{} \ ^-OOC-\overset{\overset{CH_3}{|}}{\underset{\underset{H}{|}}{C}}-\overset{\overset{O}{\|}}{C}-CoA$$

succinyl-CoA

L-methylmalonyl-CoA

Conversion of valine to succinyl-CoA

methylmalonyl-CoA, succinyl-CoA. The former reaction requires biotin. The latter reaction requires a VITAMIN B$_{12}$-dependent enzyme, *methylmalonyl-CoA mutase.*

An inborn error of metabolism in the oxidative decarboxylation step in the degradation of valine (as well as of ISOLEUCINE and LEUCINE) results in maple syrup urine disease, named for the odor, color, and viscosity of the urine. See also: MAPLE SYRUP URINE DISEASE.

SUGGESTED READINGS

Staten, M. A., D. M. Bier, and D. E. Matthews. 1984. Regulation of valine metabolism in man: A stable isotope study. *Am. J. Clin. Nutr.* 40:1224–1234.

See suggested readings for BRANCHED-CHAIN AMINO ACIDS; INBORN ERRORS OF METABOLISM.

valinemia. Results from the absence of the enzyme *valine aminotransferase* causing the accumulation of valine in blood and other body fluids. Symptoms include vomiting, weight loss, and mental retardation.

SUGGESTED READINGS

See suggested readings for BRANCHED-CHAIN AMINO ACIDS; INBORN ERRORS OF METABOLISM.

van der Waals bonds. An attractive, weak force between two atoms that is dependent on the distance between the atoms. The attractive force is greatest at the "contact distance," which is dependent on the distribution of the electronic charge around the atoms; at a closer distance, repulsion will occur because of the negativity of the two electron clouds. Although van der Waals bonds are much weaker than electrostatic or hydrogen bonds, they are very important in biologic systems.

very high density lipoproteins (VHDL). LIPOPROTEINS that have a high percentage of protein and low percentage of LIPIDS, and are usually included in the grouping of high density lipoproteins (HDL). See also: LIPOPROTEINS.

very low density lipoproteins (VLDL). LIPOPROTEINS synthesized primarily in the liver and used to transport lipids, mostly triacylglycerols, to peripheral tissues. See also: LIPOPROTEINS.

VHDL (very high density lipoproteins). See LIPOPROTEINS; VERY HIGH DENSITY LIPOPROTEINS.

vitamin A (all-*trans*-retinol). A fat-soluble vitamin that is essential for growth, healthy epithelial cells, and good vision, particularly night vision. It is found in animal foods, such as fish oils, eggs, and butter, and is stored in the liver. It is not found in plants; however, many deep orange and yellow vegetables contain beta carotene (β-carotene), a precursor of vitamin A. In the body, 6 μg of β-carotene are thought to produce about 1 μg of vitamin A, a rather inefficient conversion.

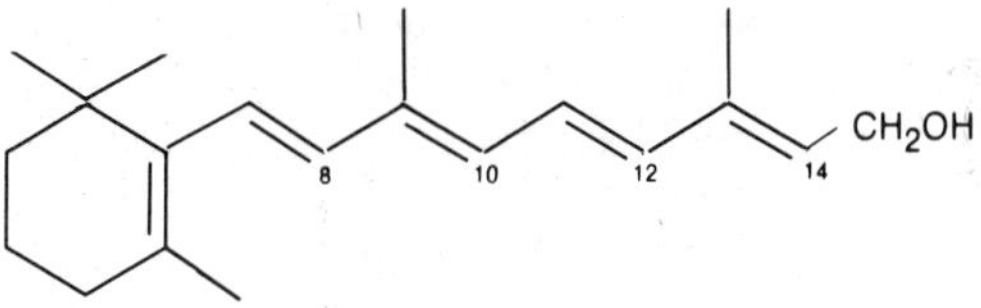

vitamin A (retinol)

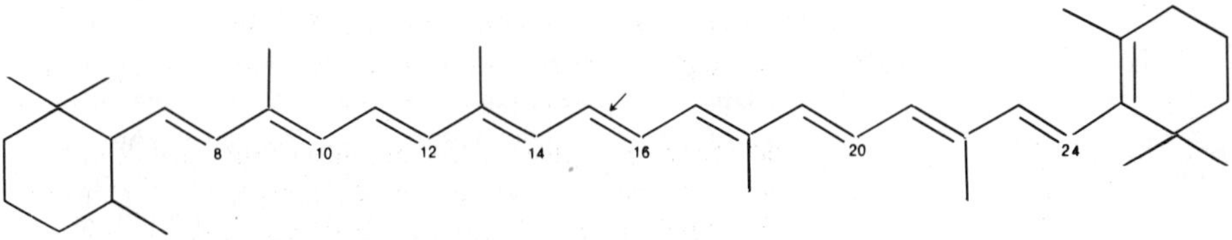

β-carotene

Cleavage of β-carotene between C-15 and C-16
results in two molecules of vitamin A

In the upper gastrointestinal tract, esterified vitamin A and β-carotene are hydrolyzed by *pancreatic esterases* to yield free vitamin A and free β-carotene. Absorption of these compounds requires the presence of fat and bile.

Within the intestinal cell, most β-carotene is converted through a series of reactions to retinol, or retinal. The vitamin A is then usually re-esterified with FATTY ACIDS and incorporated into a chylomicron, which is transported through the lymph and then into the blood for uptake by the liver.

Vitamin A from the liver is released into the blood bound to retinol-binding protein. In the plasma, retinol-binding protein complexed to retinol usually then binds to prealbumin. While vitamin A is stored in the liver, some vitamin A metabolites have been shown to be excreted from the body in both the urine and the bile.

Vitamin A deficiency symptoms are seen more often in children than in adults, probably because the rapid growth of children's tissues depletes their small stored supply in the liver; on the other hand, because adults are not growing and drawing on their stores, their livers can store about a year's supply. It is possible to reach toxic levels of vitamin A because the liver avidly stores most of the excess. Usually, however, toxicity occurs when persons take supplements rather than when they eat excess vitamin A-rich foods.

Epithelial cells become keratinized without vitamin A. The mucous linings of mouth, esophagus, and all other moist surfaces lose their water content as the cells become filled with keratin, a tough, fibrous protein that is insoluble in water. The most devastating effect is on sight where the epithelial cells of the cornea become dry and hard, a condition called xerophthalmia. This is a common cause of blindness in malnourished children in developing countries.

The best researched role of vitamin A in the body is that of the chemistry of vision. Vitamin A is the precursor of a compound whose shape is changed by the absorption of light. This change triggers a nerve impulse, then, with the help of NIACIN-containing ENZYMES, most of the original compound is regenerated, ready to re-absorb light.

The retina of the eye contains two kinds of receptor membranes, rod cells and cone cells. About a billion rod cells function in dim light but do not detect color. Cone cells, which are few in number, about three million, operate in bright light and can distinguish color.

Rhodopsin, composed of opsin (a protein) and 11-*cis*-retinal, is the molecule in rod cells that has the ability to absorb photons of light. After the absorption of light, a change from a *cis* to a *trans* double bond between C-11 and C-12 of 11-*cis*-retinal changes its shape to that of all-*trans*-retinal, and thus the nerve impulse is triggered.

opsin +

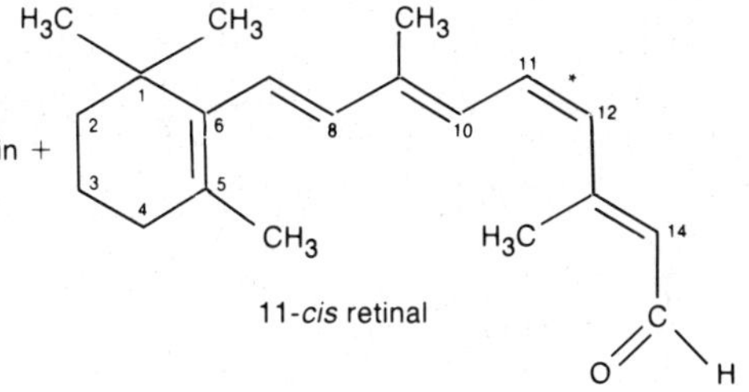

11-*cis* retinal

*note that four bonds in side chain are
trans and one is cis

Compositon of rhodopsin
(opsin + 11-cis retinal)

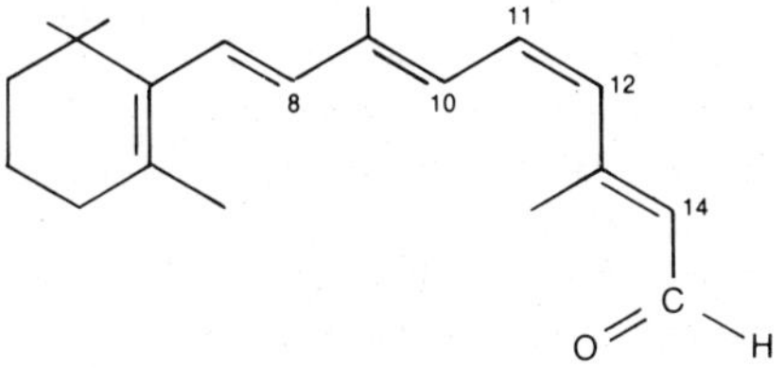

11-*cis*-retinal

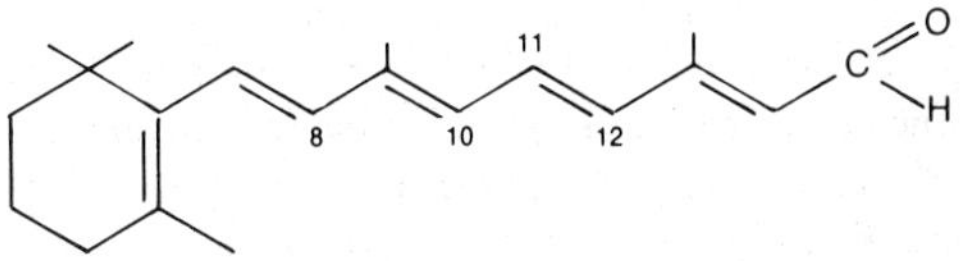

all-*trans*-retinal

With light absorption 11-cis-retinal is
transformed to all-trans-retinal

The energy of the nerve impulse alters the permeability of the membrane so that CALCIUM ions flow out of the vesicle. In this way calcium ions are the coupling agents that deliver the original impulse from light to the nerves, which can take the information to the brain. (This mechanism is akin to the way calcium ions deliver a message from the brain to contracting muscles.)

Since the all-*trans*-retinal shape is altered, it is separated from the opsin momentarily. Then, by means of reactions that involve niacin coenzymes, the all-*trans*-retinal is re-converted to the original 11-*cis*-retinal that recombines with opsin to form rhodopsin. The regeneration is now complete and the ability to see clearly is restored. See also: CIS-, TRANS-BONDS; CALCIUM.

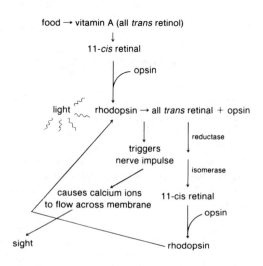

Summary of the reactions of vision

SUGGESTED READINGS

Bowmaker, J. K., and H. J. A. Dartnall. 1980. Visual pigments of rods and cones in a human retina. *J. Physiol.* 298:501–511.

Gleghorn, E. E., et al. 1986. Observations of vitamin A toxicity in three patients with renal failure receiving parenteral nutrition. *Am. J. Clin. Nutr.* 44:107–112.

Goodman, D. S. 1984. Vitamin A and retinoids in health and disease. *N. Engl. J. Med.* 310:1023–1031.

Ong, D. E. 1985. Vitamin A-binding proteins. *Nutr. Rev.* 43:225–232.

Takase, S., D. E. Ong, and F. Chytil. 1979. Cellular retinol binding protein allows specific interaction of retinol with the nucleus in vitro. *Proc. Natl. Acad. Sci.* 76:2204–2208.

vitamin B-complex. See B-VITAMIN TERMINOLOGY.

vitamin B₁. See THIAMIN.

vitamin B₂. See RIBOFLAVIN.

vitamin B_6 (pyridoxine). A water-soluble vitamin that appears in three forms: pyridoxine, pyridoxal (an aldehyde), and pyridoxamine (an amine).

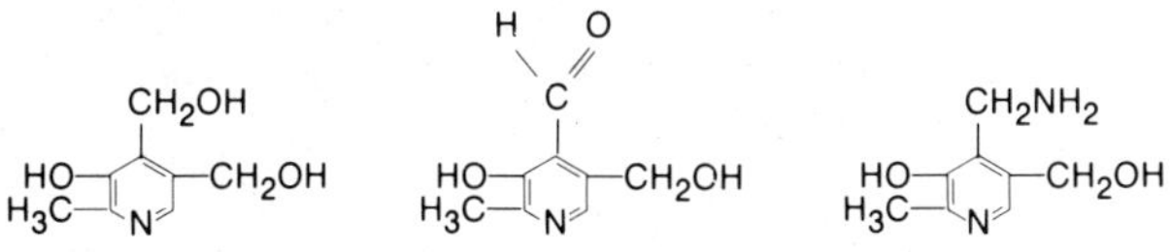

pyridoxine pyridoxal pyridoxamine

The forms of vitamin B_6

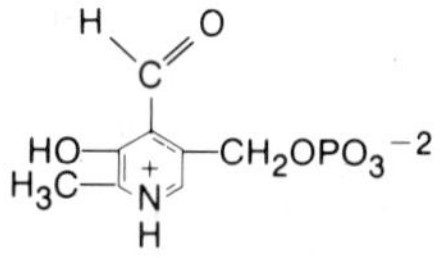

Pyridoxal phosphate (PLP)

In the body vitamin B_6 functions as a coenzyme, mostly for reactions involving AMINO ACIDS. The active coenzyme form is pyridoxal phosphate (PLP), best known for its actions with the *transaminases* that transfer NH_2 groups from an α-amino acid to an α-keto acid forming a new amino acid and a new keto acid. By transamination a nonessential amino acid can be synthesized when it is not present and is needed by a cell.

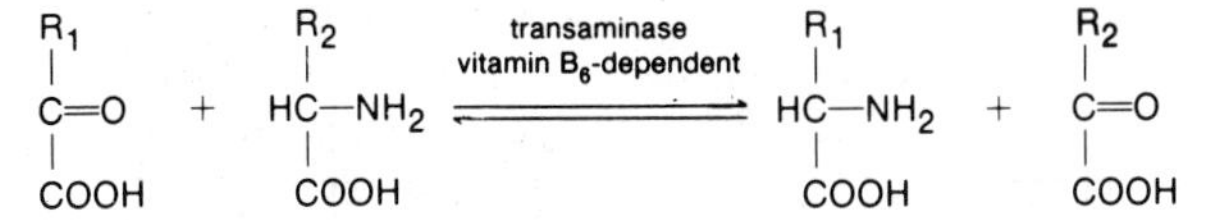

keto acid 1 amino acid 2 amino acid 1 keto acid 2

Vitamin B_6-dependent enzyme moves NH_2 group to keto acid, transforming it to an amino acid

Pyridoxal phosphate also plays key roles in aminations, deaminations, and decarboxylations. For example, aminations are important in such activities as carrying an ammonium ion to the UREA CYCLE for removal and synthesizing a nonessential amino acid for incorporation in a growing protein chain. Deaminations are important in the degradation of amino acids so that their carbon backbone can be used for other purposes, such as energy production. Examples of decarboxylations, which involve the removal of a carboxyl group from a molecule, include conversion of DOPA to dopamine in CATECHOLAMINE synthesis, degradation of HISTIDINE to histamine, and production of serotonin from TRYPTOPHAN.

Vitamin B$_6$ coenzymes are also important in the synthesis of CYSTEINE from METHIONINE, the synthesis of porphyrin (the iron-carrying portion of HEME), and the synthesis of NIACIN from tryptophan. In carbohydrate METABOLISM, vitamin B$_6$ is needed for the activity of *glycogen phosphorylase*, which is responsible for GLYCOGEN catabolism.

Deficiency symptoms of vitamin B$_6$ include anemia, irritability, and seizures. Excellent sources of vitamin B$_6$ include liver, muscle meats, legumes, and whole grain cereals. See also: CATECHOLAMINES; GAMMA AMINOBUTYRATE; GLUTAMATE; GLYCINE; HEME; HOMOCYSTINURIA; LEUCINE; METHIONINE; PHENYLALANINE; SERINE; SEROTONIN; SGOT; SGPT; TRYPTOPHAN; TYROSINE for reactions involving vitamin B$_6$.

SUGGESTED READINGS

Anderson, B. B., et al. 1971. Conversion of vitamin B$_6$ compounds to active forms in the red blood cell. *J. Clin. Invest.* 50:1901–1909.

Bottomley, S. S. 1983. Iron and vitamin B$_6$ metabolism in the sideroblastic anemias. In *Nutrition and hematology*, ed. J. Lindenbaum, 203–224. New York: Churchill Livingstone.

Dreon, D. M., and G. E. Butterfield. 1986. Vitamin B$_6$ utilization in active and inactive young men. *Am. J. Clin. Nutr.* 43:816–824.

Mehansho, H., and L. M. Henderson. 1980. Transport and accumulation of pyridoxine and pyridoxal by erythrocytes. *J. Biol. Chem.* 255:11901–11907.

Tarr, J. B., T. Tamura, and E. L. R. Stokstad. 1981. Availability of vitamin B$_6$ and pantothenate in an average American diet in man. *Am. J. Clin. Nutr.* 34:1328–1337.

vitamin B$_{12}$ (cyanocobalamin). A vitamin that cannot be synthesized by plants or animals, only by microorganisms. An unbelievably small amount (about 3 μg) is needed daily, and even at that, strict vegetarians are at long-term risk for developing a deficiency since vitamin B$_{12}$ is found almost exclusively in animal flesh or products.

In food, vitamin B$_{12}$ is bound to proteins. For absorption in the ileum, vitamin B$_{12}$ must be freed by *proteases* from the proteins and must bind to intrinsic factor, a glycoprotein made by gastric parietal cells. Consequently, vitamin B$_{12}$ made by colon bacteria is usually unavailable for absorption.

The structure of vitamin B$_{12}$ is characterized by the presence of cobalt. The cobalt is surrounded by a corrin ring consisting of four nitrogen-containing rings that are linked

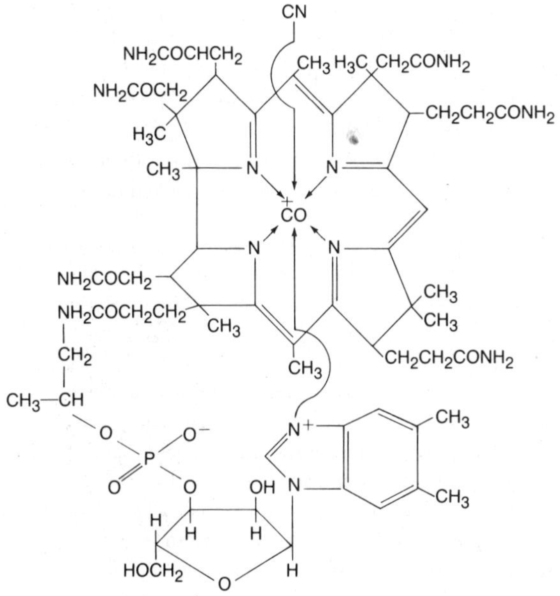

Vitamin B$_{12}$

through methylene bridges. A methyl group or a 5'-adenosyl group is attached to the cobalt to form either of the two coenzyme forms of vitamin B$_{12}$.

In the blood, vitamin B$_{12}$ is bound mainly to trans-cobalamin. In cells, vitamin B$_{12}$ functions as a coenzyme involved in two reactions. In the first, methylcobalamin is required for the methylation of homocysteine to re-form METHIONINE. This reaction also requires FOLACIN as N^5-methyltetrahydrofolate and is important in the regeneration not only of methionine but also of tetrahydrofolate. In the second reaction, 5'-adenosylcobalamin is required for the action of *methylmalonyl mutase,* which converts methylmalonyl-CoA to succinyl-CoA. This reaction is necessary for the degradation of some AMINO ACIDS and for the degradation of odd-chain FATTY ACIDS.

When intrinsic factor is missing, pernicious anemia results. This genetic condition is characterized by poorly formed, large red blood cells (megaloblastic anemia) and demyelinization of the sheaths of nerve cells. Control of the deficiency is by injection or consumption of large amounts of vitamin B$_{12}$—enough to overcome the problem of absorption. Even though the link between vitamin B$_{12}$ and pernicious anemia was not known at the time, Minot and Murphy received the Nobel prize in medicine (1934) for their discovery that large daily servings of liver would keep pernicious anemia patients alive.

The experimental work, that was to lead eventually to the definition of the role of vitamin B$_{12}$ in pernicious anemia, was hampered by several factors. First, there were two substances, not one, to be isolated and linked to the disease; and, second, these are found in the body both separated and bound together. It took many years to uncover that Vitamin B$_{12}$ is combined with the glycoprotein in the lumen and then bound by a specific receptor in the lining of the intestinal ileum. After binding, the two compounds are separated and vitamin B$_{12}$ is actively transported into the bloodstream. Another complicating factor was that one of the identifying pernicious anemia symptoms, macrocytic (large-cell), megaloblastic anemia, can be masked by generous quantities of folacin, such as might be eaten by a vegetarian. It was necessary then to be able to isolate both vitamin B$_{12}$ (cyanocobalamin) and folacin (pteroylglutamic acid) before either's roles could be studied.

Folacin, however, only clears up the macrocytic anemia of a vitamin B$_{12}$ deficiency and does nothing to stop demyelinization of nerve sheaths, which is the insidious and permanent damage resulting from this deficiency. See also: CHOLINE; COENZYME B$_{12}$; FOLACIN; METHIONINE; METHYLMALONIC ACIDEMIA.

SUGGESTED READINGS

Carmel, R. 1983. Clinical and laboratory features of the diagnosis of megaloblastic anemia. In *Nutrition and hemotology*, ed. J. Lindenbaum, 1–32. New York: Churchill Livingstone.

Chanarin, I. 1980. Cobalamins and nitrous oxide: A review. *J. Clin. Pathol.* 33:909–916.

Chanarin, I., et al. 1980. Vitamin B$_{12}$ regulates folate metabolism by the supply of formate. *Lancet* 2:505–507.

Herbert, V. 1981. Vitamin B$_{12}$. *Am. J. Clin. Nutr.* 34:971–972.

Jacob, E., S. J. Baker, and V. Herbert. 1980. Vitamin B$_{12}$-binding proteins. *Physiol. Rev.* 60:918–960.

Kanazawa, S., and V. Herbert. 1983. Mechanism of enterohepatic circulation of Vitamin B$_{12}$; movement of Vitamin B$_{12}$ from bile R binder to intrinsic factor due to the action of pancreatic trypsin. *Clin. Res.* 31:531A.

Kanazawa, S., B. Herzlich, and V. Herbert. 1982. Enhancing effect of human bile on the uptake of free vitamin B$_{12}$ and intrinsic factor-B$_{12}$ by receptors on the small bowel epithelial cells. *Blood* 60:30a.

Mahoney, M. J., and L. E. Rosenberg. 1980. Inherited defects of B_{12} metabolism. *Am. J. Med.* 48:584–593.

Marcoullis, G., and S. P. Rothenberg. 1983. Macromolecules in the assimilation and transport of cobalamin. In *Nutrition and hematology,* ed. J. Lindenbaum, 59–120. New York: Churchill Livingstone.

Scott, J. M., et al. 1981. The methyl-folate trap and the supply of S-adenosylmethionine. *Lancet* 2:755.

Sennett, C., L. E. Rosenberg, and I. S. Mellman. 1981. Transmembrane transport of cobalamin in prokaryotic and eukaryotic cells. *Ann. Rev. Biochem.* 50:1053–1086.

Shane, B., and E. L. R. Stokstad. 1985. Vitamin B_{12}-folate interrelationships. *Ann. Rev. Nutr.* 5:115–141.

Shin, Y. L., K. U. Buhring, and E. L. R. Stokstad. 1975. The relationships between vitamin B_{12} and folic acid and the effect on methionine on folate metabolism. *Mol. Cell Biochem.* 9:97–108.

Teo, N. H., et al. 1980. Effect of bile on Vitamin B_{12} absorption. *Br. Med. J.* 281:831–833.

Weir, D. G., and J. M. Scott. 1983. Interrelationships of folates and cobalamins. In *Nutrition and hematology,* ed. J. Lindenbaum, 121–142. New York: Churchill Livingstone.

vitamin B_{12}, the coenzyme. See COENZYME B_{12}.

vitamin C (ascorbic acid, dehydroascorbic acid). A water-soluble, highly unstable sugar acid that is an essential nutrient. Its reduced form is readily oxidized thus serving as an antioxidant and reducing agent. This reversibility is probably the key to its importance as a vitamin.

Most animals can synthesize vitamin C; however, humans and other primates, guinea pigs and a few other species lack the necessary ENZYMES to synthesize it and thus require a dietary source, such as fruits or vegetables.

The deficiency disease of vitamin C is scurvy. One of the tragic stories in the history of nutrition is the slowness with which the knowledge was accepted that citrus fruits would prevent and cure scurvy. As early as 1747 an experiment devised by James Lind, a British physician, showed that citrus fruits would cure the disease that commonly killed two-thirds of a ship's crew on long sea voyages. Sadly, it was to take fifty years before the British navy would rule that all crewmen should eat a lime a day. Today, scurvy is rarely seen except in a few isolated groups of persons, such as alcoholics or the elderly, who cannot care for themselves properly.

The symptoms of scurvy point to the role of vitamin C in the synthesis of COLLAGEN fibers. Muscular weakness that

ascorbic acid

dehydroascorbic acid

Active forms of vitamin C

progresses to an inability to stand is evidence of malformed collagen. Also the petechiae (tiny hemorrhages around hair follicles) that are seen on the skin of victims show that the integrity of blood vessels has been damaged. Another symptom is the loss of teeth as the cartilage holding them in place is weakened. Before that happens, however, the gums bleed profusely showing again the loss of integrity of capillary walls.

The malformation of collagen is due to the fact that vitamin C is required for hydroxylation of PROLINE to hydroxyproline. *Prolyl hydroxylase,* the enzyme that catalyzes this reaction, must have a ferrous IRON atom at its active site in order to function. Vitamin C is necessary to keep the iron in the ferrous (reduced) state. Unless hydroxylation occurs, collagen will not have its necessary strength.

Other hydroxylations in which vitamin C participates include the conversion of TRYPTOPHAN to 5-hydroxytryptophan in the synthesis of serotonin and the conversion of 3,4-dihydroxyphenylethylamine to norepinephrine in the synthesis of the CATECHOLAMINES. The synthesis of several steroid hormones also requires vitamin C.

The two active forms of vitamin C (dehydroascorbic acid and ascorbic acid) enable it to function both as a receiver and a donor of electrons in oxidation-reduction reactions. Vitamin C is essential for holding iron in its reduced state during many reactions and is important in facilitating the absorption of nonheme iron from the intestine. Vitamin C is important for the conversion of FOLACIN to tetrahydrofolate, its active form. The degradations of PHENYLALANINE, TYROSINE, and histamine also depend on vitamin C.

Daily consumption of vitamin C-rich foods is recommended since vitamin C is water soluble and not stored in the body to any great extent. Citrus fruits are the best sources, but other fruits and vegetables also contribute, depending on their freshness and post-harvest handling. The instability of the vitamin molecule requires careful handling—it is deactivated by cooking and exposure to air.

Vitamin C is absorbed from the intestine by active transport; it is found primarily in the adrenal and pituitary glands with small amounts distributed among other organs. Vitamin C and its metabolites (for example, diketogulonic acid, oxalic acid, and ascorbate 2-sulfate) are excreted primarily in the urine.

Ingestion of large (mega) doses of vitamin C has resulted in uricosuria, excessive iron absorption, impaired leukocyte activity, and hypoglycemic-type effects. Abrupt withdrawal of megadoses of vitamin C can result in symptoms resembling scurvy. There is no definitive evidence that megadoses of the vitamin prevent or cure the common cold, although a few studies have suggested that vitamin C may reduce the frequency and severity of such colds.   See also: PHENYLALANINE; TYROSINE.

SUGGESTED READINGS

Chalmers, T. C. 1975. Effects of ascorbic acid on the common cold: An evaluation of the evidence. *Am. J. Med.* 58:532–536.

Dykes, M. H. M., and P. Meier. 1975. Ascorbic acid and the common cold: Evaluation of its efficacy and toxicity. *JAMA* 231:1073–1079.

Finley, E. B., and F. L. Cerklewski. 1983. Influence of ascorbic acid supplementation on copper status in young adult men. *Am. J. Clin. Nutr.* 37:553–556.

Hogenkamp, H. P. C. 1980. The interaction between vitamin B_{12} and vitamin C. *Am. J. Clin. Nutr.* 33:1–3.

Honig, D. 1975. Metabolism of ascorbic acid. *World Rev. Nutr. Diet.* 23:225–258.

McCay, P. B. 1985. Vitamin E: Interactions with free radicals and ascorbate. *Ann. Rev. Nutr.* 5:323–340.

Mengel, C. E., and H. L. Greene, Jr. 1976. Ascorbic acid effects on erythrocytes. *Ann. Intern. Med.* 84:490.

Myllyla, R., E. R. Kuitti-Savolainen, and K. Kivirikko. 1978. The role of ascorbate in the prolyl hydroxylase reaction. *Biochem. Biophys. Res. Commun.* 83:441–448.

Shilotri, P. G., and K. S. Bhat. 1977. Effect of mega doses of vitamin C on bactericidal activity of leukocytes. *Am. J. Clin. Nutr.* 30:1077–1081.

Stein, H. G., A. Hasan, and I. H. Fox. 1976. Ascorbic acid-induced uriocosuria: A consequence of megavitamin therapy. *Ann. Intern. Med.* 84:385–388.

vitamin D (cholecalciferol, D_3). The fat-soluble vitamin, derived from CHOLESTEROL, that is responsible for the deposition of CALCIUM and PHOSPHORUS in bones and teeth. Vitamin D_2, also called calciferol or ergocalciferol, is found in plants.

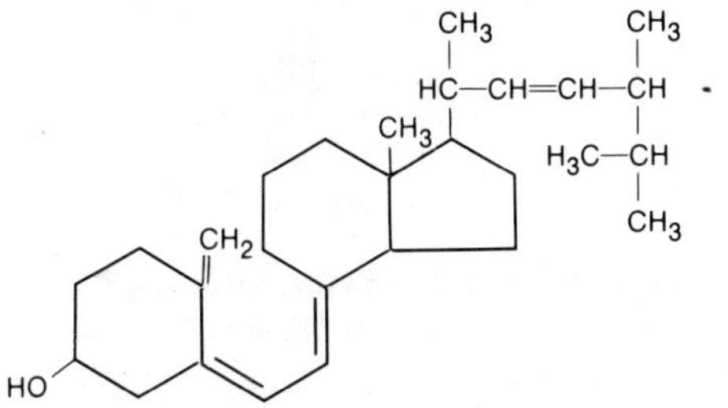

vitamin D_2 (calciferol or ergocalciferol)

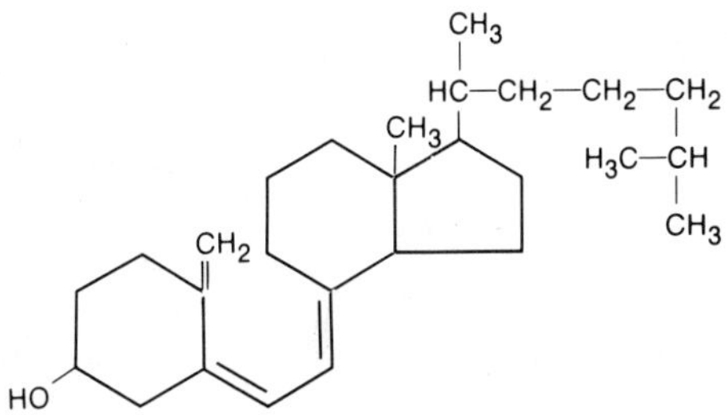

vitamin D_3 (cholecalciferol)

There are few dietary sources of vitamin D other than fish liver oils, egg yolk, and, in the United States, fortified milk. The body's main source is by the exposure of the skin to sunlight. In humans 7-dehydrocholesterol in the skin is converted by ultraviolet radiation to pre-vitamin D$_3$ that is hydroxylated, first in the liver and then in the kidney, to the active form 1,25-dihydroxy vitamin D$_3$ (also called calcitrol). 1,25-dihydroxy vitamin D$_3$ is considered to be a hormone since its action is on distant target tissues. Other metabolites of vitamin D$_3$ (1,24,25-trihydroxy vitamin D$_3$, 24,25-dihydroxy vitamin D$_3$, and 25,26-dihydroxy vitamin D$_3$) are also produced in the kidney from 25-hydroxy vitamin D$_3$. The actions of these metabolites are under investigation.

The synthesis of the active vitamin D (1,25-dihydroxy vitamin D$_3$) is stimulated by low plasma levels of calcium

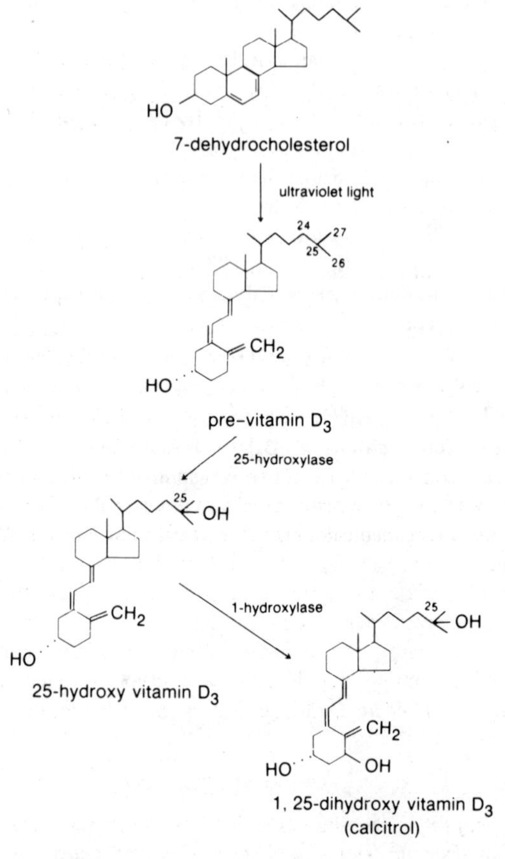

The synthesis of active vitamin D$_3$ from the action of ultraviolet light on 7-dehydrocholesterol in skin

and phosphorus. The fall in blood level of calcium stimulates the parathyroid gland to release parathyroid hormone (PTH) that, by activation of vitamin D_3, stimulates the active transport of calcium and phosphorus across the intestinal mucosa. This action is thought to result from a vitamin D-induced synthesis of a calcium-binding protein in the intestinal cell. 1,25-dihydroxy vitamin D_3 can increase calcium reabsorption from the kidney as well as stimulate the mobilization of calcium from bones. When the plasma calcium level rises to normal, the synthesis of PTH and 1,25-dihydroxy vitamin D_3 is slowed. If the blood level should rise above normal, calcitonin, a hormone secreted by the thyroid gland, will reverse the actions of PTH and the vitamin-hormone, bringing the blood level back toward normal. In this way, vitamin D plays a major role in the homeostatic control of calcium and, along with it, phosphorus.

Vitamin D deficiency affects the mineralization of bones and teeth and causes the disease rickets in children and osteomalacia in adults. Both diseases are characterized by soft bones that bend under the weight of the body. Early observations of rickets in children in northern climates led to the discovery of vitamin D and the use of cod liver oil to prevent and cure the disease.

Because the most important source of this vitamin-hormone is through the action of sunlight on skin, anything that interferes with the short rays of the sun will limit vitamin D production. For example, long winters of dark days of the northern part of the Northern hemisphere, smoke-filled skies of industrial cities, keeping the skin covered as some cultures demand of women, or indoor living as experienced by institutionalized elderly persons could severely limit the amount of vitamin D obtained from this source.

Supplements of vitamin D are not necessary for persons who get a reasonable amount of irradiation of the skin. Because vitamin D accumulates in the liver, it can reach toxic levels. It has been observed that some children (mostly in England) have experienced vitamin D toxicity from the ingestion of vitamin D-fortified children's foods in combination with vitamin D supplements. Symptoms of toxicity include hypercalcemia and deposition of calcium in soft tissues.

SUGGESTED READINGS

Adams, J. S., et al. 1982. Vitamin-D synthesis and metabolism after ultraviolet irradiation of normal and vitamin-D-deficient subjects. *N. Engl. J. Med.* 306:722–725.

Fraser, D. R. 1980. Regulation of the metabolism of vitamin D. *Physiol. Rev.* 60:551–613.

Halloran, B. P., and H. F. DeLuca. 1980. Calcium transport in small intestine during pregnancy and lactation. *Am. J. Physiol.* 239:E64–E68.

DeLuca, H. F. 1982. New developments in the vitamin D endocrine system. *J. Am. Diet. Assoc.* 80:231–236.

DeLuca, H. F., and H. K. Schnoes. 1983. Vitamin D: Recent advances. *Ann. Rev. Biochem.* 52:411–439.

Malluche, H. H., et al. 1980. Effects and interactions of 24,25(OH)$_2$D$_3$ and 1,25(OH)$_2$D$_3$ on bone. *Am. J. Physiol.* 238:E494–E498.

Norman, A. W., et al. 1980. Vitamin D deficiency inhibits pancreatic secretion of insulin. *Science* 209:823–825.

vitamin E (α-tocopherol). A fat-soluble vitamin that, chemically, is one of eight naturally occurring compounds. Vitamin E compounds may be classified as tocopherols or tocotrienols. The tocopherols contain a 16-carbon, saturated isoprenoid side chain; the tocotrienols contain three unsaturated bonds in the side chain. The number and position of the methyl groups bonded to the ring structure form the basis for the designations α, β, γ, and δ. α-Tocopherol is the most widely distributed and most biologically active vitamin E compound.

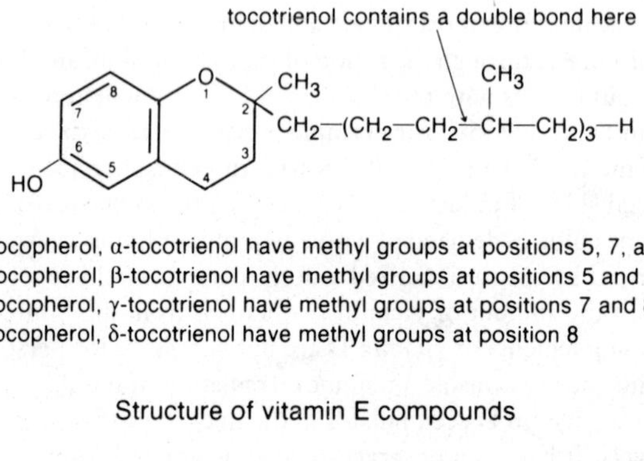

α-tocopherol, α-tocotrienol have methyl groups at positions 5, 7, and 8
β-tocopherol, β-tocotrienol have methyl groups at positions 5 and 8
γ-tocopherol, γ-tocotrienol have methyl groups at positions 7 and 8
δ-tocopherol, δ-tocotrienol have methyl groups at position 8

Structure of vitamin E compounds

Over the years much research has been conducted to find the function or functions of vitamin E in biologic tissues. The most widely accepted theory is that vitamin E functions as an antioxidant of polyunsaturated FATTY ACIDS and other conjugated molecules, such as VITAMIN A, in the tissues. As an antioxidant, vitamin E protects the polyunsaturated fatty acids in MEMBRANES from oxidation.

The best sources of vitamin E are vegetable oils, particularly safflower, corn, soybean, and cottonseed. Since vitamin E is stored in abundance in the fat tissues of humans, human vitamin E deficiency is relatively uncommon.

Research on animals has shown that vitamin E deficiency results in reproductive dysfunction: in male rats atrophied, brown, flabby testes and lowered spermatogenesis results; in female rates fetal resorption occurs. Another deficiency symptom observed in animals is nutritional muscular dystrophy. However, studies have failed to show that in humans these same conditions may be improved or cured by vitamin E.

SUGGESTED READINGS

Ali, M., G. G. Gudbranson, and J. W. D. McDonald. 1980. Inhibition of human platelet cyclooxygenase by alpha-tocopherol. *Prostaglandins Med.* 4:79–85.

Bieri, J. G., L. Corash, and V. S. Hubbard. 1983. Medical uses of vitamin E. *N. Engl. J. Med.* 308:1063–1071.

Farrell, P. M. 1979. Vitamin E deficiency in premature infants. *J. Pediatr.* 95:869–872.

Hoekstra, W. G. 1975. Biochemical function of selenium and its relation to vitamin E. *Fed. Proc.* 34:2083–2089. 34:2083–2089.

Kligman, A. M. 1982. Vitamin E toxicity. *Arch. Dermatol.* 118:289.

McCay, P. B. 1985. Vitamin E: Interactions with free radicals and ascorbate. *Ann. Rev. Nutr.* 5:323–340.

McLaughlin, P. J., and J. L. Weihrauch. 1979. Vitamin E content of foods. *J. Am. Diet. Assoc.,* 75:647–665.

Roberts, H. J. 1981. Perspectives on vitamin E therapy. *JAMA* 246:129–131.

Scott, M. L. 1980. Advances in our understanding of vitamin E. *Fed. Proc.* 39:2736–2739.

vitamin K. The "K" comes from the Danish word "Koagulation" signifying the importance of this vitamin in blood clotting. Vitamin K plays a prominent role in the formation of prothrombin (factor II) and other blood-clotting factors (VII, IX, and X). Prothrombin is the precursor of thrombin, the enzyme in blood that converts fibrinogen to fibrin. Fibrin is the insoluble substance that forms a "net" to seal in the vital fluid after an injury causes bleeding.

Investigations of prothrombin and factors VII, IX, and X, demonstrated that they contain a series of glutamic acid residues. Vitamin K is needed for the carboxylation of these residues. Once carboxylated, the glutamates are referred to as γ-carboxyglutamic acid (GLA). This alteration is necessary for prothrombin to bind CALCIUM, a necessary step in the clotting process.

Chemically, vitamin K is not a single substance but a group of quinones that can be grouped according to their source: phylloquinones (vitamin K_1) come from plants;

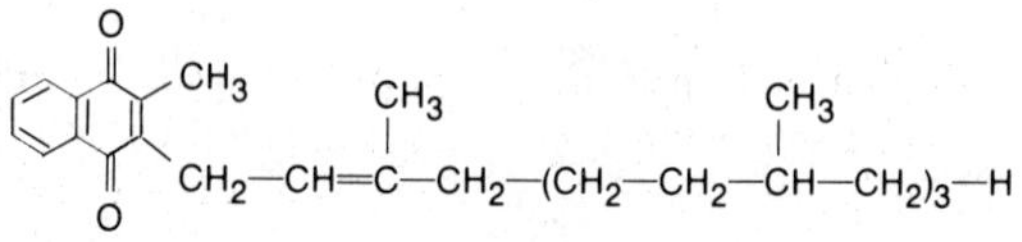

phylloquinone (K₁)

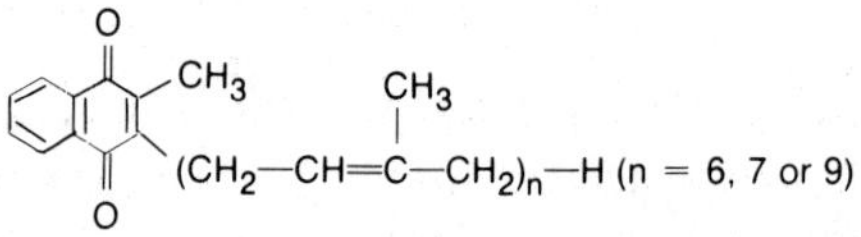

menaquinone (K₂)

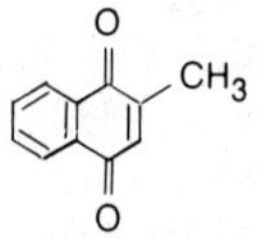

menadione

Vitamin K compounds

menaquinones (vitamin K_2) are found in bacteria. In addition, there are synthetic vitamin K compounds, notably menadione.

Vitamin K, a fat-soluble vitamin, is found in leafy, green vegetables, notably turnip greens, broccoli, and other members of the cabbage family. It is also synthesized by bacteria in the small intestine.

Bile and pancreatic juice are needed for the absorption of vitamin K in the ileum. Therefore any situation, such as obstructive jaundice, that hinders these from getting to the small intestine would also reduce the absorption of the available vitamin K. Diseases such as sprue, pellagra, ulcerative colitis, and any others that upset the normal action of the intestine, would induce a deficiency; in these diseases the contents pass through the ileum too quickly for the vitamin to be absorbed. In addition, any condition that contributes to the malabsorption of lipids would decrease the vitamin K absorbed. Antibiotics such as ones given prior to intestinal surgery that destroy the intestinal flora may cause a temporary vitamin K deficiency.

Because of the widespread availability of vitamin K, deficiencies are not common. However, babies are sometimes born without sufficient vitamin K because it is not readily transmitted by the placenta during gestation and at birth babies have a sterile intestine. It takes only a few days, however, for the bacterial flora to become established and begin supplying vitamin K to the infant. In many hospitals a single dose of water-soluble synthetic vitamin K is given at birth to prevent the occurrence of "hemorrhagic disease of the newborn."

One well-known antagonist of vitamin K is dicoumarol, the substance in wet sweet clover *(Melilotus)* that causes a fatal hemorrhagic disease in cattle. Dicoumarol is used as an anticoagulant to prevent clotting in patients who are at risk for blood clots. Warfarin, another antagonist, has commercial use as a rat poison. These substances inhibit the carboxylation of blood clotting proteins, which hampers calcium-binding, a necessary step in blood clotting.

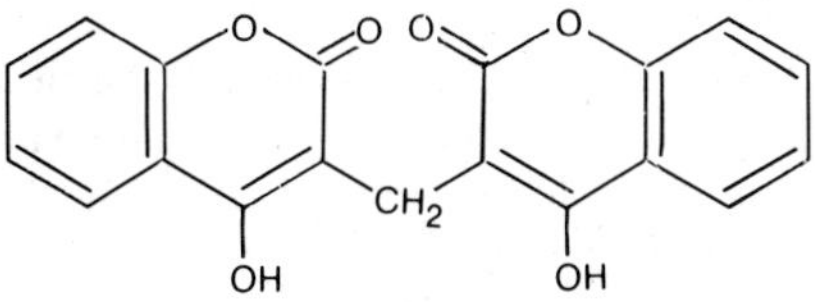

dicoumarol

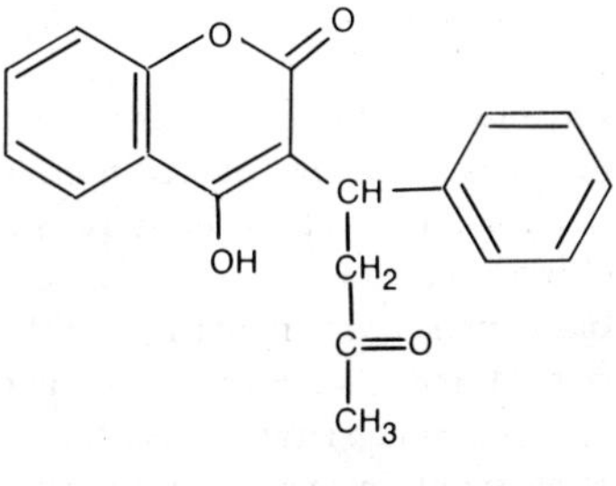

warfarin

Antagonists of vitamin K

SUGGESTED READINGS

Ansell, J. E., R. Kuman, and D. Deykin. 1977. The spectrum of vitamin K deficiency. *JAMA* 238:40–42.

DiScipio, R. G., et al. 1977. A comparison of human prothrombin, factor IX (Christmas factor), factor X (Stuart factor), and protein S. *Biochemistry* 16:698–706.

Jackson, C. M., and Y. Nemerson. 1980. Blood coagulation. *Ann. Rev. Biochem.* 49:765–811.

Nelsestuen, G. L., T. H. Zytkovicz, and J. B. Howard. 1973. The mode of action of vitamin K. Isolation of a peptide containing the vitamin K-dependent portion of prothrombin. *Proc. Natl. Acad. Sci. USA* 70:3366–3370.

Nelsestuen, G. L., T. H. Zytkovicz, and J. B. Howard. 1974. The mode of action of vitamin K. Identification of γ-carboxyglutamic acid as a component of prothrombin. *J. Biol. Chem.* 249:6347–6350.

Olson, R. E., and J. W. Suttie. 1978. Vitamin K and γ-carboxyglutamate biosynthesis. *Vitamin Horm.* 35:59–108.

Stenflo, J., et al. 1974. Vitamin K-dependent modifications of glutamic acid residues in prothrombin. *Proc. Natl. Acad. Sci. USA* 71:2730–2733.

Stenflo, J., and J. W. Suttie. 1977. Vitamin K-dependent formation of γ-carboxyglutamic acid. *Ann. Rev. Biochem.* 46:157–172.

Suttie, J. W. 1983. Current concepts of the mechanism of action of vitamin K and its antagonists. In *Nutrition and hematology*, ed. J. Lindenbaum, 245–270. New York: Churchill Livingstone.

Suttie, J. W. 1985. Vitamin K-dependent carboxylase. *Ann. Rev. Biochem.* 54:459–477.

Suttie, J. W., and C. M. Jackson. 1977. Prothrombin structure, activation, and biosynthesis. *Physiol. Rev.* 57:1–70.

vitamins. Organic substances needed by the body in tiny amounts, the dietary absence of which can cause specific metabolic defects. These substances may in some instances be synthesized by humans, but may not be synthesized in sufficient quantity to support normal health.

Vitamins A, D, and NIACIN can be made in the body from other substances although it is not accurate to say that the body can synthesize them. VITAMIN A can be made by cleavage of beta-carotene; VITAMIN D can be formed from the action of sunlight on 7-dehydrocholesterol in the skin; and niacin is a normal degradative product of the amino acid TRYPTOPHAN. BIOTIN and VITAMIN K technically are not synthesized by humans, but by bacteria living in the human gut; however, humans can use this source. VITAMIN B_{12} is also made by the action of intestinal bacteria, but not enough of this source is absorbed to meet human requirements.

A deficiency disease produced by the lack of a vitamin is specific for that vitamin. In popular nutrition literature authors frequently attribute various health problems to lack of certain vitamins. In valid scientific reporting, however, a disease is attributed to a vitamin deficiency only after controlled experiments show that a metabolic disease developed when the vitamin (and nothing else) was withdrawn from the diet. In addition, the disease must disappear after the vitamin (and nothing else) is reintroduced into the diet.

Overdosing with vitamin supplements may cause toxicity symptoms, but rarely can the consumption of foods containing the vitamin cause toxicity. An exception to this general statement is vitamin A toxicity that has been reported by Artic hunters who have eaten liver from polar bears. The consumption of megadoses of vitamin supplements, a relatively recent phenomenon, is being watched for signs of toxicity.   See also: B-VITAMIN TERMINOLOGY; FAT-SOLUBLE VITAMINS; WATER-SOLUBLE VITAMINS; topics listed under individual vitamin names.

VLDL (very low density lipoproteins).   See LIPOPROTEINS; VERY LOW DENSITY LIPOPROTEINS.

von Gierke's disease (glycogen storage disease: type I).   A condition in which excessive amounts of GLYCOGEN are stored in the liver causing it to enlarge. The body is unable to use this glycogen for glucose production and overproduction of KETONE BODIES results. The disorder stems from a recessively inherited deficiency of the enzyme, *glucose 6-phosphatase.*

SUGGESTED READINGS

Howell, R. R., and J. C. Williams. 1983. The glycogen storage diseases. In *The metabolic basis of inherited disease,* 5th ed., ed. J. B. Stanbury et al., 141–166. New York: McGraw-Hill.

warfarin. A VITAMIN K antagonist. See also: VITAMIN K.

water-soluble vitamins. BIOTIN, CYANOCOBALAMIN (B_{12}) FOLACIN, NIACIN, PANTOTHENATE, RIBOFLAVIN (B_2), THIAMIN (B_1), VITAMIN B_6, and VITAMIN C.

Wilson's disease. A hereditary syndrome transmitted as a recessive trait in which liver proteins cause increased binding of COPPER. This binding causes a decrease in synthesis of ceruloplasmin and a decrease in excretion of bile copper. There is also an accumulation of copper in the brain, liver, kidney, and cornea. Patients are treated with drugs that bind copper and increase its excretion by the kidneys.

SUGGESTED READINGS

Danks, D. M. 1983. Hereditary disorders of copper metabolism in Wilson's disease and Menkes' disease. In *The metabolic basis of inherited disease*, 5th ed., ed. J. B. Stanbury et al., 1251–1268. New York: McGraw-Hill.

Z

zinc (Zn⁺⁺). A metallic ion that is necessary for the action of many ENZYMES. Zinc atoms can activate (play a catalytic role in) and/or stabilize (play a structural role in) enzymes. In many cases, other divalent metals seem to perform these roles about as well as zinc, which may explain why a zinc-deficient diet does not always depress the activities of all zinc-containing enzymes.

A zinc metalloenzyme in red blood cells, *carbonic anhydrase*, plays a vital role at the end of all energy-producing reactions. The enzyme changes the carbon dioxide end product (CO_2) to a bicarbonate ion (HCO_3^-), which can be carried safely in the blood to the lungs for excretion of its carbon dioxide portion. The zinc ion in the enzyme is complexed with three HISTIDINE residues and a molecule of water. The strong positive ion repulses the hydrogen from the water molecule, leaving a hydroxide. Then the carbon dioxide joins with the hydroxyl ion on the enzyme to form a bicarbonate ion, which is freed from the enzyme complex.

Another zinc metalloenzyme, *alcohol dehydrogenase*, catalyzes the conversion of ethanol to ACETALDEHYDE, the first step in one of the pathways for the breakdown of beverage alcohol. Here, zinc is complexed with three AMINO ACIDS (two CYSTEINES and one histidine) and a molecule of ethanol. Again, the strong positive zinc ion repulses other positive charges and loosens their bonds. In this case a hydride ion is transferred from alcohol to the NIACIN coenzyme NAD^+ forming acetaldehyde, which enters the GLUCOSE-to-energy pathway in the complex step between pyruvate and ACETYL-COA.

Zinc is also involved in *carboxypeptidase,* which hydrolyzes proteins, and in *alkaline phosphatase,* which removes phosphates from various molecules. It is important in the storage of insulin and in the senses of taste and smell. Zinc is essential for the activity of *thymidine kinase* and it plays roles in the transcription and translation of hereditary information.

Although zinc is widely distributed throughout the tissues of the human body, it is concentrated in the liver, kidneys, pancreas, and brain. Zinc absorption is thought to occur by an active process in the small intestine. In the blood, it is bound to albumin, α_2-macroglobulin, and amino acids, such as histidine or cysteine. Zinc is excreted primarily through the gastrointestinal tract with lesser amounts found in the urine and sweat.

The best dietary sources of zinc are oysters, lean beef, and beef liver. The poorest sources are fruits and vegetables with dairy products being of moderate value. It should not be surprising then that in modern society zinc deficiencies are more often found in the poorest segment, since the middle- and upper-income groups are able to afford the meats that donate large quantities. Strict vegetarians, and especially their children during rapid growth periods, may also develop zinc deficiencies.

Populations that subsist primarily on whole grain cereals (especially unleavened breads) may develop zinc deficiencies. In this case, both the fiber and the phytates in the cereals may complex with the zinc and make it unavailable. In yeast breads an enzyme in the yeast and changes in PH are thought to break the bonds that hold the zinc-phytate complex together and render some of the zinc available for absorption.

Acrodermatitis enteropathica, an inherited disease, results in severe zinc deficiency as absorption is thought to be impaired. Pharmacologic doses of zinc may be prescribed during treatment.

The overt symptoms of zinc deficiency are loss of taste, poor appetite, poor wound healing, low growth rate, and delayed sexual development. Much is known about these symptoms, but the responsible metabolic defects are as yet little understood.

SUGGESTED READINGS

Abbasi, A. A., et al. 1980. Experimental zinc deficiency in man. Effect in testicular function. *J. Lab. Clin. Med.* 96:544–550.

Apgar, J. 1985. Zinc and reproduction. *Ann. Rev. Nutr.* 5:43–68.

Cousins, R. J. 1979. Regulatory aspects of zinc metabolism in liver and intestine. *Nutr. Rev.* 37:97–103.

Ghishan, F. K., et al. 1986. Intestinal transport of zinc and folic acid: A mutual inhibitory effect. *Am. J. Clin. Nutr.* 43:258–262.

Greger, J. L., and S. M. Snedeker. 1980. Effect of dietary protein and phosphorus levels on the utilization of zinc, copper and manganese by adult males. *J. Nutr.* 110:2243–2253.

Istfan, N. W., M. Janghorbani, and V. R. Young. 1983. Absorption of stable ^{70}Zn in healthy young men in relation to zinc intake. *Am. J. Clin. Nutr.* 38:187–194.

Klevay, L. M. 1980. Interactions of copper and zinc in cardiovascular disease. *Ann. N.Y. Acad. Sci.* 355:140–151.

Prasad, A. S. 1985. Clinical manifestations of zinc deficiency. *Ann. Rev. Nutr.* 5:341–363.

Prasad, A. S., et al. 1978. Hypocupremia induced by zinc therapy. *JAMA* 240:2166–2168.

Roth, H. P., and M. Kirchgessner. 1980. Zinc metalloenzyme activities. *World Rev. Nutr. Diet.* 34:144–160.

Sandstead, H. H., et al. 1982. Zinc nutriture in the elderly in relation to taste acuity, immune response, and wound healing. *Am. J. Clin. Nutr.* 36:1046–1059.

Solomons, N. W., and R. A. Jacob. 1981. Studies on the bioavailability of zinc in humans: Effects of heme and nonheme iron on the absorption of zinc. *Am. J. Clin. Nutr.* 34:475–482.

Solomons, N. W., et al. 1983. Studies on the bioavailability of zinc in humans: Mechanism of the intestinal interaction of non-heme iron and zinc. *J. Nutr.* 113:337–349.

Spencer, H., et al. 1984. Effect of calcium and phosphorus on zinc metabolism in man. *Am. J. Clin. Nutr.* 40:1213–1218.

Valberg, L. S., P. R. Flanagan, and M. J. Chamberlain. 1984. Effects of iron, tin and copper on zinc absorption in humans. *Am. J. Clin. Nutr.* 40:536–541.

Weismann, K., and H. Hoyer. 1985. Serum alkaline phosphatase and serum zinc levels in the diagnosis and exclusion of zinc deficiency in man. *Am. J. Clin. Nutr.* 41:1214–1219.

zymogens. An inactive enzyme that becomes active only in the presence of its substrate. A zymogen is nature's answer to the question: What keeps an enzyme, whose task is to degrade a protein, from degrading the proteins in the tissue that is synthesizing the enzyme? This question troubled researchers for many years and still is frequently asked by a curious student.

Some of the digestive ENZYMES are synthesized outside the digestive tract in organs such as the pancreas and, upon stimulation by hormones, are released into the digestive tract. If these enzymes were allowed to be active while outside the digestive tract, they could disrupt the structure of the cells responsible for their own synthesis. Instead, the DNA instructions in the cells that produce the enzyme call for the production of an enzyme identical to the active enzyme except that the active site is chemically altered or blocked. This "inactive" enzyme is the zymogen and because the active site is unavailable, no chemical action will take place.

When the zymogen enters the digestive tract, its conformation will be shifted by a simple maneuver, perhaps a slight shift in PH or the action of another enzyme in the gastrointestinal tract, and the active site will become available. The substrate, protein from food for example, will be able to fit into the active site and the chemical action will then take place. Once the active site has been exposed, however, there is no way that it can be blocked again to deactivate the enzyme.

Chymotrypsinogen, a good example of a zymogen, becomes the enzyme *chymotrypsin* specific for the peptide bonds on the carboxyl side of TYROSINE, TRYPTOPHAN, and

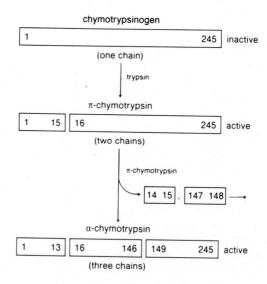

Formation of chymotrypsin

PHENYLALANINE, and of large hydrophobic residues such as those of METHIONINE. *Chymotrypsinogen,* produced in the pancreas, does no harm to the structure of the pancreas. Upon a hormonal signal that protein food will be arriving in the duodenum, *chymotrypsinogen* is secreted into the duodenum where it will be activated by the enzyme *trypsin.*

Chymotrypsinogen is a single-stranded protein molecule made up of 245 amino acids and held in its conformation by five disulfide bridges. When the peptide bond holding together amino acids 15 and 16 is broken by *trypsin,* π-*chymotrypsin* is formed, which can act on itself to release α-*chymotrypsin.* Both π-*chymotrypsin and* α-*chymotrypsin* are active, but the latter is more stable. Other examples of zymogens include *trypsinogen, procarboxy peptidase, proelastase,* and *pepsinogen.*

Subject Groupings of Topics

The following lists provide a guide for the student or professional who wishes to review multiple topics for a thorough understanding of a subject. Due to the style of this text, the names of topics suggested under a given subject may not appear appropriate; however, the text written under the topic contributes to an understanding of the subject. There are many additional topics which may prove helpful which are not included in these subjects.

AMINO ACIDS

acidic amino acids
alanine
aliphatic amino acids
amide bond
amides of acidic amino acids
amino acid biosynthesis
amino acid degradation
amino acid pool
amino acids
amino transferases
anomeric carbon
arginine
aromatic amino acids
asparagine
aspartate
basic amino acids
beta alanine
branched-chain amino acids
cysteine
essential amino acids
glucogenic amino acids
glutamate
glutamine
glycine
histidine
hydroxylysine
hydroxyproline
isoleucine
ketogenic amino acids
leucine
lysine
methionine
nonessential amino acids
phenylalanine
proline
serine
sulfur-containing amino acids
threonine
tryptophan
tyrosine
valine

CARBOHYDRATE

acetyl-CoA
blood glucose level
carbohydrate digestion
carbohydrate structures
Cori cycle
fiber
fructose
galactose
glucagon
gluconeogenesis
glucose
glycogen
glycogenesis
glycogenolysis

ribose
ribosome
RNA
sickle cell anemia
transcription
transfer RNA
translation

LIPIDS

acetyl-CoA
beta oxidation
bile salts
carnitine
cholesterol
chylomicron
cis-, trans-bonds
diacylglycerol
eicosanoids
emulsion
enterohepatic circulation
essential fatty acids
fat-soluble vitamins
fatty acids
fatty acid nomenclature
fatty acid oxidation
fatty acid synthesis
glycerol
glycolipid
glycerol phosphate shuttle
glycolipid
glycolysis
high density lipoprotein
lecithin
lipids
lipid digestion
lipogenesis
lipolysis
lipoproteins
low density lipoprotein
membranes
micelle
monoacylglycerol
monounsaturated fatty acid
phospholipid
polyunsaturated fatty acid
saturated fatty acids

sterols
triacylglycerols
unsaturated fatty acids
very high density lipoproteins
very low density lipoproteins

METABOLIC DISORDERS

albinism
alkaptonuria
analbuminemia
Andersen's disease
argininemia
argininosuccinic acidemia
citrullinemia
Cori's disease
Cushing's disease
cystathioninuria
cystinuria
diabetes mellitus
erythropoietic porphyria
Fanconi's syndrome
favism
galactosemia
Gaucher's disease
glycogen storage diseases
hemochromotosis
Hers' disease
histidinemia
homocystinuria
hyperammonemia type I
hyperammonemia type II
Lesch-Nyhan syndrome
maple sugar urine disease
McArdle's disease
methylmalonic aciduria
Nieman-Pick disease
PKU
Pompe's disease
sickle-cell anemia
Tangier disease
Tarui's disease
Tay-Sachs disease
thalessemia
valinemia
von Gierke's disease
Wilson's disease

Appendix

METABOLIC PATHWAYS
acetyl-CoA
amino acid degradation
Cori cycle
cytochromes
fatty acid oxidation
fatty acid synthesis
gluconeogenesis
glycerol phosphate shuttle
glycogenesis
glycogenolysis
glycolysis
ketone bodies
lipogenesis
lipoic acid
lipolysis
malate-aspartate shuttle
pentose phosphate pathway
protein biosynthesis
respiratory chain
TCA cycle
urea cycle

MINERALS
calcium
chloride
chromium
copper
fluoride
iodide
iron
magnesium
manganese
molybdenum
phosphorus
potassium
selenium
sodium
sulfur
zinc

PROTEIN
(Also see the grouping under amino acids.)
acetyl-CoA
amide bond
collagen
complete protein

denaturation
elastin
enzyme
glycoprotein
hemoglobin
isoelectric point
lipoproteins
mutual supplementation
nitrogen
nitrogen balance
peptide bond
protein
protein biosynthesis
protein digestion
protein structure
sickle cell anemia
stereoisomer
TCA cycle
zymogens

VITAMINS and COENZYMES
B-vitamin terminology
beta carotene
biotin, the coenzyme
biotin, the vitamin
coenzyme A
coenzyme B_{12}
cofactor
FAD, FMN
fat-soluble vitamins
folacin
NAD^+, $NADP^+$
niacin
pantothenic acid
pyridoxal phosphate
riboflavin
tetrahydrofolate
thiamin
thiamin pyrophosphate
vitamins
vitamin A
vitamin B_6
vitamin B_{12}
vitamin C
vitamin D
vitamin E
vitamin K
water-soluble vitamins